# Yogāvatāraṇam

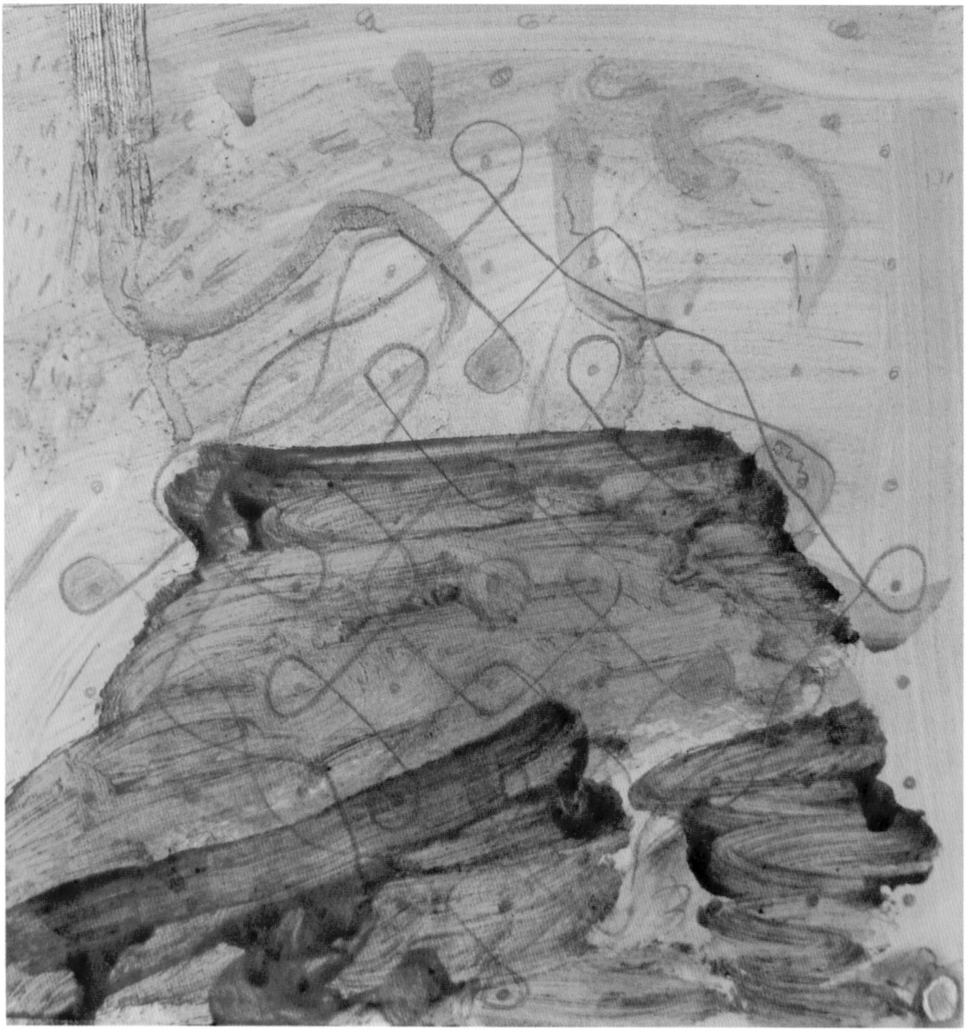

# YOGĀVATĀRAṆAM

## *The Translation of Yoga*

Zoë Slatoff-Ponté

Art by Ben Ponté

North Point Press
A division of Farrar, Straus and Giroux
New York

North Point Press
A division of Farrar, Straus and Giroux
18 West 18th Street, New York 10011


Printed in China
First edition, 2015

Grateful acknowledgment is made for permission to reprint "The Opening of Eyes" by David Whyte.


Library of Congress Cataloging-in-Publication Data
Slatoff-Ponté, Zoë, author.
Yogavataranam : the translation of yoga : a new approach to Sanskrit, integrating traditional and academic methods and based on classic yoga texts for university courses, yoga programs, and self study / Zoë Slatoff-Ponté ; illustrated by Ben Ponté. — First edition.
pages cm
Includes bibliographical references.
ISBN 978-0-86547-754-4 (paperback) — ISBN 978-1-4299-5583-6 (e-book)
1. Yoga—Translating. 2. Sanskrit language—Study and teaching. 3. Sanskrit language—Translating. I. Ponté, Ben, illustrator. II. Title.

B132.Y6S573 2015
491'.282421—dc23

2014044609

Designed by Newgen KnowledgeWorks



3 5 7 9 10 8 6 4 2

*I dedicate this book to my teacher*
*Śrī K. Pattabhi Jois,*
*in loving memory and gratitude*

गणानां त्वा गणपतिगं हवामहे कविं कवीनामुपमश्रवस्तमम् ।
ज्येष्ठराजं ब्रह्मणा ब्रह्मणस्पत आ नः शृण्वन्नूतिभिस्सीद सादनम् ॥

**gaṇānāṃ tvā gaṇapati-gaṃ havāmahe**
**kaviṃ kavīnām upamaśra-vastamam |**
**jyeṣṭha-rājaṃ brahmaṇā brahmaṇas-pata**
**ā naḥ śṛṇvann ūtibhis sīda sādanam ||**

We honor you, Ganeśa, leader of all the hosts of gods,
Poet among poets, of the highest renown.
King among elders, lord of sacred words,
Hearing us, sit down in this place, with your kindness and riches.

# CONTENTS

*List of Illustrations* *xiii*
*"The Opening of Eyes"* *xv*
*Preface* *xvii*
*How to Use This Book* *xxiii*
*Found in Translation: A Note on the Images* *xxvii*

**Part I**

1. The *Devanāgarī* Alphabet ***3***

2. Verbs: Present Tense, *Parasmaipada*, First, Fourth, Sixth, and Tenth Class; Pronouns: Nominative Case; *Sandhi* Review ***25***

3. Nouns: Masculine and Neuter Nouns Ending in अ; Examples of Cases ***41***

4. Verbs: Present Tense, *Ātmanepada*, First, Fourth, Sixth, and Tenth Class; Feminine Nouns Ending in आ and ई; *Sandhi* Review ***65***

5. Masculine and Feminine Nouns Ending in इ and उ; Verbs: Imperative and Optative ***85***

6. Familial and Agent Nouns Ending in ऋ; Past Imperfect Tense; Verbal Prefixes; Gerunds and Infinitives ***103***

7. Verbs: Future Tense; Pronouns, Relative and Correlative Pronouns; Pronominal Adjectives ***119***

*Sandhi* Review ***139***

Part I Review: *Gurvaṣṭakam* by Ādi Śaṅkarācārya ***145***

*Viṣkambha*: Interlude ***149***

## Part II

8. Nouns Ending in Simple Consonants; Vowel Strength; Verb Conjugations: Second and Third Class ***153***

9. Nouns Ending in अन्; Verb Conjugations: Fifth and Eighth Class; Quotations and the Particle इति ***171***

10. Nouns Ending in स्; Verb Conjugations: Seventh and Ninth Class; Causative Verbs ***183***

11. Compounds: *Dvandva*; Passive Voice; Past Passive Participles ***197***

12. Compounds: *Tatpuruṣa*, *Karmadhāraya* ***211***

13. Compounds: *Bahuvrīhi*; Possessive Nouns Ending in मत् or वत्; Present Participles ***227***

14. Compounds: *Avyayībhāva*; the Suffix इन्; Gerundives; Locative and Genitive Absolute ***243***

Part II Review: *Bhagavadgītā*, Chapter 12 ***257***

## Part III

15. Sanskrit Numerals; Degrees of Comparison; आदि, अद्य, and प्रभृति ***263***

16. Perfect Tense; Periphrastic Perfect; Periphrastic Future; Perfect Active Participle ***279***

17. Desideratives; Intensive/Frequentative Verbs; Denominatives ***293***

18. Demonstrative Pronouns इदम् and अदस्; Past Active Participles; Neuter Nouns Ending in इ and उ; Irregular Declensions ***303***

19. Nominal Derivation: कृत् and तद्धित Suffixes; Pronoun: एनम् ***317***

20. The Aorist ***327***

21. Conditional and Benedictive Mode; Composite Verbs and च्वि Formation; Directional Words with the Suffix -अञ्च् ***341***

Part III Review: *Chāndogyopaniṣat* 4.4–9 ***353***

*Notes on the Translations* *357*
*Answer Key: Translations* *359*
*Abbreviations* *439*
*Glossary* *441*
*Bibliography* *491*
*Acknowledgments* *495*

# Illustrations

All works are oil and mixed media on paper on board.

Threshold *Frontispiece*

Translation I *1*

Articulation Points *7*

Chart *10*

Da *12*

Pat Pat Pat *28*

Sama *37*

Field of Dharma *58*

Sūryanamaskāra *61*

Nāsāgra *74*

Śiva's Hair *76*

The Third Step of Vāmana *127*

Translation II *151*

Soul and Spirit *173*

Elephant *225*

Rabbit Moon *231*

Growing Down *234*

Translation III *261*

Secondhand Knowledge *269*

Load of Dharma *274*

## THE OPENING OF EYES

That day I saw beneath dark clouds
the passing light over the water
and I heard the voice of the world speak out,
I knew then, as I had before
life is no passing memory of what has been
nor the remaining pages in a great book
waiting to be read.

It is the opening of eyes long closed.
It is the vision of far off things
seen for the silence they hold.
It is the heart after years
of secret conversing,
speaking out loud in the clear air.

It is Moses in the desert
fallen to his knees before the lit bush.
It is the man throwing away his shoes
as if to enter heaven
and finding himself astonished,
opened at last,
fallen in love with solid ground.

—David Whyte,
from *Songs for Coming Home*

# Preface

अज्ञानतिमिरान्धस्य ज्ञानाञ्जनशलाकया ।
चक्षुरुन्मीलितं येन तस्मै श्रीगुरवे नमः ॥

**ajñāna-timirāndhasya jñānāñjana-śalākayā |**
**cakṣur unmīlitaṃ yena tasmai śrī-gurave namaḥ ||**

I bow to that sacred guru,
By whom the eyes,
Of one who was blind because of the darkness of ignorance,
Were opened, with the collyrium* pencil of knowledge.

योगहीनं कथं ज्ञानं मोक्षदं भवति ध्रुवम् ॥
योगो हि ज्ञानहीनस्तु न क्षमो मोक्षकर्मणि ।
तस्माज्ज्ञानं च योगं च मुमुक्षुर्दृढमभ्यसेत् ॥

**yoga-hīnaṃ kathaṃ jñānaṃ mokṣadam bhavati dhruvam ||**
**yogo hi jñāna-hīnas tu na kṣamo mokṣa-karmaṇi |**
**tasmāj jñānaṃ ca yogaṃ ca mumukṣur dṛḍham abhyaset ||**

Without yoga, how can there be knowledge,
Which surely bestows liberation.
But yoga, without knowledge, is not enough,
As an action leading toward liberation.
Therefore, one desiring freedom,
Should steadily practice both yoga and knowledge.

—*Yogatattvopaniṣat* 14cd–15

*A black pigment applied to the eyes, an eye-salve, cleanser for the eyes.

The first time I heard Guruji, Śrī K. Pattabhi Jois, chant the opening mantra of Ashtanga yoga, followed by the long trail of Sanskrit words that only he seemed to know, I felt something deep within me awaken. I was twenty years old and had been practicing Ashtanga yoga for a few years, but those mornings practicing in the skylight ballroom of the Puck building in downtown New York City, listening to Guruji counting in "the language of the gods," hundreds of people breathing in unison, I was filled with a sense of deep contentment, a peace I had never experienced before. Later that year, I left my engineering degree and went to Mysore, South India, for the first time. In the afternoons, Guruji would sit in his little front room, reading the paper, telling us stories, answering questions, and reciting and explaining verses from various texts. He had this remarkable way of making the Sanskrit come to life, of making these ancient enigmatic teachings simple and understandable. I listened to him reciting Sanskrit verses and was intrigued by the powerful vibration and lyrical quality inherent in the language. I started studying Sanskrit on that trip, walking around singing the alphabet, loving the feeling of the new sounds rolling off my tongue.

I continued to study Sanskrit on my own when I returned home, renewing my inspiration every time I went to Mysore. Finally, I decided to immerse myself completely and returned to school at Columbia University to study Sanskrit. After years of studying both in the traditional method of *śruti paramparā*, chanting and memorizing verses, and amid the quiet rigor of Western academia, I have learned the benefits of both methods. This book is my attempt to build a bridge between those two worlds, to join my experience and scholarship together. Through this, I hope to share the love for Sanskrit that Guruji inspired in me and to provide a welcoming pathway into Sanskrit and yoga philosophy.

Yoga is considered to be one of the six *darśanas*, or philosophical viewpoints of Hinduism; it is both a practical and theoretical method for living in and transcending this world. The word *darśana* can be translated as seeing; it also has the connotation of knowing. The practice of yoga therefore implies contemplation, as well as a focused gaze. The word "yoga" is usually translated as *samādhi* (meditative absorption), union, or the yoking of one's awareness; however, within the context of the study of grammar, it can also mean the connection between words or the connection of a word with its root. Awareness of the context in which a word is used is imperative to its individual interpretation and therefore to our understanding of the work as a whole.

This book is an invitation to go beyond reading works in translation, to join practice together with theory, and to be active participants rather than outside observers. Translation is a dynamic act of observing, perceiving, and understanding. It is both a collision and collaboration between the literal and the imaginary; the point where

where our inner and outer worlds meet. It is a dance between the "facts" we see before our eyes and the "fictions" sprouting in our minds, loosening the boundaries that attempt to hold these worlds apart. Translation is a continuous process, one that we are constantly engaged in, knowingly and unknowingly. I look at the tree outside my window, and my experience is immediately translated into thoughts and words. The linguistic choices we make (or that are made for us) influence our perspective, which in turn creates our experience; word and meaning constantly inform each other, merging into each other until they are almost inextricable. When we read a text in translation, we are inevitably viewing it through the subjective lens of the translator as well as our own.

Each Sanskrit word has dozens of possible meanings; each *sūtra* and each verse has limitless possibilities. For example, the word *guru* is usually translated as "teacher" and often referred to as "one who removes darkness." But a more literal meaning of the word is "heaviness"—a teacher is someone who is weighty with knowledge, who has a solid presence. It is no contradiction that *guru* means both light and heavy; there was an old joke at Harvard that every Sanskrit word means itself, its opposite, the name of a god, and a sexual position.* The sacred and the profane are intimately and inseparably woven together in the fabric of Indian thought. The word "yoga" itself is given at least seventy-eight different definitions in V. S. Apte's dictionary.† If the word "yoga" is this complex, how can we even imagine that there could be a singular definitive meaning for any text?

There are numerous translations of fundamental texts, such as the *Yogasūtra* and the *Bhagavadgītā*; some are so different that it is difficult to believe that they stem from the same works. The translator is constantly making choices—which words to translate and which to leave in the original. Should the same word be translated

*Wendy Doniger, *The Hindus: An Alternative History* (New York: Penguin Group, 2009), 44.

†Including: joining, uniting, union, junction, combination, contact, touch, connection, employment, application, use, mode, manner, course, means, a yoke, conveyance, vehicle, carriage, armor, consequence, result, fitness, propriety, suitableness, occupation, work, business, trick, fraud, device, expedient, plan, means, endeavor, zeal, diligence, assiduity, remedy, cure, charm, spell, incantation, magic, gaining, acquisition, equipment of an army, fixing, putting on, practice, side, argument, occasion, opportunity, possibility, occurrence, wealth, substance, rule, precept, dependence of one word on another, etymology or derivation of the meaning of a word, deep and abstract meditation, concentration of the mind, contemplation of the Supreme Spirit, system of philosophy established by Patañjali, conjunction, combination of stars, devotion, spy, secret agent, traitor, violator of truth or confidence, an attack, ability, power, equality, and sameness. (Vaman Shivaram Apte, *The Practical Sanskrit English Dictionary* [Delhi: Motilal Banarsidass Publishers, 2007], 1316–17.)

differently in different contexts? Are some words untranslatable? For once something is named as a recognizable, defined, unquestionable entity, it takes on a specific shape from which it is very hard to return to its original multifaceted potential.

The philosophy and practice of yoga are limitless; yoga cannot be owned or contained by anyone. And because it is so immense, there can be no definitive meaning for any of these texts. This is clearly evident from the long-standing custom of questioning and debate—a vibrant practice in existence since before these texts were even written down—recorded in the numerous commentaries that have grown up alongside the texts themselves. I hope to participate in this movement toward discussion, to welcome and encourage a living, breathing practice that is constantly transforming and growing to support the modern world, with thoughtfulness and consideration.

The question arises as to what is our *dharma*, our duty, as yoga students so removed from the original context in which these texts and practices first arose. How can we actively participate in this tradition, while still honoring its roots, as well as our own? It seems that the only way to do this is by engaging directly with the original texts, by questioning for ourselves whether these statements still make sense thousands of years later, in different countries and different contexts. This investigation into words and meaning is really a path of self-exploration. It takes flexibility and a willingness to walk the edge of uncertainty in order to explore the depths below the surface, rather than taking translations at face value. Translation is a risky undertaking—if we question our definitions, we are questioning the very fabric of our being: our spiritual and ethical values, our beliefs, our thought patterns, our emotions, and our perceptions, all of which are lenses for viewing and relating to our world.

When I speak of yoga texts, I am not speaking only of the corpus of *haṭhayoga* texts, or of Patañjali's *Yogasūtra*, but of the rich philosophical fabric—the *Upaniṣads*, the epics, and the poetry—from which the yoga tradition has been born. Modern yoga, despite the attempts of many to distance it from its history and remake it according to their own desires, can never be severed from its roots. Contained within the most despiritualized *āsana* class are the echoes of tradition. I have written this book in the hope that more people will try to explore rather than ignore that heritage.

Unlike other Sanskrit textbooks, this one will give you the challenge and the opportunity to work with real texts right from the beginning. However, it is important to remember that you are reading these verses out of context. The verses in each chapter have been chosen based on their level of grammatical difficulty as well as their interest and relevance for yoga students. The verses have been rearranged by text in the Answer Key and notes on each text have been provided throughout the book, in order to give the reader a greater sense of the work as a whole and the context from which it emerged. When translating, it is helpful to try to place oneself within the context in which the text was written and to try, as much as possible, to imagine and re-create the spirit in which the author was writing.

The most important ingredient in this process is a "re-spect" for the work you are translating.* "Re-spect" derives from the Latin *respectus*, from the verb *respicere*, "look back at, regard," consisting of *re-*, "back" + *specere*, "look at" or "look back." So, to read a text with "re-spect" literally means to look again, to keep looking with increasingly sensitive eyes. The text must be handled delicately, its subtleties appreciated. Doing so requires an acknowledgment of one's own limitations. At the same time, by puzzling over the text yourself, you will come closer to the meaning than you ever will through reading a translation and accepting it at face value. There is a tendency when reading texts in translation to latch on to a false ideal of simplicity that never existed in the original. One of the reasons it is so important to engage with these texts ourselves is to give us a place to acknowledge the complexity of these ideas and to grapple with them.

It is in this spirit that I am proposing translation as a form of yoga. To translate literally means "to carry across"; translation is both a tool and a meditation in itself. The word *avatāraṇam* means "translation" as well as "descent" or "incarnation." It is important to acknowledge that by translating we are giving life to these texts in a new incarnation, as well as participating in an old tradition. Because we live in a different time and in a different place, parts of these texts may be directly relevant and other pieces may not make sense to us today. Rather than our trying to adapt the meaning of the text to say something that feels relevant, it is important to read the texts as they are, to acknowledge the differences, and to try to make sense of those differences in relation to our present experience.

Part of my intention in this book is to integrate the oral tradition with the written, to help reignite an interest in the relation of sound and meaning, to open an ear to listening. When I started studying Sanskrit on my first trip to India, it was a world with no cell phones, no Internet, no television, no digital screens of any kind. I would walk through the streets chanting the alphabet, immersed in sounds, sights, and smells I had never experienced before. The texts I began to memorize were woven together with women selling flower *mālās* (garlands), men walking around with baskets of fruit and vegetables yelling "Pa-pay-a! Pa-pay-a! Pa-pay-a!," cows eating garbage, and temple bells ringing.

---

* James Hillman. *The Thought of the Heart and the Soul of the World* (Putnam, Conn.: Spring Publications, 1992), 129.

The stories, drawings, and audio that I provide are my attempt to give you a bit of that experience. The stories that I tell throughout the text are a mix of fact and fiction, myth and reality, for in translation that boundary blurs. If a myth is alive in people's imaginations, then it is real for all intents and purposes. If you were to study with a teacher in India, you would be told stories interwoven with conjugations and declensions. The polytheism pervasive in India is the backdrop for these texts and it is important to try to read them through a lens that gives space for multiplicity. The myths are important because they keep the imagination alive and remind us not to get stuck in a monocentric, dualistic, or literalistic approach.

Translation is necessarily practice mixed together with theory, a fine line walked down the middle of the two. While it is important to understand the grammar and follow it, this theoretical approach must be seen through your own experience and made sense of in practice. At the crossroads between knowledge and intuition, translation becomes poetry. Translating can create a bridge between mind and heart, Soul and Spirit, and the worldly and the transcendent. By acknowledging the limitations inherent in our own definitions, we can escape being trapped by them. At its heart, translation is an exploration of the immensity of knowledge, a homage to tradition, as well as an enlivening of the imagination. The wisdom inherent in these texts transcends time and space, and has the potential to guide us into transformation. Our task is to keep our eyes open, to capture the space between these ancient words with our own words, and to make the intangible essence dance and come alive on the page through our own understanding.

# How to Use This Book

This book is for anyone with the desire to learn Sanskrit, from those who want to dip their toes in to those who are seeking a full immersion. It can be used by teachers in an academic class or a yoga course, for private or small study groups, or for *svādhyāya*, "self-study." Of course, as with yoga practice, it is important to have the guidance of a teacher along the way, whenever possible; however, practice can also be undertaken or maintained on one's own.

The text is divided into three segments—the first, which teaches reading, with basic grammar, is suitable for anyone beginning Sanskrit study. The second part covers more extensive grammar, and the third section covers complex grammar, enough to begin to look at and understand more complex texts, such as the *Upaniṣads*. It is important to listen to the audio recording for each chapter, as proper pronunciation is essential to understanding the true meaning of these texts. The audio files can be found at http://us.macmillan.com/yogavataranamthetranslationofyoga/zoeslatoffponte, where you can also download *sandhi*, verb, and noun charts and other supplemental materials and writing.

By the end of the book, students will be capable of reading, somewhat fluently, whatever text they choose. My hope with this book is to invite the student in, to build a bridge that provides an entry into these texts and the worlds they encompass, at any level one desires.

## FOR SELF STUDY

Whether you are brand-new to studying Sanskrit or have some experience, whether you are interested in learning proper pronunciation, reading the *devanāgarī* script, delving into meaning and grammar, or in just deepening your yoga practice, this book is appropriate for all levels. The study of Sanskrit at any level will deepen your yoga practice both on and off the mat, opening your heart, mind, and soul to greater levels of subtle awareness, concentration, and understanding.

This book is to be approached slowly, over time. In Chapter 1, you will learn to read the alphabet, the foundation of Sanskrit study, which is akin to learning sun salutations, *sūryanamaskāra*. You will learn to read through familiar words, such as *āsana* (yoga posture) names, and key words from the *Yogasūtra*, the *Bhagavadgītā*, and other yogic texts. By the end of Chapter 1, small excerpts from these texts and familiar *mantras* (chants) will be given as reading practice. Grammar will be taught, as well, through yogic philosophy. At any stage, one can flip through and read the stories alongside the text or accompanying the illustrations, or read the translations at the end of the book, but for the most part, the text develops progressively, each section building on the last.

Each section is subdivided into chapters, with detailed examples and exercises illustrating each grammatical concept. There is a review at the end of each chapter, as well as a full answer key at the end of the book. It is important to try to translate each exercise on your own before looking at the translations. Each verse is both a little puzzle to be solved and a meditation. Even if the meaning is obscure to begin with, with time, patience, and concentration, the essence will become clear.

## FOR TEACHERS

This book began out of my desire for a book I could teach from myself—one that integrates traditional and academic methods of learning and allows students to read texts as soon as possible. I have tried to incorporate the stories I might tell and the tips I might give into the text itself, but of course, a book is always enriched by a human touch. I hope that the text can be used as a vehicle, to which you can add your own knowledge and tales and go through examples with students when necessary. I have had to choose a select number of verses as examples and exercises, but of course, there are many more possible examples, and you may want to add verses where you feel that students need more practice. You may also want to quiz students on the grammatical rules and conjugations at various junctures throughout the course of study.

In a nonacademic setting, it can be helpful to teach a mixed-levels class, teaching students individually within a group setting. I recommend beginning and ending the class by chanting together as a group, emphasizing the primacy of oral learning in Sanskrit study. During class, students can be broken into groups according to level of ability and given individual instruction and assignments. This allows students to learn at their own pace, with support as necessary, and allows for new students to join the group at any time. It also enables students to work together and learn from one another. The new students are inspired by hearing the more advanced students reading and translating verses together; the more advanced students are reminded of the importance of the fundamentals by hearing the beginners chanting the alphabet and reading simple words. Throughout the class, the common thread (or *sūtra*) is the indescribable essence that weaves through all of Sanskrit study—the echoes of tradition and the promise of new meaning.

# Found in Translation: A Note on the Images

## *Ben Ponté*

Art plays an *unknowing* game with ultimate things . . .
—Paul Klee

When Zoë first asked me if I would like to illustrate this book, I was immediately faced with issues of translation. While feeling honored that she would ask, I was reluctant to enter such well-tended philosophical and spiritual territory—territory where questions inevitably arise . . .

How can one appreciate the subtle meaning of a text without imposing upon it an interpretation borne from one's own culture and experience? How can one pay homage to the culture in which a text is rooted while recognizing the limitations of one's own knowledge in relation to it? Is there a way between or beyond lingering tendencies of exotic orientalism on the one hand and detached objective literalism on the other? What is the relationship between word and meaning? What is the relationship between symbol and form? And is it possible to *translate* the verbal into the visual without diminishing the innate qualities of either medium?

Through the process of contemplating and working with the materials, I began to feel that the only way to approach these questions was to acknowledge, rather than attempt to get beyond, my own cultural heritage. As an artist I am largely indebted to Western traditions of image making and particular movements that oscillate between the figurative and the abstract. This relationship became the ground upon which these works were cultivated. Paradoxically, once I embraced the subjectivity involved in my own art practice, the works seemed to take on a form of their own.

I began placing works upon one another, overlapping and transposing images and words. Images fell within images, text within images, images within text, and as they did, the images, the materials, and the text began another kind of conversation. As the conversation deepened, the idea of "illustration" started to fall away, and as it did the works became less literally descriptive and more concerned with the issue of translation itself. The relationship among the image as an illusory two-dimensional space, the text as a symbolic form, and the materials upon which they rest became suggestive of both the meaning we carry with us into the world and the wider background of meaning that carries us. The apex where these worlds meet was ripe with implication.

The word "attention" comes from the Latin *attendere*, which literally means "to stretch." As we pay attention to, and therefore stretch, the interval in the mind between seeing and interpreting, knowing and understanding, perceiving and reacting, the world becomes a very different place. That difference requires us to stretch the mind further still, beyond the frames that keep our practical and theoretical worlds divided and out into a world where such divisions ultimately seem futile. I have come to see that liminal moment of attention as a moment of *translation*, the practice of being in that moment as *yoga*, and the work that may or may not emerge from it as *art*.

In that space I saw an image of this book as condensation on the window of Zoë's life. The droplets of wisdom and the trails of insight that were left on the glass came not only from her broad theoretical knowledge but from lived and felt experience, and from something innate in Zoë's soul—an unknowing and seeing presence intuitively apparent to everybody and *everysoul* she has taught. Zoë lives and breathes her theory and her practice to a point in which they are inseparable. I feel very fortunate to be invited into her process in this way and grateful she is now opening that window for us all.

# PART I

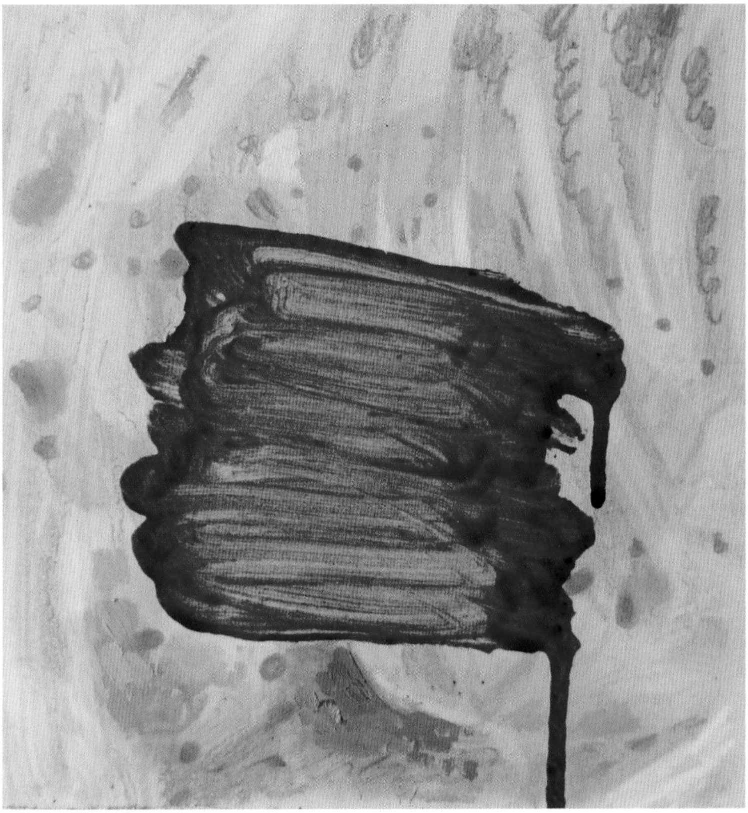

# 1
# THE *DEVANĀGARĪ* ALPHABET

स तु दीर्घकालनैरन्तर्यसत्कारासेवितो दृढभूमिः ॥ १.१४ ॥
**sa tu dīrgha-kāla-nairantarya-satkārāsevito dṛḍha-bhūmiḥ**
And that practice attains firm ground when cultivated for a long time, without interruption, and with devotion.
|| *Yogasūtra* 1.14 ||

## THE SANSKRIT LANGUAGE

Sanskrit, or *saṃskṛta*, means "refined, polished, well formed." It is derived from the root *kṛ* (to do or make), combined with the prefix *saṃ* (together), to create *saṃskṛ*, "to adorn, refine, polish, form well." This is also the root of *saṃskāra*, a word you might be familiar with, meaning "refining, perfection, impression." Sanskrit is an Indo-Aryan language, a sub-branch of Indo-Iranian, which itself is a branch of the Indo-European language family that includes Latin, Greek, English, and most European languages.

Classical Sanskrit, which we will study in this book, was codified by Pāṇini around 500 B.C.E., in his *Aṣṭādhyāyī*, or "Eight Chapters," made up of almost four thousand terse *sūtras* defining the rules of correct grammar. Classical Sanskrit was preceded by Vedic Sanskrit, the language of the *Vedas*, which can be dated to around 1500 B.C.E. and was preserved through oral tradition. Even in India today, there is an emphasis on the oral transmission of texts, and students often memorize texts in their entirety before being taught their meaning. It is not known exactly when Sanskrit stopped being a spoken language, but at a certain point it gave way to the *Prākṛta*, or "natural" languages, which evolved into the vernacular languages, such as Hindi, spoken in Northern India today, leaving Sanskrit as a primarily literary and religious ritual–oriented language.

Although you do not need to memorize this textbook before commencing study, it is my hope to keep alive a certain focus on orality, and I encourage you to listen to the audio recording and recite the letters, paradigms, and verses aloud whenever possible. The *sūtra* at the top of this page applies as much to Sanskrit study as it does to yoga practice. A similar level of consistency and concentration is necessary to reach fluency as to attain fluidity in *āsana* practice, and within that consistency, a meditative, contemplative state can arise, leading to deeper understanding.

# THE *DEVANĀGARĪ* ALPHABET

The Sanskrit language can be written in multiple scripts; however, we will learn it in its most common script today, *devanāgarī*, the "script of the gods." Traditionally, the Sanskrit language was written in the local script; however, with the advent of printing, *devanāgarī* became the standard script for Sanskrit texts.

The *devanāgarī* alphabet consists of forty-nine different sounds, which correspond to forty-nine different "letters" arranged systematically, according to the point of articulation, like all Indian scripts. Unlike in English, where two different letters can represent the same sound and the same letter can represent multiple sounds (as in "cat" and "lake" or "peace" and "sea" or "ocean" and "shell"), in Sanskrit there is a one-to-one correspondence between each sound and letter. These letters are divided into vowels (*svara*, or sounds) and consonants (*vyañjana*, or signs). The vowels exist in two different forms. As freestanding letters, they can only occur at the beginning of a word. When following a consonant they take on different combining forms. Consonants cannot exist or be pronounced without an accompanying vowel.

## Vowels (*Svara*)

The first nine vowels are considered simple vowels, consisting of four pairs of short sounds, followed by their long equivalents (represented in transliteration with a line on top of the letter), plus one last vowel, ḷ, which is quite uncommon in usage, pronounced as l + ṛ. The last four vowels are often categorized as diphthongs (although, technically, this is not quite accurate): sounds comprised of two simple vowel sounds combined, which are all considered long.

| | | | | | |
|---|---|---|---|---|---|
| अ a | आ ā | इ i | ई ī | उ u | ऊ ū |
| ऋ ṛ | ॠ ṝ | ऌ ḷ | | | |
| ए e | ऐ ai | ओ o | औ au | | |

## Consonants (*Vyañjana*)

All of the consonants are learned and pronounced with the vowel अ (a) attached. Thus, "letters" in Sanskrit are actually short syllables. The majority of the consonants are divided into five groups, reading across, according to where the sound is articulated in the mouth. See the diagram on page 7.

These groups are:

| | |
|---|---|
| Guttural: | pronounced at the back of the throat |
| Palatal: | pronounced with a slight smile, at the soft palate |
| Retroflex or Cerebral: | pronounced by curling the tongue to touch the roof of the mouth behind the teeth |
| Dental: | pronounced with the tongue between the teeth |
| Labial: | pronounced at the lips |

Within each of the five groups, the consonants are further ordered according to the following criteria:

- unvoiced, unaspirated stop
- unvoiced, aspirated stop
- voiced, unaspirated stop
- voiced, aspirated stop
- voiced, nasal

A stop or plosive is a sound that blocks the flow of air within the vocal tract. A voiced sound is one that uses the vocal cords in pronunciation; an aspirated sound creates an explosion of breath as the sound is articulated. Nasals are voiced sounds that allow the air to pass through the nose. Although these distinctions may appear confusing at first, as you listen, you will start to hear the differences between these sounds. These distinctions are important to learn, not only for pronunciation of each individual letter, but also for understanding how letters and words combine together through *sandhi* (conjunction).

| | Unvoiced | | Voiced | | Voiced |
|---|---|---|---|---|---|
| | Unaspirated | Aspirated | Unaspirated | Aspirated | Nasal |
| Guttural | क ka | ख kha | ग ga | घ gha | ङ ṅa |
| Palatal | च ca | छ cha | ज ja | झ jha | ञ ña |
| Retroflex | ट ṭa | ठ ṭha | ड ḍa | ढ ḍha | ण ṇa |
| Dental | त ta | थ tha | द da | ध dha | न na |
| Labial | प pa | फ pha | ब ba | भ bha | म ma |

Semivowels are voiced sounds, considered somewhere between a consonant and a vowel, but treated as consonants. Sibilants are unvoiced. ह (ha) is guttural, aspirated, and voiced.

| | Palatal | Retroflex | Dental | Labial | Guttural |
|---|---|---|---|---|---|
| Semivowels (Voiced): | य ya | र ra | ल la | व va | |
| Sibilants (Unvoiced): | श śa | ष ṣa | स sa | (Voiced): | ह ha |

There are two other syllabic sounds—*anusvāra*, a nasalization of the preceding vowel, represented by the symbol "ं" and written in transliteration as "ṃ," and *visarga*, pronounced as an aspiration of the preceding vowel, or as an "h" followed by an echo of the preceding vowel, represented by the symbol "ः" and written as "ḥ" in transliteration. Both of these sounds can be added on to any vowel. Below they are presented attached to the letter अ.

| | Anusvāra | Visarga |
|---|---|---|
| Add-on sounds: | अं aṃ | अः aḥ |

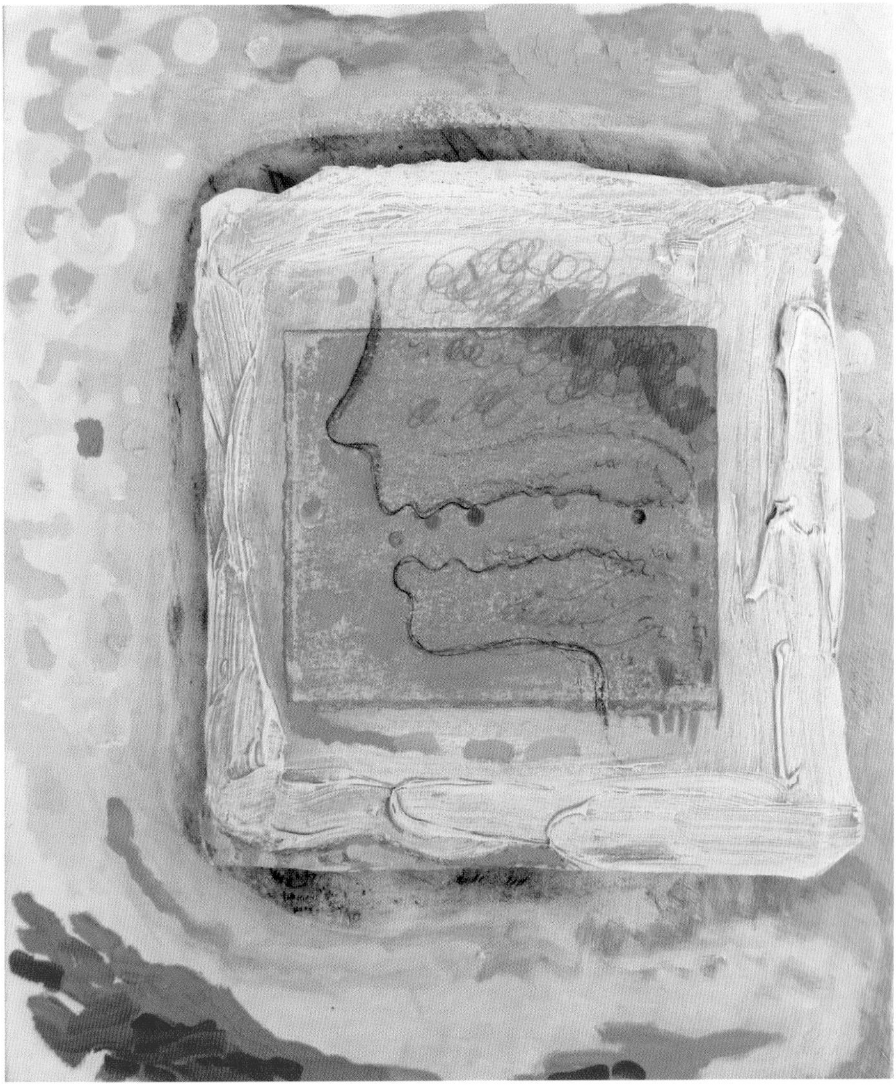

- कण्ठ्य *Kaṇṭhya* Guttural
- तालव्य *Tālavya* Palatal
- मूर्धन्य *Mūrdhanya* Retroflex
- दन्त्य *Dantya* Dental
- ओष्ठ्य *Oṣṭhya* Labial

अ a आ ā इ i ई ī उ u ऊ ū

ऋ ṛ ॠ ṝ ऌ ḷ

ए e ऐ ai ओ o औ au अं aṃ अः aḥ

क ka ख kha ग ga घ gha ङ ṅa

च ca छ cha ज ja झ jha ञ ña

ट ṭa ठ ṭha ड ḍa ढ ḍha ण ṇa

त ta थ tha द da ध dha न na

प pa फ pha ब ba भ bha म ma

य ya र ra ल la व va

श śa ष ṣa स sa ह ha

अ आ इ ई उ ऊ

ऋ ॠ ऌ

ए ऐ ओ औ अं अः

क ख ग घ ङ

च छ ज झ ञ

ट ठ ड ढ ण

त थ द ध न

प फ ब भ म

य र ल व

श ष स ह

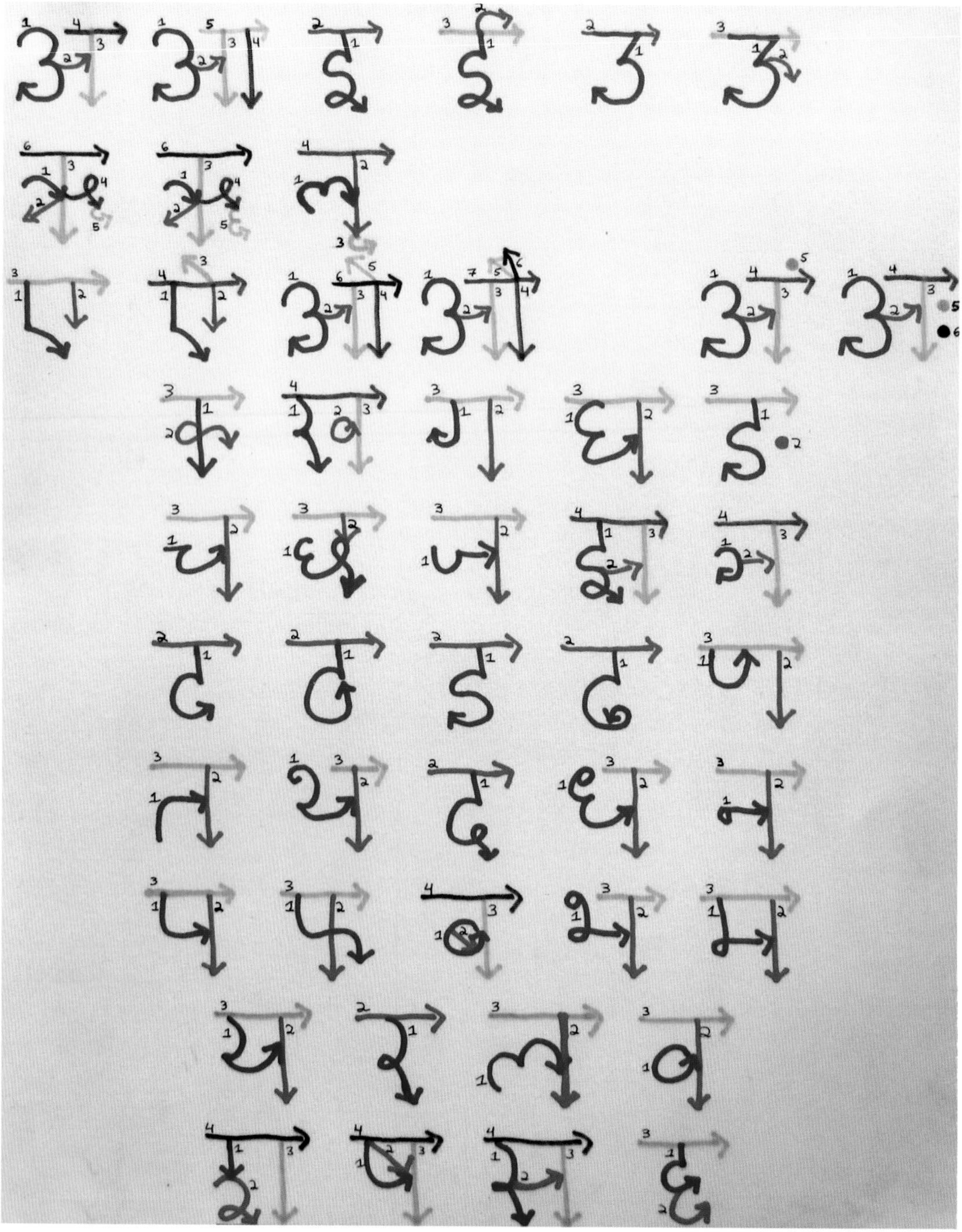

## Writing Practice

The easiest way to learn the alphabet is to write it out every day (as shown on page 9). First thing in the morning, when your mind is fresh, is a good time, although anytime you have a few quiet minutes is fine. Listen to the audio recording as much as possible and recite the alphabet aloud as you write it.

Write the alphabet from left to right, one row at a time. When you write each letter, go from left to right and top to bottom, putting the top line on last, like a hat (as shown on page 10). Note that, as in any language, handwritten letters will look slightly different from the printed ones. As we start to join letters together to make words, there will be one long top line that covers all (or most) of the letters in a word. Interestingly, this top line is called a *sūtra*, as it is the "thread" that strings the letters in a word together.

### A. Simple Words

Copy in *devanāgarī* and write in transliteration. Many of these are words you will already be familiar with; see if you can determine their meanings. The transliterations, as well as the definitions of the words, can be found in the Answer Key at the end of the book. It is a good idea to memorize these words and their meanings, as they are important vocabulary, which we will encounter later on, in various verses.

1. आसन
2. यम
3. अथ
4. हठ
5. हल
6. जप
7. बक
8. पद्
9. जय
10. जन
11. कफ
12. रस

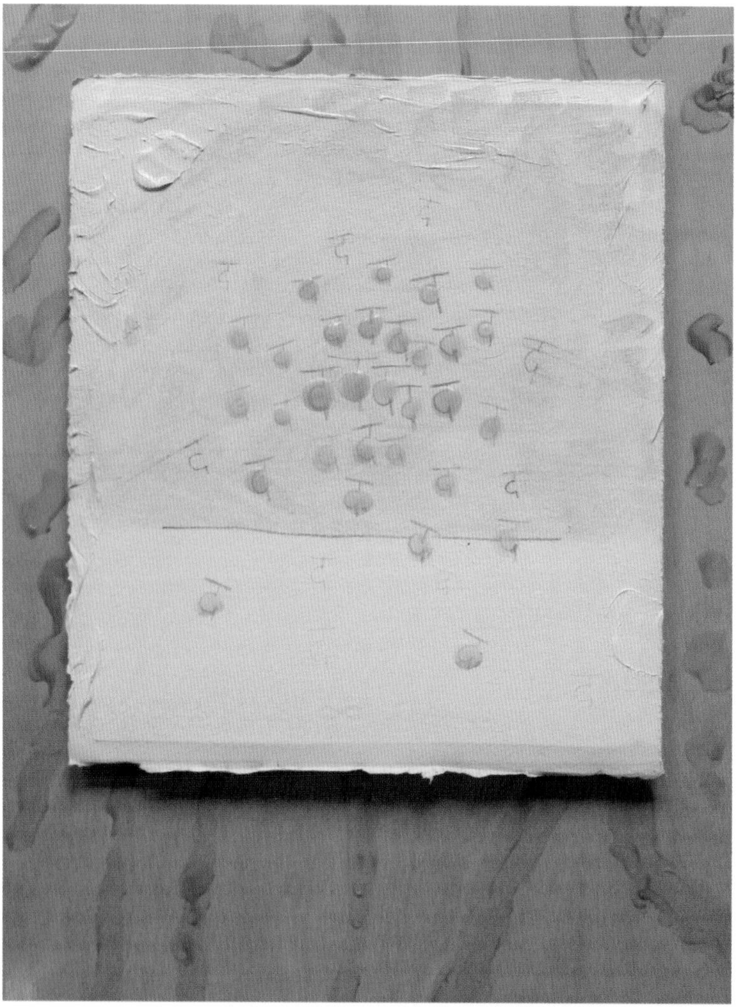

In the *Bṛhadāraṇyakopaniṣat (Bṛhadāranyaka Upaniṣad)*, 5.2.1–3, the three types of beings—gods, humans, and demons—went to the creator, Prajāpati, and asked for instruction.
To the gods, he said द्, which they took to mean *dāmyata*, "be self-controlled."
To the humans he said द्, which they took to mean *datta*, "be generous."
To the demons he said द्, which they took to mean *dayadhvam*, "be compassionate."
द् द् द्, like the divine sound of thunder; this one single syllable contains these three teachings: be self-controlled; be generous; be compassionate.

Traditionally, every letter of the alphabet is learned with the vowel "a" affixed to it, as seen in the alphabet chart. To attain the letter by itself, a mark called a *virāma* (्) is placed below the letter, for example, क् = k. In general, these forms are only found at the end of a line of verse, a sentence, or a *sūtra*, or in the middle of a phrase if a word ends in a consonant and the rules of *sandhi* are not applied to join it to the following word.

### B. Transliterate the Following Words

1. सत्
2. असत्
3. तपस्
4. तमस्
5. रजस्
6. नमस्
7. मनस्
8. एकम्

The vowel आ, when not the first letter of a word, is written as a vertical line (ा) attached to any consonant (e.g., का = kā).

### C. Write in Transliteration

1. साधन
2. पाद
3. साधन पाद
4. धारणा
5. वात
6. अपान
7. आकाश
8. माला
9. हालाहल
10. हलासन
11. पाशासन
12. शलभासन
13. बकासन

Note the similarity between the following letters:

घ gha, ध dha
ट ṭa, ठ ṭha, ढ ḍha
थ tha, य ya
ब ba, व va
भ bha, म ma
ख kha, र + व = रव rava

14. राग
15. राज
16. राम
17. रामायण
18. महाभारत
19. राधा
20. अनाहत

## Vowel Combination

The vowels you learned at the beginning of the chapter are used only when a vowel is the first letter of a freestanding word. When vowels are found in any other position in a word, they are written in a different combining form. Below, the vowels are added to the letter क्.

| | | |
|---|---|---|
| क् + अ ⇒ क | क् + ऋ ⇒ कृ | क् + अं ⇒ कं |
| क् + आ ⇒ का | क् + ॠ ⇒ कॄ | क् + अः ⇒ कः |
| क् + इ ⇒ कि | क् + ए ⇒ के | |
| क् + ई ⇒ की | क् + ऐ ⇒ कै | |
| क् + उ ⇒ कु | क् + ओ ⇒ को | |
| क् + ऊ ⇒ कू | क् + औ ⇒ कौ | |

Note that in the table on the following pages, the added vowels are shown in red. First read through the table, going from left to right across each line, and then write out the forms for each letter, reciting as you write. For the most part, this chart is a repetition of the simple pattern shown above, as represented with the dummy letter "x" on the second line. The starred forms indicate letters that have slightly unusual representations and, thus, are deviations from this pattern. The letter ऌ has been omitted as it only occurs in the verb क्लृ, *kḷ*, "to be fit for, bring about, accomplish."

| +अ | +आ | +इ | +ई | +उ | +ऊ | +ऋ | +ॠ | +ए | +ऐ | +ओ | +औ | +अं | +अः |
|---|---|---|---|---|---|---|---|---|---|---|---|---|---|
| X | Xा | िX | Xी | Xु | Xू | Xृ | Xॄ | Xे | Xै | Xो | Xौ | Xं | Xः |
| क | का | कि | की | कु | कू | कृ | कॄ | के | कै | को | कौ | कं | कः |
| ख | खा | खि | खी | खु | खू | खृ | खॄ | खे | खै | खो | खौ | खं | खः |
| ग | गा | गि | गी | गु | गू | गृ | गॄ | गे | गै | गो | गौ | गं | गः |
| घ | घा | घि | घी | घु | घू | घृ | घॄ | घे | घै | घो | घौ | घं | घः |
| ङ | ङा | ङि | ङी | ङु | ङू | ङृ | ङॄ | ङे | ङै | ङो | ङौ | ङं | ङः |
| च | चा | चि | ची | चु | चू | चृ | चॄ | चे | चै | चो | चौ | चं | चः |
| छ | छा | छि | छी | छु | छू | छृ | छॄ | छे | छै | छो | छौ | छं | छः |
| ज | जा | जि | जी | जु | जू | जृ | जॄ | जे | जै | जो | जौ | जं | जः |
| झ | झा | झि | झी | झु | झू | झृ | झॄ | झे | झै | झो | झौ | झं | झः |
| ञ | ञा | ञि | ञी | ञु | ञू | ञृ | ञॄ | ञे | ञै | ञो | ञौ | ञं | ञः |
| ट | टा | टि | टी | टु | टू | टृ | टॄ | टे | टै | टो | टौ | टं | टः |
| ठ | ठा | ठि | ठी | ठु | ठू | ठृ | ठॄ | ठे | ठै | ठो | ठौ | ठं | ठः |
| ड | डा | डि | डी | डु | डू | डृ | डॄ | डे | डै | डो | डौ | डं | डः |
| ढ | ढा | ढि | ढी | ढु | ढू | ढृ | ढॄ | ढे | ढै | ढो | ढौ | ढं | ढः |
| ण | णा | णि | णी | णु | णू | णृ | णॄ | णे | णै | णो | णौ | णं | णः |
| त | ता | ति | ती | तु | तू | तृ | तॄ | ते | तै | तो | तौ | तं | तः |
| थ | था | थि | थी | थु | थू | थृ | थॄ | थे | थै | थो | थौ | थं | थः |
| द | दा | दि | दी | दु | दू | दृ | दॄ | दे | दै | दो | दौ | दं | दः |
| ध | धा | धि | धी | धु | धू | धृ | धॄ | धे | धै | धो | धौ | धं | धः |
| न | ना | नि | नी | नु | नू | नृ | नॄ | ने | नै | नो | नौ | नं | नः |
| प | पा | पि | पी | पु | पू | पृ | पॄ | पे | पै | पो | पौ | पं | पः |
| फ | फा | फि | फी | फु | फू | फृ | फॄ | फे | फै | फो | फौ | फं | फः |
| ब | बा | बि | बी | बु | बू | बृ | बॄ | बे | बै | बो | बौ | बं | बः |
| भ | भा | भि | भी | भु | भू | भृ | भॄ | भे | भै | भो | भौ | भं | भः |
| म | मा | मि | मी | मु | मू | मृ | मॄ | मे | मै | मो | मौ | मं | मः |
| य | या | यि | यी | यु | यू | यृ | यॄ | ये | यै | यो | यौ | यं | यः |
| र | रा | रि | री | *रु | *रू | *र्ऋ | *र्ॠ | रे | रै | रो | रौ | रं | रः |

| | | | | | | | | | | | | | |
|---|---|---|---|---|---|---|---|---|---|---|---|---|---|
| ल | ला | लि | ली | लु | लू | लृ | लॄ | ले | लै | लो | लौ | लं | लः |
| व | वा | वि | वी | वु | वू | वृ | वॄ | वे | वै | वो | वौ | वं | वः |

| | | | | | | | | | | | | | |
|---|---|---|---|---|---|---|---|---|---|---|---|---|---|
| श | शा | शि | शी | शु | शू | शृ | शॄ | शे | शै | शो | शौ | शं | शः |
| ष | षा | षि | षी | षु | षू | षृ | षॄ | षे | षै | षो | षौ | षं | षः |
| स | सा | सि | सी | सु | सू | सृ | सॄ | से | सै | सो | सौ | सं | सः |
| ह | हा | हि | ही | हु | हू | *हृ | हॄ | हे | है | हो | हौ | हं | हः |

### D. Transliterate the Following Words

1. योग
2. नियम
3. समाधि
4. अनुशासनम्
5. गुरु
6. वीर
7. सीता
8. सुख
9. दुःख
10. शौच
11. दोष
12. लोक
13. शोक
14. वेद
15. मूल
16. अहिंसा
17. गुण
18. शिव
19. दैवत
20. अमृत
21. विभूति
22. पृथिवी
23. हृदय
24. भगवद् गीता
25. असतो मा सद् गमय ।
26. हेयं दुःखम् अनागतम् ॥ *Yogasūtra* 2.16 ॥

The most well-known and referenced text on yoga, the *Yogasūtra*, often known as the *Yoga Sūtras*, was systematized by Patañjali, sometime between the second century B.C.E and the second century C.E. It consists of 195 *sūtras*, literally "threads," or terse aphorisms, divided into four books, for easy memorization at a time when oral tradition was the main means of transmission. It describes an eight-limbed (*aṣṭāṅga*) yoga, culminating in *samādhi*, or "meditative absorption." The goal is the realization of the *puruṣa* (Soul) as separate from *prakṛti* (Nature), and its liberation through various meditative techniques.

*Sandhi* (Conjunction) Rule #1: When two similar simple vowels, either short or long (अ, आ, इ, ई, उ, ऊ, ऋ, ॠ), are joined together, they combine to become the long vowel of the pair. This occurs both internally, within a word, and externally, when two separate words are written in sequence in a sentence.

अ / आ + अ / आ ⇒ आ
इ / ई + इ / ई ⇒ ई
उ / ऊ + उ / ऊ ⇒ ऊ
ऋ / ॠ + ऋ / ॠ ⇒ ॠ

27. वीर् + आसन = वीरासन
28. कपोत + आसन = कपोतासन
29. मायुर + आसन = मायुरासन
30. भुजपीड + आसन = भुजपीडासन
31. योग + अनुशासनम् = योगानुशासनम्
32. अथ योगानुशासनम् ॥ *Yogasūtra* 1.1 ॥

## Compound Consonants

When two letters are joined together in a compound, the first letter usually loses its right-hand vertical line. Thus, you will see half of the first letter joined to the whole second letter.

### Examples

स् + त = स्त
त् + य = त्य
न् + ध = न्ध
ध् + य = ध्य

### E. Transliterate

1. नमस्ते
2. अभ्यास
3. वैराग्य
4. ध्यान
5. सत्य
6. अस्तेय
7. सन्तोष

8. स्वाध्याय
9. शान्ति
10. समस्थिति
11. पादहस्तासन
12. उत्कटासन
13. बन्ध
14. वन्दे
15. अरविन्द
16. वन्दे गुरूणां चरणारविन्दे ।
17. स्थिरसुखम् आसनम् ॥ *Yogasūtra* 2.46 ॥

Sometimes, letters are joined vertically, with the second letter written beneath the first. Similarly, three letters can be joined together, and sometimes even four, or, rarely, five. The following table shows the more common conjuncts. There is no need to memorize all of these combinations; it is just important to learn to recognize them. The combinations involving the letter "r" will be explained in more detail on page 21. Note the following three consonant combinations, which are important common exceptions to the normal rules of conjunction.

क् + ष = क्ष kṣa
त् + र = त्र tra
ज् + ञ = ज्ञ jña

Also note the irregular combining form of श (e.g., श् + च = श्च).

| | | | | | | | | | |
|---|---|---|---|---|---|---|---|---|---|
| क्क | क्ख | क्च | क्त | क्त्र | क्म | क्य | क्र | क्ल | क्व |
| kka | kkha | kca | kta | ktra | kma | kya | kra | kla | kva |
| क्ष | क्ष्म | क्ष्य | क्ष्व | | | | | | |
| kṣa | kṣma | kṣya | kṣva | | | | | | |
| ख्न | ख्य | ख्र | | | | | | | |
| khna | khya | khra | | | | | | | |
| ग्न | ग्य | ग्र | ग्ल | | | | | | |
| gna | gya | gra | gla | | | | | | |
| घ्न | घ्न्य | घ्य | घ्र | | | | | | |
| ghna | ghnya | ghya | ghra | | | | | | |
| ङ्क | ङ्क्त | ङ्ख | ङ्ग | ङ्घ | | | | | |
| ṅka | ṅkta | ṅkha | ṅga | ṅgha | | | | | |

| | | | | | |
|---|---|---|---|---|---|
| च्च | च्छ | च्य | | | |
| cca | ccha | cya | | | |
| ज्ज | ज्ञ | ज्म | ज्य | ज्र | ज्व |
| jja | jña | jma | jya | jra | jva |
| ञ्च | ञ्छ | ञ्ज | | | |
| ñca | ñcha | ñja | | | |

| | | | | | | |
|---|---|---|---|---|---|---|
| ट्ट | ट्य | | ठ्ठ | | | |
| ṭṭa | ṭya | | ṭhṭha | | | |
| ड्ग | ड्ड | ड्भ | ड्म | ड्य | | ढ्य |
| ḍga | ḍḍa | ḍbha | ḍma | ḍya | | ḍhya |
| ण्ट | ण्ठ | ण्ड | ण्ण | ण्य | ण्व | |
| ṇṭa | ṇṭha | ṇḍa | ṇṇa | ṇya | ṇva | |

| | | | | | | | | | | | | | | |
|---|---|---|---|---|---|---|---|---|---|---|---|---|---|---|
| त्क | त्त | त्त्य | त्त्व | त्थ | त्न | त्प | त्म | त्य | त्र | त्र्य | त्व | त्स | | |
| tka | tta | ttya | ttva | ttha | tna | tpa | tma | tya | tra | trya | tva | tsa | | |
| थ्न | थ्य | | | | | | | | | | | | | |
| thna | thya | | | | | | | | | | | | | |
| द्ग | द्ग्र | द्घ | द्द | द्ध | द्ध्य | द्ब | द्भ | द्भ्य | द्म | द्य | द्र | द्र्य | द्व | द्व्य |
| dga | dgra | dgha | dda | ddha | ddhya | dba | dbha | dbhya | dma | dya | dra | drya | dva | dvya |
| ध्न | ध्म | ध्य | ध्र | ध्व | | | | | | | | | | |
| dhna | dhma | dhya | dhra | dhva | | | | | | | | | | |
| न्त | न्त्र | न्थ | न्द | न्ध | न्न | न्म | न्य | न्र | न्व | न्स | | | | |
| nta | ntra | ntha | nda | ndha | nna | nma | nya | nra | nva | nsa | | | | |

| | | | | | | | | |
|---|---|---|---|---|---|---|---|---|
| प्त | प्न | प्प | प्म | प्य | प्र | प्ल | प्स | |
| pta | pna | ppa | pma | pya | pra | pla | psa | |
| ब्ज | ब्द | ब्न | ब्र | | | | | |
| bja | bda | bna | bra | | | | | |
| भ्न | भ्य | भ्र | | | | | | |
| bhna | bhya | bhra | | | | | | |
| म्न | म्प | म्ब | म्भ | म्म | म्य | म्र | म्ल | म्व |
| mna | mpa | mba | mbha | mma | mya | mra | mla | mva |

| | | | | | | | | | |
|---|---|---|---|---|---|---|---|---|---|
| य्य | ल्क | ल्प | ल्म | ल्य | ल्ल | ल्व | व्न | व्य | व्र |
| yya | lka | lpa | lma | lya | lla | lva | vna | vya | vra |

| | | | | | | | |
|---|---|---|---|---|---|---|---|
| श्च | श्न | श्म | श्य | श्र | श्ल | श्व | श्श |
| śca | śna | śma | śya | śra | śla | śva | śśa |
| ष्ट | ष्ट्व | ष्ठ | ष्ण | ष्प | ष्म | ष्य | ष्व |
| ṣṭa | ṣṭva | ṣṭha | ṣṇa | ṣpa | ṣma | ṣya | ṣva |

| | | | | | | | | | | | | |
|---|---|---|---|---|---|---|---|---|---|---|---|---|
| स्क | स्त | स्त्र | स्थ | स्न | स्प | स्फ | स्म | स्य | स्र | स्ल | स्व | स्स |
| ska | sta | stra | stha | sna | spa | spha | sma | sya | sra | sla | sva | ssa |
| ह्ण | ह्न | ह्म | ह्य | ह्र | ह्ल | | | | | | | |
| hṇa | hna | hma | hya | hra | hla | | | | | | | |

### F. Transliterate

1. अष्टाङ्ग
2. पद्म
3. सहस्र
4. ईश्वर
5. श्वेत
6. भक्ति
7. मन्त्र
8. चित्त
9. पित्त
10. सत्त्व
11. ज्ञान
12. मोक्ष
13. सूत्र
14. पतञ्जलि
15. शङ्ख
16. विघ्न
17. युद्ध
18. क्षेत्र

## The Letter "R"

The letter "r" can be joined in two ways. When following a consonant, the letter "r" is usually written as a diagonal line and appears differently depending on which consonant it attaches to (see the chart of conjunct consonants). When it precedes a consonant it is written as "र्" and is placed on top. It is always placed as far to the right as possible, while still attached to the same syllable.

Example: कूर्म = *kūrma* (the "r" is written on top of the "ma")
but कूर्मासन = *kūrmāsana* (the "r" is written above the vertical line representing "ā," because it is the vowel of the syllable "mā")

### G. Transliterate

1. कर्म
2. धर्म
3. सर्व
4. चर्य
5. शिर्षासन
6. प्राण
7. प्रमाण
8. प्रणिधान
9. चक्र
10. क्रिया
11. अपरिग्रह
12. वीरभद्रासन
13. नासाग्र
14. ब्रह्मचर्य
15. धर्मक्षेत्रे कुरुक्षेत्रे समवेता युयुत्सवः । *Bhagavadgītā* 1.1ab ।

> Contained within the *Bhīṣma Parvan*, the sixth book of the *Mahābhārata* (approximately fourth century B.C.E.), the *Bhagavad Gītā*, or "Song of the Beloved Lord," is a dialogue between Arjuna, one of the five Pāṇḍava brothers, and the god Kṛṣna. Through Arjuna's external conflict over whether to fight his cousins, the Kauravas, in battle, the internal struggle in his Soul is revealed. Kṛṣṇa responds by teaching him yoga, both as a means to journey inward toward the ultimate stage of union with the Divine and as a way of learning to act and to fulfill one's *dharma* in the world.

## Review Exercises

Copy in *devanāgarī* and transliterate.

1. *Hitopadeśa*

विद्या ददाति विनयं विनयाद्याति पात्रताम् ।
पात्रत्वाद्धनमाप्नोति धनाद्धर्मस्ततः सुखम् ॥

Knowledge gives humility,
From humility proceeds honor.
From honor, wealth is obtained,
From wealth, good works.
From that, happiness.

2. *Śivasaṃhitā* 3.53

सन्त्यत्र बहवो विघ्नाः दारुणा दुर्निवारणाः ।
तथापि साधयेद्योगी प्राणैः कण्ठगतैरपि ॥

Here, in yoga practice, there are many obstacles,
Frightful and difficult to ward off.
Nevertheless, the yogī should practice,
Even if he is at his last breath.

3. *Yogasūtra* 2.35–36

अहिंसाप्रतिष्ठायां तत्सन्निधौ वैरत्यागः ।
सत्यप्रतिष्ठायां क्रियाफलाश्रयत्वम् ।

When one is established in nonviolence, hostility is abandoned in his presence.
When one is established in truthfulness, he rests in the fruits of his actions.

4. *Bhagavadgītā* 6.20–22

यत्रोपरमते चित्तं निरुद्धं योगसेवया ।
यत्र चैवात्मनात्मानं पश्यन्नात्मनि तुष्यति ॥

सुखमात्यन्तिकं यत्तद् बुद्धिग्राह्यमतीन्द्रियम् ।
वेत्ति यत्र न चैवायं स्थितश्चलति तत्त्वतः ॥

यं लब्ध्वा चापरं लाभं मन्यते नाधिकं ततः ।
यस्मिन् स्थितो न दुःखेन गुरुणापि विचाल्यते ॥

When the mind becomes quiet,
Stilled by the practice of yoga.
And when, seeing the Soul with the Soul,
One is content in the Soul, alone.

One who knows that infinite happiness,
Which is grasped by understanding and beyond the senses.
And, established there,
Does not move away from Truth.

And when, having attained this,
One cannot imagine a higher gain.
Established in this, one is not agitated,
Even by great sorrow.

# 2
# VERBS: PRESENT TENSE, *PARASMAIPADA*, FIRST, FOURTH, SIXTH, AND TENTH CLASS; PRONOUNS: NOMINATIVE CASE; *SANDHI* REVIEW

तपःस्वाध्यायेश्वरप्रणिधानानि क्रियायोगः ॥ २.१ ॥
**tapaḥ-svādhyāyeśvara-praṇidhānāni kriyā-yogaḥ**
The yoga of action consists of discipline, self-study,
and surrender to the Divine.
॥ *Yogasūtra* 2.1 ॥

In this chapter, we will begin to explore Sanskrit verbs in the present tense, as well as some simple pronouns and a few basic *sandhi* rules. The verbal root is called a धातु, the same word used in Āyurveda for the seven "constituent elements" of the body. Verbal roots are marked by the radical sign √. Although the verbal root is actually a fictional construction invented by the grammarians, for the most part, all verbal forms and nouns are understood as deriving from these verbal roots.

For example:
योग (union, the act of yoking) comes from the root √युज्, "to join, unite, yoke, harness."
क्रिया and कर्म (action) both come from the root √कृ, "to do, make, perform."

## VERBS

A finite verb (one that has a subject, either expressed or implied, and is essential to any independent clause) is the main component of a Sanskrit sentence, whether it is included or assumed. All finite verbs are differentiated according to person (first, second, and third) and number (singular, dual, and plural), as well as tense, mode, and voice. These distinctions will be explained as they arise. We will begin by learning verbs in the present tense, active voice. The active voice is called परस्मैपद, "word for another," which indicates an action that is directed outward and can act on an object other than the agent of the action.

## Present Tense Verbs, *Parasmaipada* Conjugations

### Endings

| | Singular | Dual | Plural |
|---|---|---|---|
| 3rd person (He/She/It/They) | -ति | -तः | -अन्ति |
| 2nd person (You) | -सि | -थः | -थ |
| 1st person (I/we) | -मि | -वः | -मः |

*You might know the word गण (*gaṇa*) from the words गणेश (*Gaṇeśa*) or गणपति (*Gaṇapati*), the elephant-headed god who removes obstacles, literally the "lord of the groups."

These endings are attached to a verbal stem in slightly different ways, depending upon which group the verb belongs to. There are ten गण* (groups) of verbs, divided into thematic and athematic verbs. The first, fourth, sixth, and tenth groups are similar and are all considered "thematic" verbs, because they all share a *gaṇa* sign that is or ends with the thematic vowel अ. Additionally, for these four *gaṇas*, once their verbal stem is formed, it remains unchangeable throughout all conjugations.

### First Class *Parasmaipada* (4P) Verbs

The first group is called *bhvādi*, meaning "beginning with √भू (to be)," which is the first verb of the group. Verbal forms consist of a verbal stem (verbal base + specific *gaṇa* sign) + endings. In the first group, the *gaṇa* sign अ is added to the base before second- and third-person endings, and is lengthened to आ before first-person endings. Note that the *gaṇa* sign is lost before endings beginning with अ, for example, the third-person plural form.

**√पत् (root) to fall ⇒ पत् (base)**

| | Verbal Stem | | | | | | |
|---|---|---|---|---|---|---|---|
| | Base | | Gaṇa Sign | | Ending | | |
| 3rd person singular | पत् | + | अ | + | ति | ⇒ | पतति |
| 3rd person plural | पत् | + | अ | + | अन्ति | ⇒ | पतन्ति |
| 1st person singular | पत् | + | आ | + | मि | ⇒ | पतामि |

| | Singular | Dual | Plural |
|---|---|---|---|
| 3rd person | पतति<br>He/she/it falls | पततः<br>They two fall | पतन्ति<br>They all fall |

| | | | |
|---|---|---|---|
| 2nd person | पतसि<br>You fall | पतथः<br>You both fall | पतथ<br>You all fall |
| 1st person | पतामि<br>I fall | पतावः<br>We both fall | पतामः<br>We all fall |

For some verbal roots, as seen above, the root and the base are the same. However, some verbal roots change when they are conjugated, according to the rules of internal *sandhi* (which you need not be concerned about at this point). When you learn a new verb, it is important to remember both the root and the third-person singular conjugation, which indicates the verbal base and stem form.

**√भू (root) to be, to become ⇒ भव् (base)**

| | Verbal Stem | | | | | | |
|---|---|---|---|---|---|---|---|
| | Base | | Gaṇa Sign | | Ending | | |
| 3rd person singular | भव् | + | अ | + | ति | ⇒ | भवति |
| 1st person singular | भव् | + | आ | + | मि | ⇒ | भवामि |

| | Singular | Dual | Plural |
|---|---|---|---|
| 3rd person | भवति | भवतः | भवन्ति |
| 2nd person | भवसि | भवथः | भवथ |
| 1st person | भवामि | भवावः | भवामः |

**Conjugate**

When you are conjugating, or doing any Sanskrit exercise, it is important that you recite the words aloud as well as write out the paradigm. Note the starred verbs below, which have a verbal base that differs from the root.

| Root | | Base | 3rd pers. singular |
|---|---|---|---|
| √खाद् | to eat | खाद् | खादति |
| √गम् | to go | *गच्छ् | गच्छति |
| आ√गम् | to come | *आगच्छ् | आगच्छति |
| √जि | to conquer | *जय् | जयति |
| √त्यज् | to abandon | त्यज् | त्यजति |
| √दृश् | to see | *पश्य् | पश्यति |
| √नम् | to bow | नम् | नमति |
| √पठ् | to read, study | पठ् | पठति |

Note that letters before the root sign (√) represent a prefix that can alter (to varying degrees) the meaning of the verb.

The word दृष्टि, "gazing point," derives from the root √दृश्. Note, however, that √दृश् uses the base पश्य् for its present tense conjugations.

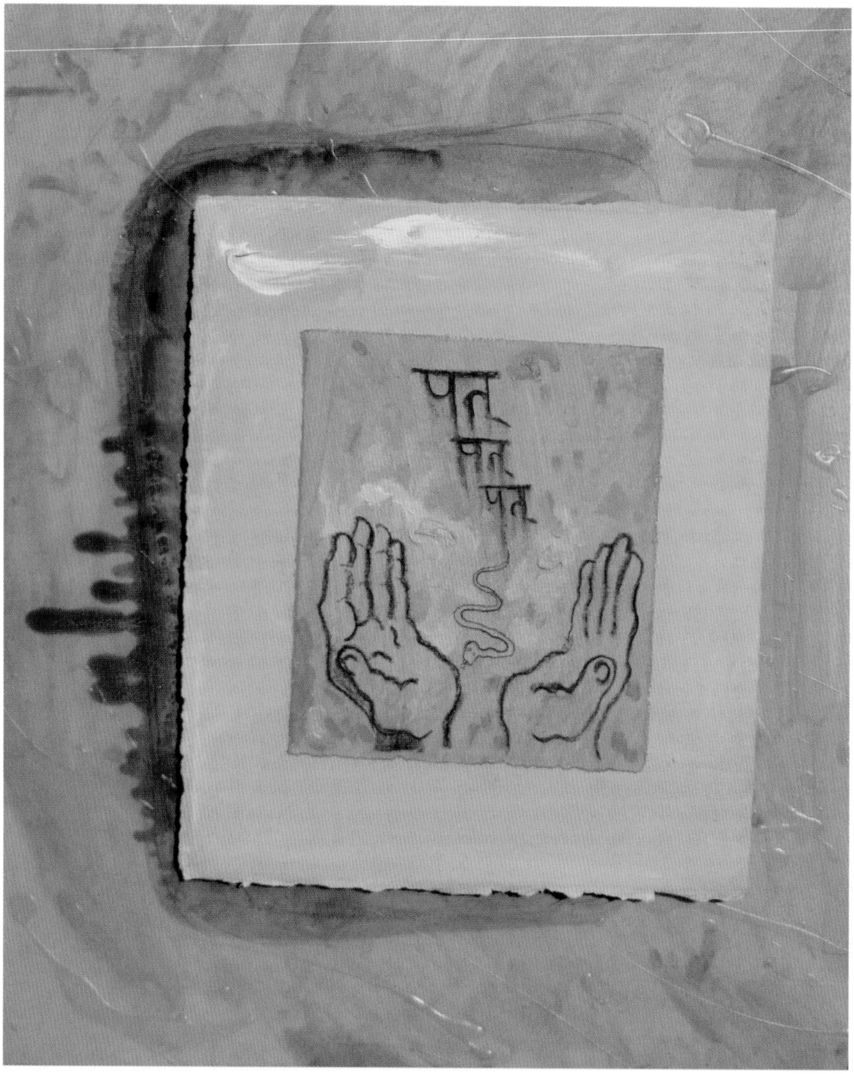


Around the second century C.E., when diseases of body, mind, and speech were pervading the world, the sages prayed to Lord Viṣṇu for help. Viṣṇu sent the sacred serpent, Ādiśeṣa, upon whom he'd been resting, to incarnate in the world as Patañjali to write treatises to purify body, mind, and speech. The yoginī Goṇikā had been praying to the Sun God for a son and was graced by a tiny snake falling into her open palms. The root पत् (*pat*) is the basis of the name पतञ्जलि (*Patañjali*), the author of the *Yogasūtra*, whose name means "fallen into the hollow of the hands," अञ्जलि, *añjali*.

| | | | |
|---|---|---|---|
| √बुध् | to know | *बोध् | बोधति |
| √वद् | to speak | वद् | वदति |
| √सद् | to sit, sink down | *सीद् | सीदति |

> The root √नम् is the origin of the word नमस्ते, which means "I bow to you" or "salutations to you."

## PRONOUNS

In Sanskrit there is an extensive system of pronouns, called सर्वनामन्, used, as in English, as substitutes for specific nouns. The first and second person refer to forms of "I" and "you," respectively. The third person is divided into three genders—masculine, feminine, and neuter. The pronouns we will consider now are all in the nominative or subject case, meaning they are used to designate the agent of action.

### Nominative (Subject) Case

| | | Singular | | Dual | | Plural | |
|---|---|---|---|---|---|---|---|
| 3rd person | Masculine | सः | he | तौ | they two (m.) | ते | they (m.) |
| | Feminine | सा | she | ते | they two (f.) | ताः | they (f.) |
| | Neuter | तत् | it | ते | they two (n.) | तानि | they (n.) |
| 2nd person | | त्वम् | you | युवाम् | you two | यूयम् | you all |
| 1st person | | अहम् | I | आवाम् | we two | वयम् | we all |

#### A. Translate

1. अहं पश्यामि ।
2. सा गच्छति ।
3. त्वं पठसि ।
4. ते बोधन्ति ।
5. युवां पतथः ।
6. वयं सीदामः ।

> *Sandhi* Rule: When an म् is the last letter of a word and is followed by a word beginning with a consonant, it becomes an *anusvāra* (ं).
>
> Example: अहम् पश्यामि ⇒ अहं पश्यामि

## INDECLINABLES

च and
न no/not

The conjunction च can occur either after each word it is connecting, or just once after the last word in the series. The particle न usually occurs directly before the verbal action it is negating. See the following exercises.

### B. Translate

1. अहं पश्यामि च नमामि च ।
2. सा गच्छति खादति च ।
3. त्वं न पठसि ।
4. ते बोधन्ति च वदन्ति च ।
5. युवां न पतथः ।
6. वयं न सीदामः ।

### C. Simple Sentences

Write five simple sentences using the pronouns, verbs, and indeclinables given. For now, do not worry about *sandhi* rules when you are writing sentences.

## FOURTH, SIXTH, AND TENTH CLASS VERBS

As mentioned earlier, these three classes plus the first class verbs detailed above form the group of "thematic" verbs.

### Fourth Class *Parasmaipada* (4P) Verbs

Fourth class verbs are conjugated exactly like first class verbs, except that the *gaṇa* sign य is added to the verbal base before second- and third-person endings, and is lengthened to या before first-person endings. The fourth class is called *divādi*, meaning "beginning with √दिव् (to play)," the first verb of the group.

**√नृत् (root) to dance ⇒ नृत् (base)**

| | Verbal Stem | | | | | | |
|---|---|---|---|---|---|---|---|
| | Base | | Gaṇa Sign | | Ending | | |
| 3rd person singular | नृत् | + | य | + | ति | ⇒ | नृत्यति |
| 1st person singular | नृत् | + | या | + | मि | ⇒ | नृत्यामि |

| | Singular | Dual | Plural |
|---|---|---|---|
| 3rd person | नृत्यति | नृत्यतः | नृत्यन्ति |
| 2nd person | नृत्यसि | नृत्यथः | नृत्यथ |
| 1st person | नृत्यामि | नृत्यावः | नृत्यामः |

**Conjugate**

| Root | | Base | 3rd person singular |
|---|---|---|---|
| √तुष् | to be pleased/content | तुष् | तुष्यति |
| √दिव् | to play | दिव् | दिव्यति |
| √नश् | to be lost/destroyed | नश् | नश्यति |
| √पुष् | to be nourished | पुष् | पुष्यति |

√तुष् is the root of the word सन्तोष, "contentment," the second नियम, "observance," the second limb of अष्टाङ्गयोग.

## Sixth Class *Parasmaipada* (6P) Verbs

For sixth class verbs, the *gaṇa* sign is अ before second- and third-person endings and आ before first-person endings. Although this is the same rule as for first class verbs, the difference is that in this case, the verbal root and the verbal base are almost always identical. The sixth class is called *tudādi*, meaning "beginning with √तुद् (to push)," the first verb of the group.

**√विश् (root) to enter ⇒ विश् (base)**

| | Verbal Stem | | | | | | |
|---|---|---|---|---|---|---|---|
| | Base | | Gaṇa Sign | | Ending | | |
| 3rd person singular | विश् | + | अ | + | ति | ⇒ | विशति |
| 1st person singular | विश् | + | आ | + | मि | ⇒ | विशामि |

| | Singular | Dual | Plural |
|---|---|---|---|
| 3rd person | विशति | विशतः | विशन्ति |
| 2nd person | विशसि | विशथः | विशथ |
| 1st person | विशामि | विशावः | विशामः |

**Conjugate**

| Root | | Base | 3rd person singular |
|---|---|---|---|
| √क्षिप् | to throw | क्षिप् | क्षिपति |
| √तुद् | to push | तुद् | तुदति |
| √दिश् | to show | दिश् | दिशति |
| √स्पृश् | to touch | स्पृश् | स्पृशति |

### Tenth Class *Parasmaipada* (10P) Verbs

Tenth class verbs add the *gaṇa* sign अय before second- and third-person endings, which is lengthened to अया before first-person endings. The tenth class is called *curādi*, meaning "beginning with √चुर् (to steal)," the first verb of the group.

**√चिन्त् (root) to think, contemplate ⇒ चिन्त् (base)**

| | Verbal Stem | | | | | | |
|---|---|---|---|---|---|---|---|
| | Base | | Gaṇa Sign | | Ending | | |
| 3rd person singular | चिन्त् | + | अय | + | ति | ⇒ | चिन्तयति |
| 1st person singular | चिन्त् | + | अया | + | मि | ⇒ | चिन्तयामि |

| | Singular | Dual | Plural |
|---|---|---|---|
| 3rd person | चिन्तयति | चिन्तयतः | चिन्तयन्ति |
| 2nd person | चिन्तयसि | चिन्तयथः | चिन्तयथ |
| 1st person | चिन्तयामि | चिन्तयावः | चिन्तयामः |

#### Conjugate

| Root | | Base | 3rd person singular |
|---|---|---|---|
| √कथ् | to tell | कथ् | कथयति |
| √गण् | to count | गण् | गणयति |
| √चुर् | to steal | *चोर् | चोरयति |
| √पूज् | to honor, worship | पूज् | पूजयति |

## *SANDHI* (CONJUNCTION)

Just as in English, our pronunciation of the last letters of a word may change depending on the word that follows, so too in Sanskrit does the pronunciation of a word change depending on the following word. However, in Sanskrit, not only does the pronunciation change, but the spelling itself is actually altered to allow for smoother pronunciation. An elaborate set of rules of conjunction or *sandhi* exists in Sanskrit, with the intention of making reading and pronunciation easier and creating euphony—a pleasing effect to the ear. These rules will be introduced as they arise. Try to learn each rule as you come across it and be able to recognize the *sandhi* changes it produces.

There is a review at the end of this chapter and at the end of Chapter 4. Also, see pages 139–44 for charts and explanations of all other *sandhi* rules.

D. Translate

1. ते नृत्यतः ।
2. स* दिव्यति च क्षिपति च ।
3. तानि न नश्यन्ति ।
4. यूयं चिन्तयथ कथयथ च ।
5. तौ न स्पृशतः ।
6. आवां तुष्यावः ।

> *Sandhi* Rule: The *visarga* in सः, when followed by a consonant, must be dropped, except at the end of a sentence or when followed by अ.

## HOW TO APPROACH A VERSE

Reading a verse is like solving a puzzle. It is important to keep a simultaneous awareness of the specific parts of the verse as well as of the whole. Sometimes the verse will make logical sense and sometimes you will need to use your imagination to fill in the gaps. Begin by copying the verse by hand. As you go through the verse, write down a provisionary translation or translations for each word, separating the words that are joined by *sandhi*. You may find it helpful to identify the different parts of speech, particularly the subject or agent of action and the verb or action word.

The meter of a verse is categorized according to the number of syllables per *pāda*, or quarter. Within this categorization, different meters are distinguished according to the pattern of लघु (light) and गुरु (heavy) syllables. A syllable is considered लघु if it contains a short vowel (अ, इ, उ, ऋ, ऌ) followed by a single consonant. A syllable is considered गुरु if it contains a long vowel (आ, ई, ऊ, ॠ, ए, ऐ, ओ, औ) or a short vowel followed by a conjunct consonant, an *anusvāra* or a *visarga*. For each meter, there is a unique pattern of light and heavy syllables that makes it recognizable.

The most common meter for verse is called *anuṣṭubh* or *śloka* meter. In this meter, each verse consists of four *pādas*, or quarters, of eight syllables each. When you are translating a verse, you can usually think of each *pāda* as a separate phrase and decipher each one separately, although in some cases you may need to rearrange words or even *pādas* in order for the verse to make sense in English. Once you've gone through the whole verse, go back to the beginning and try to put the *pādas* together and make sense of the verse in its entirety.

**Please note:** All vocabulary for the verses will be provided below the verse, unless we have previously encountered the word. If a word is being used with a different meaning than we have seen before, the new meaning will be given as well. If you don't remember a word's meaning, you will find it in the glossary at the end of the book. The underlined words are examples of the specific grammatical constructs learned in the preceding section and should be given particular attention. In the examples, these specific words will be shown in bold in the English translations.

### Example: *Bhagavadgītā* 6.30

*Kṛṣṇa* is speaking to Arjuna.

यो मां पश्यति सर्वत्र सर्वं च मयि पश्यति ।
तस्याहं न प्रणश्यामि स च मे न प्रणश्यति ॥

Note the eight syllables in each *pāda*:

1. यो / माम् / पश् / य / ति / सर् / व / त्र
2. सर् / वम् / च / म / यि / पश् / य / ति
3. तस् / या / हम् / न / प्र / णश् / या / मि
4. स / च / मे / न / प्र / णश् / य / ति

Vocabulary

यः who
माम् me
सर्वत्र everywhere
सर्वम् everything
मयि in me
तस्य of/to him
प्र√णश् 4P, to be lost/destroyed
मे of/to me

*Sandhi* Rule: If a *visarga* (ः) is preceded by अ and followed by a voiced consonant, then अः becomes ओ.

Example: यः माम् ⇒ यो माम्

*Sandhi* Rule: (Remember from Chapter 1) Two like vowels, short or long, combine to form the long version of the vowel.

Example: तस्य अहम् ⇒ तस्याहम्

| यो | मां | पश्यति | सर्वत्र | सर्वं | च | मयि | पश्यति । |
|---|---|---|---|---|---|---|---|
| who | me | **sees** | everywhere | everything | and | in me | **sees** |

| तस्य | अहं | न | प्रणश्यामि | स | च | मे | न | प्रणश्यति ॥ |
|---|---|---|---|---|---|---|---|---|
| to him | I | not | **am lost** | he | and | to me | not | **is lost** |

Who (यो) **sees** (पश्यति) me (माम्) everywhere (सर्वत्र),
And (च) sees (पश्यति) everything (सर्वम्) in me (मयि).
To him (तस्य) I (अहम्) **am** not (न) **lost** (प्रणश्यामि),
And (च) he (स) **is** not (न) **lost** (प्रणश्यति) to me (मे).

## THE VERB √अस्, TO BE

This is one of the most important verbs in Sanskrit. It is actually a second class verb, but because it is so commonly used and also conjugated irregularly, you should memorize its paradigm now. It is also often understood, but not written, in sentences consisting of two nouns, or a noun and an adjective.

**√अस् to be**

| | Singular | Dual | Plural |
|---|---|---|---|
| 3rd person | अस्ति | स्तः | सन्ति |
| 2nd person | असि | स्थः | स्थ |
| 1st person | अस्मि | स्वः | स्मः |

### Example: *Mahāvākyas*

According to the Advaita Vedanta school of thought, the *mahāvākyas* are "great statements" from the *Upaniṣads*, which express the ultimate equation of *Ātman*, the individual Soul, and *Brahman*, the universal Spirit.

1. तत् त्वम् असि ⇒ तत्त्वमसि ।
   You are that.

2. अहम् ब्रह्म अस्मि ⇒ अहं ब्रह्मास्मि ।
   I am *Brahman*.

3. सः अहम् ⇒ सोऽहम् [अस्मि] ।
   I [am] that.

*Sandhi* Rule: When a word ends in a consonant and the next word begins in a vowel, the two words are combined together.

Example: त्वम् असि ⇒ त्वमसि
Note also that तत् and त्वम् join together to form तत्त्वम्.

*Sandhi* Rule: If a *visarga* is preceded by अ and followed by अ, then अः becomes ओ and the second अ disappears and is replaced by an *avagraha* (ऽ).

Example: सः अहम ⇒ सोऽहम्

### E. "No Equal"

This is a *subhāṣita*, or "good saying," similar to a proverb. Note that I have given the *subhāṣitas* names for easy reference. Translate each *pāda* as a separate sentence.

नास्ति विद्यासमं चक्षुर् नास्ति सत्यसमं तपः ।
नास्ति रागसमं दुःखं नास्ति त्यागसमं सुखम् ॥

> नास्ति = न + अस्ति.
> There is no . . .

Vocabulary

विद्यासमम् equal to knowledge
    समम् equal to
चक्षुर् eye
सत्यसमम् equal to truth
तपः discipline
रागसमम् equal to attachment
दुःखम् suffering
त्यागसमम् equal to renunciation
सुखम् happiness

> The *Gheraṇḍasaṃhitā* was composed in the eighteenth century C.E., in the form of a dialogue between Gheraṇḍa and Caṇḍakāpālin. It describes a seven-fold yoga, consisting of *ṣatkarma* (cleansing actions), *āsana* (postures), *mudrā* (bodily seals), *pratyāhāra* (sensory withdrawal), *prāṇāyāma* (breath control), *dhyāna* (meditation), and *samādhi* (absorption).

### F. *Gheraṇḍasaṃhitā* 1.4

नास्ति मायासमः पाशो नास्ति योगात्परं बलम् ।
नास्ति ज्ञानात्परो बन्धुर् नाहंकारात्परो रिपुः ॥

Vocabulary

मायासमः equal to illusion
पाशः chain, fetter, noose
योगात्परम् greater than yoga
बलम् strength
ज्ञानात्परो greater than knowledge
बन्धुर् relative
अहंकारात्परो greater than ego
रिपुः enemy

> *Sandhi* Rule: If a *visarga* is preceded by अ and followed by an unvoiced consonant, there is no change.
>
> Example: मायासमः पाशः ⇒ मायासमः पाशः

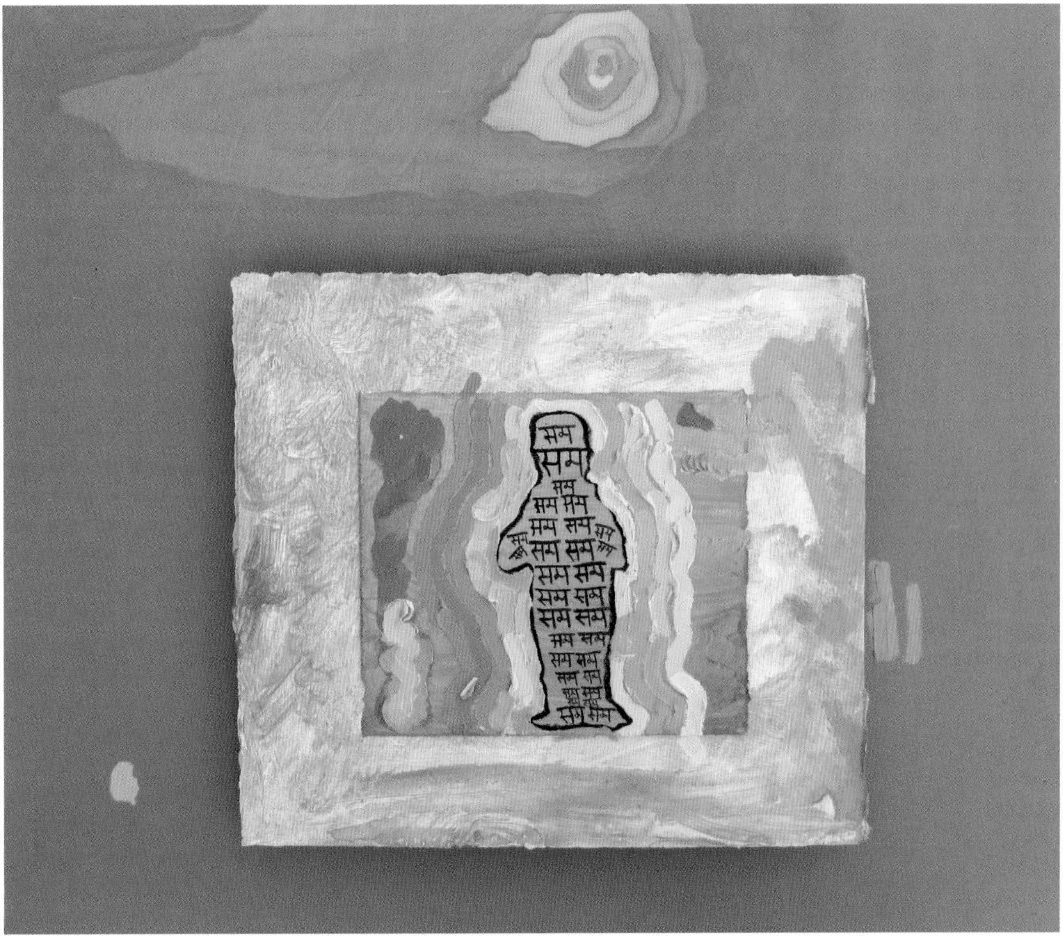

You might know the word सम from समस्थितिः, “equal standing pose.”
It is cognate with the English word “same.”

## *SANDHI* REVIEW

Below you will find all of the *sandhi* rules we have learned so far, with examples from the *Yogasūtra*. In each example, the particular rule being explained is illustrated in red or blue.

### Word Combination

In the *devanāgarī* script, when a word ends in a consonant and the next word begins in a vowel, the two words are combined together.

**Example: *Yogasūtra* 2.21**

तद् अर्थ एव दृश्यस्यात्मा ⇒ तदर्थ एव दृश्यस्यात्मा ।

### Vowel *Sandhi*

1. Two similar simple vowels, either short or long (अ, आ, इ, ई, उ, ऊ, ऋ, ॠ), combine to form the long vowel of the pair.

अ / आ + अ / आ ⇒ आ
इ / ई + इ / ई ⇒ ई
उ / ऊ + उ / ऊ ⇒ ऊ
ऋ / ॠ + ऋ / ॠ ⇒ ॠ

**Example 1: *Yogasūtra* 1.1**

अथ योग अनुशासनम् ⇒ अथ योगानुशासनम् ।

**Example 2**

ध्यानबिन्दु उपनिषद् ⇒ ध्यानबिन्दूपनिषद्

### Consonant *Sandhi*

2. When an म् is the last letter of a word and is followed by a word beginning with a consonant, it becomes an *anusvāra* (ं). When an म् is the last letter of a word and is followed by a word beginning with a vowel, the two words are joined together.

**Example: *Yogasūtra* 2.16**

हेयम् दुःखम् अनागतम् ⇒ हेयं दुःखमनागतम् ।

### *Visarga Sandhi*

3. If a *visarga* (ः) is preceded by अ and followed by an unvoiced consonant (one that does not use the vocal cords—the first two columns of consonants and the sibilants), there is no change.

**Example:** ***Yogasūtra*** **1.5**

वृत्तयः पञ्चतय्यः क्लिष्टाक्लिष्टाः ⇒ वृत्तयः पञ्चतय्यः क्लिष्टाक्लिष्टाः ।

4. If a *visarga* is preceded by अ and followed by a voiced consonant (one that uses the vocal cords—the last three columns of consonants and the semivowels), then अः becomes ओ.

**Example:** ***Yogasūtra*** **1.8**

विपर्ययः मिथ्याज्ञानमतद्रूपप्रतिष्ठम् ⇒ विपर्ययो मिथ्याज्ञानमतद्रूपप्रतिष्ठम् ।

5. If a *visarga* is preceded by अ and followed by अ, then अः becomes ओ and the second अ disappears and is replaced by an *avagraha* (ऽ).

**Example:** ***Yogasūtra*** **1.13**

तत्र स्थितौ यत्नः अभ्यासः ⇒ तत्र स्थितौ यत्नोऽभ्यासः ।

Note that the *avagraha* (ऽ) is represented by an apostrophe in transliteration.
*tatra sthitau yatnaḥ abhyāsaḥ* ⇒ *tatra sthitau yatno 'bhyāsaḥ*

6. The *visarga* after सः and एषः when followed by a consonant does not follow normal *sandhi* rules and must be dropped, except at the end of a *pāda* or sentence.

**Example:** ***Yogasūtra*** **1.14**

सः तु दीर्घकालनैरन्तर्यसत्कारासेवितो दृढभूमिः ⇒ स तु दीर्घकालनैरन्तर्यसत्कारासेवितो दृढभूमिः ।

## Review Exercises

### G. *Bhagavadgītā* 1.29

Arjuna is speaking to Kṛṣṇa about his fear of engaging in battle with his cousins. Note that मम, "my," goes with both गात्राणि and मुखम्.

सीदन्ति मम गात्राणि मुखं च परिशुष्यति ।
वेपथुश्च शरीरे मे रोमहर्षश्च जायते ॥

> *Sandhi* Rule: A *visarga* before a च or छ becomes a श्.
>
> Example: वेपथुः च ⇒ वेपथुश्च
> रोमहर्षः च ⇒ रोमहर्षश्च

Vocabulary

मम my
गात्राणि limbs
मुखम् mouth, face
परि√शुष् 4P, to dry, wither
वेपथुः quivering, trembling
शरीरे मे in my body
रोमहर्ष bristling of the hairs of the body
जायते is born, is produced

### H. *Bhagavadgītā* 1.31

The (implied) subject is अहम्, "I," and refers to Arjuna. Here, the first two *pādas* form one sentence and the third and fourth *pādas* together form another sentence.

निमित्तानि च पश्यामि विपरीतानि केशव ।
न च श्रेयोऽनुपश्यामि हत्वा स्वजनमाहवे ॥

Vocabulary

निमित्तानि signs, omens
विपरीतानि adverse, inauspicious
केशव O Handsome-haired One (Kṛṣṇa)
श्रेयस् welfare, good fortune, happiness
अनु√पश् 1P, to look at, perceive
हत्वा having killed
स्वजनम् one's own people
आहवे in battle

# 3
# Nouns: Masculine and Neuter Nouns Ending in अ; Examples of Cases

तत्र स्थितौ यत्नोऽभ्यासः ॥ १.१३ ॥
**tatra stithau yatno 'bhyāsaḥ**
Among those, practice is the effort toward stability.
॥ *Yogasūtra* 1.13 ॥

This chapter will introduce nouns and their conjugations. Unlike English, where separate prepositions—such as "by," "through," "to," "for," "from," "of," or "in"—must be added to express relational concepts, in Sanskrit these relationships are expressed simply through the addition of eight different case endings to the noun itself. All of these relationships will be exemplified by verses and *sūtras* from the *Bhagavadgītā*, *Yogasūtra*, and other yoga-related texts. Try to memorize these verses, as the verses will help you to remember the paradigms.

## NOUNS

All nouns are divided into three genders—masculine (m.), feminine (f.), and neuter (n.). Some of these distinctions will be obvious; most you will learn as you go along. When you look a word up in the dictionary, the gender will be given. Adjectives can usually belong to any of the three genders, depending upon the word that they modify, and are listed in the dictionary as mfn. The most common nouns end in अः / अम् / आ (m./n./f.). The declensions of other nouns will be presented later, but are very similar. As you learn the declensions, read aloud across each row and then down. Explanations and examples of the eight cases will be given one at a time, in sequence, later in the chapter.

## Masculine Nouns Ending in अ:

**अभ्यासः m. practice**

| | Singular | Dual | Plural |
|---|---|---|---|
| **Nominative** | अभ्यासः<br>practice (subject) | अभ्यासौ<br>the two practices (subject) | अभ्यासाः<br>the practices (subject) |
| **Accusative** | अभ्यासम्<br>practice (object) | अभ्यासौ<br>the two practices (object) | अभ्यासान्<br>the practices (object) |
| **Instrumental** | अभ्यासेन<br>by practice | अभ्यासाभ्याम्<br>by the two practices | अभ्यासैः<br>by the practices |
| **Dative** | अभ्यासाय<br>to/for practice | अभ्यासाभ्याम्<br>to/for the two practices | अभ्यासेभ्यः<br>to/for the practices |
| **Ablative** | अभ्यासात्<br>from practice | अभ्यासाभ्याम्<br>from the two practices | अभ्यासेभ्यः<br>from the practices |
| **Genitive** | अभ्यासस्य<br>of practice | अभ्यासयोः<br>of the two practices | अभ्यासानाम्<br>of the practices |
| **Locative** | अभ्यासे<br>in practice | अभ्यासयोः<br>in the two practices | अभ्यासेषु<br>in the practices |
| **Vocative** | अभ्यास<br>O practice | अभ्यासौ<br>O two practices | अभ्यासाः<br>O practices |

**योगः m. the act of yoking, union**

| | Singular | Dual | Plural |
|---|---|---|---|
| **Nominative** | योगः | योगौ | योगाः |
| **Accusative** | योगम् | योगौ | योगान् |
| **Instrumental** | योगेन | योगाभ्याम् | योगैः |
| **Dative** | योगाय | योगाभ्याम् | योगेभ्यः |
| **Ablative** | योगात् | योगाभ्याम् | योगेभ्यः |
| **Genitive** | योगस्य | योगयोः | योगानाम् |
| **Locative** | योगे | योगयोः | योगेषु |
| **Vocative** | योग | योगौ | योगाः |

Vocabulary

अर्जुनः m. hero of the *Bhagavadgītā*

अर्थः m. purpose, aim, worldly prosperity

आकाशः m. space, ether
कामः m. desire
क्रोधः m. anger
जनः m. person, people
देवः m. god
धर्मः m. right action, justice, duty
बालः m. boy
मोक्षः m. liberation
रामः m. hero of the *Rāmāyaṇa*
लोकः m. world, inhabitants of the world
वृक्षः m. tree
संशयः m. doubt

The four traditional human aims in Hinduism, पुरुषार्थाः, are all masculine nouns ending in अ: धर्मः, "right action," अर्थः, "worldly prosperity," कामः, "desire," and मोक्षः, "liberation."

#### Decline

आकाशः, कामः, देवः, and लोकः.

### Neuter Nouns Ending in अम्

Neuter nouns ending in अम् are declined exactly like masculine nouns in अः except for in the nominative, accusative, and vocative cases. The declensions for these three cases are all exactly the same, which helps with memorization; however, when reading, the only way to determine whether a word is in the nominative, accusative, or vocative case is through context.

**चित्तम् n. mind/consciousness**

| | Singular | Dual | Plural |
|---|---|---|---|
| **Nominative** | चित्तम्<br>the mind (subject) | चित्ते<br>the two minds (subject) | चित्तानि<br>the minds (subject) |
| **Accusative** | चित्तम्<br>the mind (object) | चित्ते<br>the two minds (object) | चित्तानि<br>the minds (object) |
| **Instrumental** | चित्तेन<br>by the mind | चित्ताभ्याम्<br>by the two minds | चित्तैः<br>by the minds |
| **Dative** | चित्ताय<br>to/for the mind | चित्ताभ्याम्<br>to/for the two minds | चित्तेभ्यः<br>to/for the minds |
| **Ablative** | चित्तात्<br>from the mind | चित्ताभ्याम्<br>from the two minds | चित्तेभ्यः<br>from the minds |

| | | | |
|---|---|---|---|
| **Genitive** | चित्तस्य<br>of the mind | चित्तयोः<br>of the two minds | चित्तानाम्<br>of the minds |
| **Locative** | चित्ते<br>in the mind | चित्तयोः<br>in the two minds | चित्तेषु<br>in the minds |
| **Vocative** | चित्तम्<br>O mind | चित्ते<br>O two minds | चित्तानि<br>O minds |

**शरीरम् n. body**

| | Singular | Dual | Plural |
|---|---|---|---|
| **Nominative** | शरीरम् | शरीरे | शरीराणि* |
| **Accusative** | शरीरम् | शरीरे | शरीराणि* |
| **Instrumental** | शरीरेण* | शरीराभ्याम् | शरीरैः |
| **Dative** | शरीराय | शरीराभ्याम् | शरीरेभ्यः |
| **Ablative** | शरीरात् | शरीराभ्याम् | शरीरेभ्यः |
| **Genitive** | शरीरस्य | शरीरयोः | शरीराणाम्* |
| **Locative** | शरीरे | शरीरयोः | शरीरेषु |
| **Vocative** | शरीरम् | शरीरे | शरीराणि* |

*Internal *Sandhi* Rule:
Dental न् changes to retroflex ण् if, within the same word, it is preceded by र्, ऋ, or ष् and immediately followed by a vowel, semivowel, or nasal. This rule only holds if no palatal, retroflex or dental consonant (except य्) intervenes.

Example: nom./acc./voc. pl. शरीराणि; inst. sg. शरीरेण; gen. pl. शरीराणाम्

Vocabulary

अरविन्दम् n. lotus
आसनम् n. seat
दुःखम् n. suffering
पदम् n. foot, word, grammar, state
पुस्तकम् n. book
पूर्णम् n. full, whole, entire, complete
फलम् n. fruit
भोजनम् n. food
मलम् n. dirt, impurity
मुखम् n. mouth, face
वैराग्यम् n. detachment
सत्यम् n. truth
सुखम् n. happiness
हृदयम् n. heart

### Decline

आसनम्, भोजनम्, सत्यम्, and सुखम्.

## THE EIGHT CASES

The following is an explanation of the most simple and common uses of the different cases. Other uses and exceptions will be presented in further chapters. Although most Sanskrit words have multiple meanings, in all of the examples, the vocabulary will be given with definitions specific to the verse. Focus your attention on the grammatical part of speech being specifically demonstrated (underlined in each verse); don't worry about anything that seems unfamiliar. The grammatical forms we have not learned yet will be given in parentheses, but need not be focused on at this point. Compound words will be explained in greater detail later, but for now, note that most of the individual words within the compound will be given below each compound.

### I. Nominative

The nominative case is used for naming, to represent *who* or *what* is being described or is performing an action (i.e., the subject). It is always in agreement with the finite verb in the sentence, whether it is included or implied.

The simplest type of sentence contains two words in the nominative case with an assumed or stated version of the verb अस्ति, "to be" (i.e., X is Y). Other simple sentences consist of a word in the nominative case with a verb, as we saw in Chapter 2.

#### Example 1: *Yogasūtra* 1.2

Note that although this text is most commonly called the *Yoga Sūtras*, Patañjali called each individual aphorism a *sūtra*, as well as the entire text the *Yogasūtra* or *Yogasūtram*, indicating that each individual *sūtra* is a "thread," and also that the work as a whole is a "thread," weaving through every aphorism. The Sanskrit plural *Yogasūtrāṇi* is also sometimes used for the whole text.

योगः चित्तवृत्तिनिरोधः ⇒ योगश्चित्तवृत्तिनिरोधः ।

> *Sandhi* Rule:
> A *visarga* before a च or छ becomes a श्.
> A *visarga* before a ट or ठ becomes a ष्.
> A *visarga* before a त or थ becomes a स्.

Vocabulary

योगः m. nom. sg.

चित्तवृत्तिनिरोधः m. nom. sg. stilling of the fluctuations of the mind

चित्तम् n. mind, consciousness

वृत्तिः fluctuations (f.)
निरोधः m. restraint, control, stilling, destruction

In this example, both the word "yoga" and the following compound are in the nominative case in order to imply equation. What is yoga?

**Yoga** (योगः) [is] **the stilling of the fluctuations of the mind** (चित्तवृत्तिनिरोधः).

### Example 2

लोकाः समस्ताः सुखिनो भवन्तु ।

#### Vocabulary

लोकाः m. nom. pl. worlds, inhabitants of the world
समस्ताः m. nom. pl. all
सुखिनः possessing happiness (m. nom. pl.)
भवन्तु may they be (3rd p. pl. imperative √भू)

Here, लोकाः, "the inhabitants of the world," is modified by the adjective समस्ताः, "all." These two words in the nominative case are joined together with a third nominative word by the imperative verb भवन्तु, "may they be." May **all** (समस्ताः) **the inhabitants of the world** (लोकाः) be (भवन्तु) possessed of happiness (सुखिनः). May all beings be happy.

### Translation I

Note that in the translation exercises, the sentences will be written without *sandhi* on the left and with *sandhi* on the right. The verses will only be written with *sandhi*.

1. योगः अभ्यासः भवति । ⇒ योगोऽभ्यासो भवति ।
2. योगः जयति । ⇒ योगो जयति ।
3. रामः पश्यति ।
4. अर्जुनः बोधति । ⇒ अर्जुनो बोधति ।
5. जनाः पठन्ति ।
6. पदौ गच्छतः ।
7. हृदये बोधतः ।
8. अरविन्दानि नमन्ति ।

Composed by Svātmarāma in the fifteenth century C.E., the *Haṭhapradīpikā* is the first text advocating *haṭhayoga* above all other types of yoga and is considered the root text of *haṭhayoga*. It is the first text known to include *āsana* among the practices of *haṭhayoga*, describing fifteen postures, in addition to *mudrā*, *bandha*, and *prāṇāyāma*. It is mostly a compilation, drawing from more than twenty different earlier texts.

### A. *Haṭhapradīpikā* 1.15

The main sentence of this verse is found in the fourth *pāda*—"Yoga is utterly lost by means of these six." The six conditions are given in the first three *pādas*.

अत्याहारः प्रयासश्च प्रजल्पो नियमग्रहः ।
जनसङ्गश्च लौल्यं च षड्भिर्योगो विनश्यति ॥

> *Sandhi* Rule: If a *visarga* is preceded by a vowel other than अ / आ and followed by an unvoiced consonant, there is no change. If it is followed by a voiced consonant or a vowel, it becomes र्.
>
> Ex. षड्भिः योगः ⇒ षड्भिर्योगः

Vocabulary
अत्याहारः m. eating too much
प्रयासः m. overexertion
प्रजल्पः m. talking too much
नियमग्रहः m. holding on to rules/restrictions
जनसङ्गः m. excessive socializing
लौल्यम् n. restlessness
षड्भिः by means of the six (m. inst. sg.)
वि√नश् 4P, to perish, to be utterly lost

## II. Accusative

The accusative case is used for the direct object of a transitive verb (a verb that requires one or more objects) or the goal of an action or motion. Unlike in English, where sentences are expressed in the order subject ⇒ verb ⇒ object, in Sanskrit, sentences are usually expressed in the order subject ⇒ object ⇒ verb.

### Example: *Bhagavadgītā* 9.26

*Kṛṣṇa* is speaking to Arjuna. The first two *pādas* form one sentence and the third and fourth *pādas* form another sentence. All of the words in the first *pāda* are objects of the verb in the second *pāda*.

पत्त्रं पुष्पं फलं तोयं यो मे भक्त्या प्रयच्छति ।
तदहं भक्त्युपहृतमश्नामि प्रयतात्मनः ॥

Vocabulary
पत्त्रम् n. leaf
पुष्पम् n. flower
फलम् n. fruit
तोयम् n. water
यः who (m. nom. sg.)

मे to me (m. dat. sg.)
भक्त्या with devotion/love (f. inst. sg.)
प्र√यम् 1P, to offer
तद् that (n. acc. sg.)
भक्त्युपहृतम् offered with devotion/love (n. acc. sg)
 भक्तिः devotion, love (f.)
 उपहृतम् n. offered
अश्नामि I eat, accept (1st p. sg. √अश्)
प्रयतात्मनः from one who is pious-minded, from one whose Soul is pious (m. abl. sg.)

Who (यो) offers (प्रयच्छति) to me (मे) with devotion (भक्त्या),
**A leaf** (पत्त्रम्), **a flower** (पुष्पम्), **fruit** (फलम्), [or] **water** (तोयम्).
I (अहम्) accept (अश्नामि) that (तद्), offered with devotion (भक्त्युपहृतम्),
From one whose Soul is pious (प्रयतात्मनः).

### Translation II

1. योगः संशयम् जयति। ⇒ योगः संशयं जयति।
2. रामः लोकान् पश्यति। ⇒ रामो लोकान्पश्यति।
3. अर्जुनः योगम् च धर्मम् च बोधति। ⇒ अर्जुनो योगं च धर्मं च बोधति।
4. जनाः पदान् पठन्ति। ⇒ जनाः पदान्पठन्ति।
5. हृदये सत्यम् बोधतः। ⇒ हृदये सत्यं बोधतः।
6. जनौ भोजनम् खादतः। ⇒ जनौ भोजनं खादतः।

### B. *Haṭhapradīpikā* 1.63

In this verse, the direct object is भोजनम्, "food," found along with the subject and verb in the fourth *pāda* of the verse. All other words in the verse are adjectives modifying *bhojanam*, also given in the accusative case. As mentioned above, adjectives are declined just like nouns, but can take any gender, corresponding to the noun that they are modifying.

पुष्टं सुमधुरं स्निग्धं गव्यं धातुप्रपोषणम्।
मनोभिलषितं योग्यं योगी भोजनमाचरेत्॥

Vocabulary
पुष्ट mfn. nourishing
सुमधुर mfn. very sweet
स्निग्ध mfn. oily

गव्य mfn. coming from a cow
धातुप्रपोषण mfn. nourishing the *dhātus* (the seven constituent elements of the body)
मनोभिलषित mfn. desired by the mind
योग्य mfn. suitable
योगी practitioner of yoga (m. nom. sg.)
आचरेत् one should partake, i.e., eat (3rd p. sg. optative आ√चर्)

## III. Instrumental

The instrumental case designates the instrument and is used to explain *how* things are done. It shows agency, equivalent to the English prepositions "with," "by means of," or "through." It is also used to show accompaniment, followed by the word सह, meaning "together with."

> The idea of a unified Patañjali, who wrote treatises on yoga, grammar, and Āyurveda, has been much debated. Although the idea is much older, this verse is from Śivarāma's eighteenth-century commentary on the *Vāsavadattā*, by Subandhu. And though it may be a myth, it is important, as it lives on in many people's imaginations.

### Example 1: Invocation to *Patañjali*

योगेन चित्तस्य पदेन वाचां मलं शरीरस्य च वैद्यकेन ।
योऽपाकरोत्तं प्रवरं मुनीनां पतञ्जलिं प्राञ्जलिरानतोऽस्मि ॥

Vocabulary (for the first line)
चित्तस्य of the mind (n. gen. sg)
पदः m. grammar
वाचाम् of speech (f. gen. sg.)
शरीरस्य of the body (n. gen. sg.)
वैद्यकम् n. the science of medicine

The second line of the verse can be translated first. In the first line, the word मलम्, "impurities," is applied to all three clauses.

With palms folded together (प्राञ्जलिर्), I bow respectfully (आनतोऽस्मि) to Patañjali (पतञ्जलिम्),
That (तम्) best (प्रवरम्) of sages (मुनीनाम्), who dispelled (अपाकरोत्) . . .
The impurities (मलम्) of the mind (चित्तस्य) **with yoga** (योगेन), of speech (वाचाम्) **through grammar** (पदेन),
And (च) of the body (शरीरस्य) **by means of medicine** (वैद्यकेन).

### Example 2: *Yogasūtra* 1.12

अभ्यासवैराग्याभ्यां तन्निरोधः ।

> *Sandhi* Rule: A final त् changes to न् before an initial न्.
>
> Example: तत् निरोधः ⇒ तन्निरोधः

Vocabulary

अभ्यासवैराग्याभ्याम् n. inst. dual, through/by means of practice and detachment

तन्निरोधः m. stilling of those

 तत् that (stem form for तानि, those, n. acc. pl.)

 निरोधः m. restraint, control, stilling, destruction

There is the stilling of those [fluctuations] (तन्निरोधः) **through practice and detachment (अभ्यासवैराग्याभ्याम्).**

> *Sandhi* Rule: If a *visarga* is preceded by अ and followed by a vowel other than अ, the *visarga* is dropped and the hiatus remains.
>
> Example: योगः आसनेन ⇒ योग आसनेन

### Translation III

1. अहम् योगेन संशयम् जयामि । ⇒ अहं योगेन संशयं जयामि ।
2. योगः आसनेन मलानि जयति । ⇒ योग आसनेन मलानि जयति ।
3. रामः हृदयेन लोकान् पश्यति । ⇒ रामो हृदयेन लोकान्पश्यति ।
4. अर्जुनः चित्तेन धर्मम् बोदति । ⇒ अर्जुनश्चित्तेन धर्मं बोदति ।
5. जनाः अभ्यासेनः पदान् पठन्ति । ⇒ जना अभ्यासेनः पदान्पठन्ति ।
6. जनौ भोजनं मुखाभ्याम् खादतः । ⇒ जनौ भोजनं मुखाभ्यां खादतः ।

> *Sandhi* Rule: If a *visarga* is preceded by आ and followed by a voiced consonant or vowel, the *visarga* is dropped and the hiatus remains.
>
> Example: जनाः अभ्यासेनः ⇒ जना अभ्यासेनः

### C. *Bhagavadgītā* 6.35

This verse is probably inspired by *sūtra* 1.12 above. In it, Kṛṣṇa explains how to achieve the stilling of the fluctuations of the mind that is yoga, as defined in *sūtra* 1.2. Each line is a separate sentence.

असंशयं महाबाहो मनो दुर्निग्रहं चलम् ।
अभ्यासेन तु कौन्तेय वैराग्येण च गृह्यते ॥

> *ind. stands for indeclinable. An indeclinable word is one that cannot be grammatically inflected.

Vocabulary

असंशयम् ind.* without doubt

महाबाहो O mighty-armed one, epithet of Arjuna (m. voc. sg.)

मनः mind (n. nom. sg.)
दुर्निग्रह mfn. difficult to control
चल mfn. moving, unsteady
तु ind. but
कौन्तेय O son of Kuntī, epithet of Arjuna (m. voc. sg.)
गृह्यते it is restrained (3rd p. sg. Ā passive √ग्रह्)

## IV. Dative

The dative case is used for the indirect object or purpose, to express "to," "for," or "for the sake of" something or someone. It is often used in mantras.

### Example 1

ॐ नमः शिवाय ।

Vocabulary
नमः a bow, salutations (m. nom. sg.)

Oṃ, Salutations (नमः) **to Lord Śiva** (शिवाय)!

### Example 2: *Bhagavadgītā* 4.8

The subject of this verse and the "I" of संभवामि is Kṛṣṇa. Each *pāda* can be read as a separate clause, with the main sentence in the fourth *pāda*.

परित्राणाय साधूनां विनाशाय च दुष्कृताम् ।
धर्मसंस्थापनार्थाय संभवामि युगे युगे ॥

Vocabulary
परित्राणम् n. protection
साधूनाम् of good, virtuous people (m. gen. pl.)
विनाशः m. destruction
दुष्कृताम् of evildoers (m. gen. pl.)
धर्मसंस्थापनार्थः m. the purpose of establishing justice
    संस्थापनम् n. establishing
सं√भू 1P, to arise, be born
युगे युगे in every age (n. loc sg)
    युगम् n. an age of the world

**For the protection** (परित्राणाय) of good people (साधूनाम्),
And (च) **for the destruction** (विनाशाय) of evildoers (दुष्कृताम्).
**For the purpose of establishing justice** (धर्मसंस्थापनार्थाय),
I am born (संभवामि) in every age (युगे युगे).

### Translation IV

1. त्वम् योगाय सत्यम् वदसि । ⇒ त्वं योगाय सत्यं वदसि ।
2. रामः लोकेभ्यः रावणम् जयति । ⇒ रामो लोकेभ्यो रावणं जयति ।
3. अर्जुनः धर्माय योगम् पठति । ⇒ अर्जुनो धर्माय योगं पठति ।
4. सा बालाभ्याम् पुस्तकम् पठति । ⇒ सा बालाभ्यां पुस्तकं पठति ।
5. सः मोक्षाय अर्थम् त्यजति । ⇒ स मोक्षायार्थं त्यजति ।

### D. "For the Sake of Others"

Each *pāda* is a separate sentence.

परोपकाराय फलन्ति वृक्षाः परोपकाराय वहन्ति नद्यः ।
परोपकाराय दुहन्ति गावः परोपकारार्थमिदं शरीरम् ॥

#### Vocabulary

परोपकारः m. helping others
√फल् 1P, to bear fruit
√वह् 1P, to flow
नद्यः rivers (f. nom. pl.)
दुहन्ति they give milk (3rd p. pl. √दुह्)
गावः cows (f. nom. pl.)
परोपकारार्थम् n. for the purpose of helping others
इदम् this (n. nom. sg.)

## V. Ablative

The ablative case is used to express action *from* something, to indicate the origin or source, or to express a reason. It is also often translated as "because of," or "out of."

### Example 1: *Yogasūtra* 2.42

संतोषादनुत्तमः सुखलाभः ।

Vocabulary

संतोषः m. contentment
अनुत्तम mfn. unsurpassed
सुखलाभः m. attainment of happiness

**From contentment** (संतोषाद्), [there is] the attainment of happiness (सुखलाभः) that is unsurpassed (अनुत्तमः).

### Example 2: *Bhagavadgītā* 2.62–63

The first two *pādas* form one sentence. All the remaining *pādas* are sentences unto themselves. Note that in the last *pāda* of the second verse, the implied subject is "one."

ध्यायतो विषयान्पुंसः सङ्गस्तेषूपजायते ।
सङ्गात्संजायते कामः कामात्क्रोधोऽभिजायते ॥

क्रोधाद्भवति सम्मोहः सम्मोहात्स्मृतिविभ्रमः ।
स्मृतिभ्रंशाद्बुद्धिनाशो बुद्धिनाशात्प्रणश्यति ॥

> *Sandhi* Rule: An unvoiced final consonant becomes the unaspirated voiced consonant of the same class, before an initial voiced consonant or vowel.
>
> Example: क्रोधात् भवति ⇒ क्रोधाद् भवति ⇒ क्रोधाद्भवति
>
> स्मृतिभ्रंशात् बुद्धिनाशो ⇒ स्मृतिभ्रंशाद् बुद्धिनाशो ⇒ स्मृतिभ्रंशाद्बुद्धिनाशो

Vocabulary

ध्यायतः of/for one who is contemplating (m. gen. sg)
विषयान् sense objects (m. acc. pl.)
पुंसः of/for a man, person (m. gen. sg.)
सङ्गः m. attachment
तेषु in/to them (m. loc. pl.)
उपजायते is born, appears (3rd p. sg. Ā उप√जन्)
संजायते is born, arises (3rd p. sg. Ā सं√जन्)
अभिजायते is born, produced (3rd p. sg. Ā अभि√जन्)
सम्मोहः m. delusion
स्मृतिविभ्रमः / स्मृतिभ्रंशः m. confusion/error in memory [of the teachings of the guru and scriptures]
बुद्धिनाशः m. loss of understanding/discernment

For a person (पुंसः) who is contemplating (ध्यायतो) sense objects (विषयान्),
Attachment (सङ्गः) to them (तेषु) is born (उपजायते).
**From attachment** (सङ्गात्), desire (कामः) arises (संजायते),

**From desire** (कामात्), anger (क्रोधः) is born (अभिजायते).

**From anger** (क्रोधात्) comes (भवति) delusion (सम्मोहः),
**From delusion** (सम्मोहः), [there is] error in memory (स्मृतिविभ्रमः).
**From error in memory** (स्मृतिभ्रंशात्), [there is] loss of understanding (बुद्धिनाशः),
**From loss of understanding** (बुद्धिनाशात्), [one] is lost (प्रणश्यति).

**Translation V**

1. अहम् योगात् सुखम् बोधामि। ⇒ अहं योगात्सुखं बोधामि।
2. जनाः दुःखात् सुखम् बोधन्ति। ⇒ जना दुःखात्सुखं बोधन्ति।
3. त्वम् आसनात् उत्तिष्ठसि गच्छसि च। ⇒ त्वमासनादुत्तिष्ठसि गच्छसि च।
4. अर्जुनः धर्मात् जयति। ⇒ अर्जुनो धर्माद् जयति।
5. बालः वृक्षात् पतति। ⇒ बालो वृक्षात्पतति।
6. अहम् वृक्षात् फलम् खादामि। ⇒ अहं वृक्षात्फलं खादामि।

**E. *Haṭhapradīpikā* 1.16**

The main sentence is in the fourth *pāda*. The first three *pādas* are a list of conditions for that.

उत्साहात्साहसाद्धैर्यात्तत्त्वज्ञानाच्च निश्चयात्।
जनसङ्गपरित्यागात्षड्भिर्योगः प्रसिद्ध्यति॥

*Sandhi* Rule: Before a retroflex or palatal consonant, त् changes to the corresponding unaspirated consonant.

त् + च ⇒ च्च; त् + छ ⇒ च्छ; त् + ज ⇒ ज्ज;
त् + ट ⇒ ट्ट

Example: तत्त्वज्ञानात् च ⇒ तत्त्वज्ञानाच्च

Vocabulary
उत्साहः m. effort, perseverance
साहसम् n. boldness, daring, courage
धैर्यम् n. constancy, calmness, patience
तत्त्वज्ञानम् n. knowledge of truth
  तत्त्वम् n. truth, true state
  ज्ञानम् n. knowledge
निश्चयः m. resolution, fixed intention
जनसङ्गपरित्यागः m. abandoning excessive socializing
षड्भिर् by means of these six (mfn. inst. sg.)
प्र√सिध् 4P, is accomplished, succeeds

## VI. Genitive

The genitive case is used to express possession and is usually used to relate one noun to another, represented in English by the word "of," or by "'s" or "s'." It can also be used like the dative, "to/for."

### Example: *Bhagavadgītā* 4.7

The first two *pādas* should be read together. The तदा, "then," in the fourth *pāda* correlates with the यदा यदा, "whenever," in the first *pāda*.

यदा यदा हि धर्मस्य ग्लानिर्भवति भारत ।
अभ्युत्थानमधर्मस्य तदात्मानं सृजाम्यहम् ॥

*Sandhi* Rule: As noted earlier, when a word ends in a consonant and the next word begins in a vowel, the two words are combined together.

Example: अभ्युत्थानम् अधर्मस्य ⇒ अभ्युत्थानमधर्मस्य

This example shows how important it is to recognize this rule—धर्म and अधर्म are opposites!

Vocabulary

यदा यदा ind. whenever
  यदा ind. when
हि ind. emphatic particle, "indeed"
ग्लानिर् decrease, waning (f. acc. sg.)
भारत O descendant of Bharata (i.e., Arjuna) (m. voc. sg.)
अभ्युत्थानम् n. rising up, emerging
अधर्मः m. injustice, unrighteousness
तदा ind. then
आत्मानम् self, myself (m. acc. sg.)
√सृज् 6P, to bring forth, to create, to manifest

*Sandhi* Rule: When two dissimilar vowels are next to each other and the first vowel is a simple vowel other than अ / आ, the first vowel will change into its corresponding semivowel.

इ / ई ⇒ य्; उ / ऊ ⇒ व्; ऋ / ॠ ⇒ र्

Example: सृजामि अहम् ⇒ सृजाम्यहम्

Indeed (हि), whenever (यदा यदा) there is (भवति) a waning (ग्लानिर्)
**Of justice** (धर्मस्य), O descendant of Bharata (भारत),
And a rising up (अभ्युत्थानम्) **of injustice** (अधर्मस्य),
Then (तदा) I (अहम्) manifest (सृजामि) myself (आत्मानम्).

### Translation VI

1. योगस्य अर्थः मोक्षः भवति । ⇒ योगस्यार्थो मोक्षो भवति ।
2. चित्तस्य भोजनम् ज्ञानम् अस्ति । ⇒ चित्तस्य भोजनं ज्ञानमस्ति ।

3. हृदयस्य भोजनम् सुखम् अस्ति । ⇒ हृदयस्य भोजनं सुखमस्ति ।
4. जनाः योगेन शरीराणाम् मलानि त्यजन्ति । ⇒ जना योगेन शरीराणां मलानि त्यजन्ति ।

### F. *Bhagavadgītā* 10.22

The implied subject is अहम्, "I," and refers to Kṛṣṇa. Each *pāda* can be read as a separate sentence.

वेदानां सामवेदोऽस्मि देवानामस्मि वासवः ।
इन्द्रियाणां मनश्चास्मि भूतानामस्मि चेतना ॥

*Sandhi* Rule: Remember, if a *visarga* is preceded by अ and followed by अ, then अः becomes ओ and the second अ disappears and is replaced by an *avagraha* (ऽ).

Example: सामवेदः अस्मि ⇒ सामवेदोऽस्मि

Vocabulary

वेदः m. sacred knowledge, the *Vedas*, divided into four works, known as the *Ṛg-veda*, *Yajur-veda*, *Sāma-veda*, and *Atharva-veda*
सामवेदः m. *Sāmaveda*, the *veda* of songs
वासवः m. name of Indra, Vedic chief of gods
इन्द्रियम् n. sense, sense organ
मनस् mind (n. nom. sg.)
भूतम् n. living being
चेतना consciousness, understanding, intelligence (f. nom. sg.)

## VII. Locative

The locative case expresses location in time or space and is translated as "in," "on," "at," or "among."

### Example 1: *Yogasūtra* 3.26

भुवनज्ञानं सूर्ये संयमात् ।

Vocabulary

भुवनज्ञानम् n. knowledge of the worlds
 भुवनम् n. world

The third chapter of the *Yogasūtra*, the *Vibhūtipāda*, or "Chapter on Superhuman Powers," revolves around संयमः (*saṃyama*), the conjunction of the last three limbs of *aṣṭāṅgayoga*, to reach a profound state of meditation. The third chapter is largely a list of the various *siddhis* or powers that this can achieve. However, it is important to remember that the goal of yoga, as expressed in the fourth chapter, is to move beyond these powers, to a state of absolute independence, or *kaivalya*.

सूर्यः m. sun
संयमः m. a term for *dhāraṇā* (concentration) + *dhyāna* (meditation) + *samādhi* (absorption)

From *saṃyama* (संयमात्) **on the sun** (सूर्ये), [there is] knowledge of the worlds (भुवनज्ञानम्).

### Example 2: *Bhagavadgītā* 1.1

धर्मक्षेत्रे कुरुक्षेत्रे समवेता युयुत्सवः ।
मामकाः पाण्डवाश्चैव किमकुर्वत संजय ॥

#### Vocabulary

धर्मक्षेत्रम् n. field of justice
क्षेत्रम् n. field
कुरुक्षेत्रम् n. field of the Kurus
समवेत mfn. come together, assembled
युयुत्सवः desiring to fight (m. nom. pl.)
मामक mfn. mine, that is, my sons
पाण्डवः m. son of Pāṇḍu
एव ind. indeed (particle of emphasis)
किम् ind. what
अकुर्वत they did (3rd p. sg. Ā imperfect √कृ)
संजय O Sañjaya (m. voc. sg.)

**In the field of justice** (धर्मक्षेत्रे), **in the field of the Kurus** (कुरुक्षेत्रे),
Come together (समवेताः), desiring to fight (युयुत्सवः).
My sons (मामकाः) and (च) indeed (एव) the sons of Pāṇḍu (पाण्डवाः),
What (किम्) did they do (अकुर्वत), O Sañjaya (संजय)?

### Translation VII

1. योगे अर्जुनः चित्तस्य मलम् जयति । ⇒ योगेऽर्जुनश्चित्तस्य मलं जयति ।
2. हृदये सत्यम् च सुखम् च भवतः । ⇒ हृदये सत्यं च सुखं च भवतः ।
3. सागरे त्वम् क्रोधम् त्यजसि । ⇒ सागरे त्वं क्रोधं त्यजसि ।
4. लोकेषु योगः जयति । ⇒ लोकेषु योगो जयति ।

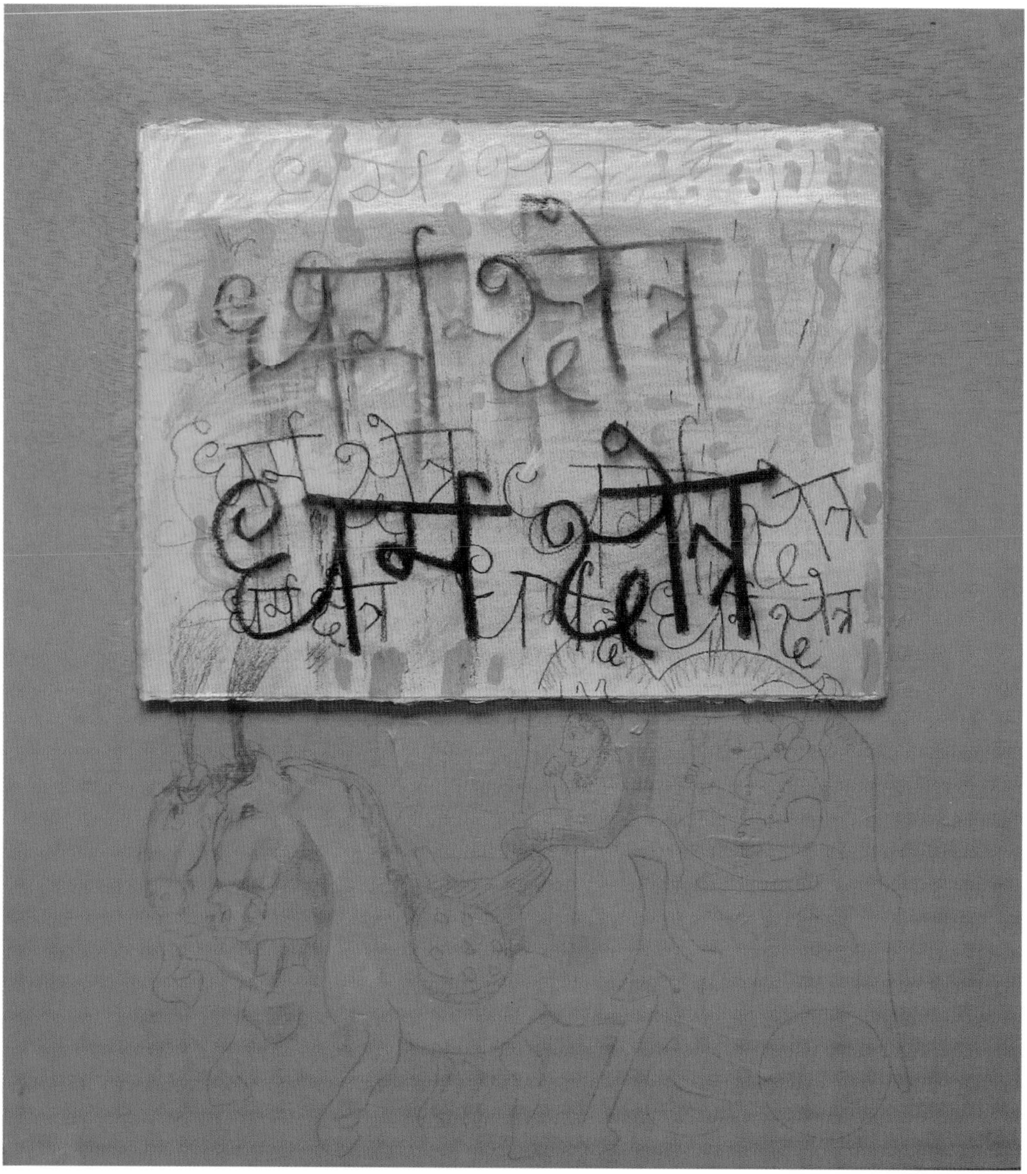


This verse sets the stage for the entire *Bhagavadgītā*. Dhṛtarāṣṭra, the blind king of the Kurus, is asking his minister, Sañjaya, to relate the story of what is happening on the epic battlefield between his children and their cousins, the Pāṇḍavas. Sañjaya proceeds to describe the entire struggle in perfect detail, which represents the age-old struggle between good and bad, right and wrong, truth and untruth, and the Soul's search for meaning.

### G. *Haṭhapradīpikā* 1.38

The first two *pādas* are separate sentences. The third and fourth *pādas* should be read together.

यमेष्विव मिताहारमहिंसां नियमेष्विव ।
मुख्यं सर्वासनेष्वेकं सिद्धाः सिद्धासनं विदुः ॥

> *Sandhi* Rule: See page 55:
> उ / ऊ ⇒ व
> यमेषु इव ⇒ यमेष्विव

Vocabulary

यमः m. restraint, first limb of *aṣṭāṅgayoga*
इव ind. like, in the same manner as, just as
मिताहारः m. moderate diet
अहिंसाम् nonviolence (f. acc sg.)
नियमः m. observance, second limb of *aṣṭāṅgayoga*
मुख्य mfn. first, principal, best
सर्वासनम् n. all postures
एकम् one, unique, special (n. nom. sg.)
सिद्धः m. an inspired sage or seer
सिद्धासनम् n. name of a seated posture
विदुः they (the seers) know (3rd. p. pl. perfect √विद्)

## VIII. Vocative

The vocative case is used for addressing a person, a god, or a personified object.

### Example: *Ādityahṛdayam* 3

राम राम महाबाहो शृणु गुह्यं सनातनम् ।
येन सर्वानरीन्वत्स समरे विजयिष्यसि ॥

Vocabulary

महाबाहो O Mighty-Armed One (m. voc. sg.)
शृणु listen (3rd p. sg. imperative, √श्रु)
गुह्यम् n. secret, mystery
सनातन mfn. eternal, everlasting

येन by which (m. inst. sg.)
सर्वान् all (m. nom. pl.)
अरीन् enemies (m. nom. pl.)
वत्सः m. calf, child
समरः m. battle, struggle
विजयिष्यसि you will succeed, conquer, be victorious (2nd p. sg. future वि√जि)

**Rāma** (राम), **O Mighty-Armed Rāma** (राम महाबाहो),
Listen (शृणु) to the everlasting (सनातनम्) secret (गुह्यम्).
By which (येन), **my dear child** (वत्स),
You will conquer (विजयिष्यसि) all (सर्वान्) [of your] enemies (अरीन्) in battle (समरे).

### Translation VIII

1. हे योग सुखम् भवसि । ⇒ हे योग सुखं भवसि ।
2. देवाः क्रोधम् त्यजथ । ⇒ देवाः क्रोधं त्यजथ ।
3. हे राम सत्यम् वदसि । ⇒ हे राम सत्यं वदसि ।

> The word हे is a vocative particle and means "O."

### H. *Gaṇeśa Mantra*

The first line is a series of epithets that go with the noun देव, all of which are in the vocative case. The देव here is Gaṇeśa, the elephant-headed god, the remover of obstacles.

वक्रतुण्ड महाकाय सूर्यकोटिसमप्रभ ।
निर्विघ्नं कुरु मे देव सर्वकार्येषु सर्वदा ॥

Vocabulary

वक्रतुण्डः m. one with a curved trunk
महाकायः m. one with great stature
सूर्यकोटिसमप्रभः m. one whose brilliance is equal to ten million suns
    कोटिः f. ten million
निर्विघ्नः m. without obstacles, freedom from obstacles
    विघ्नः m. obstacle
कुरु you make, do, grant (2nd p. sg. imperative √कृ)
मे to me (dat. sg.)
सर्वकार्यम् n. all things
सर्वदा ind. always, at all times

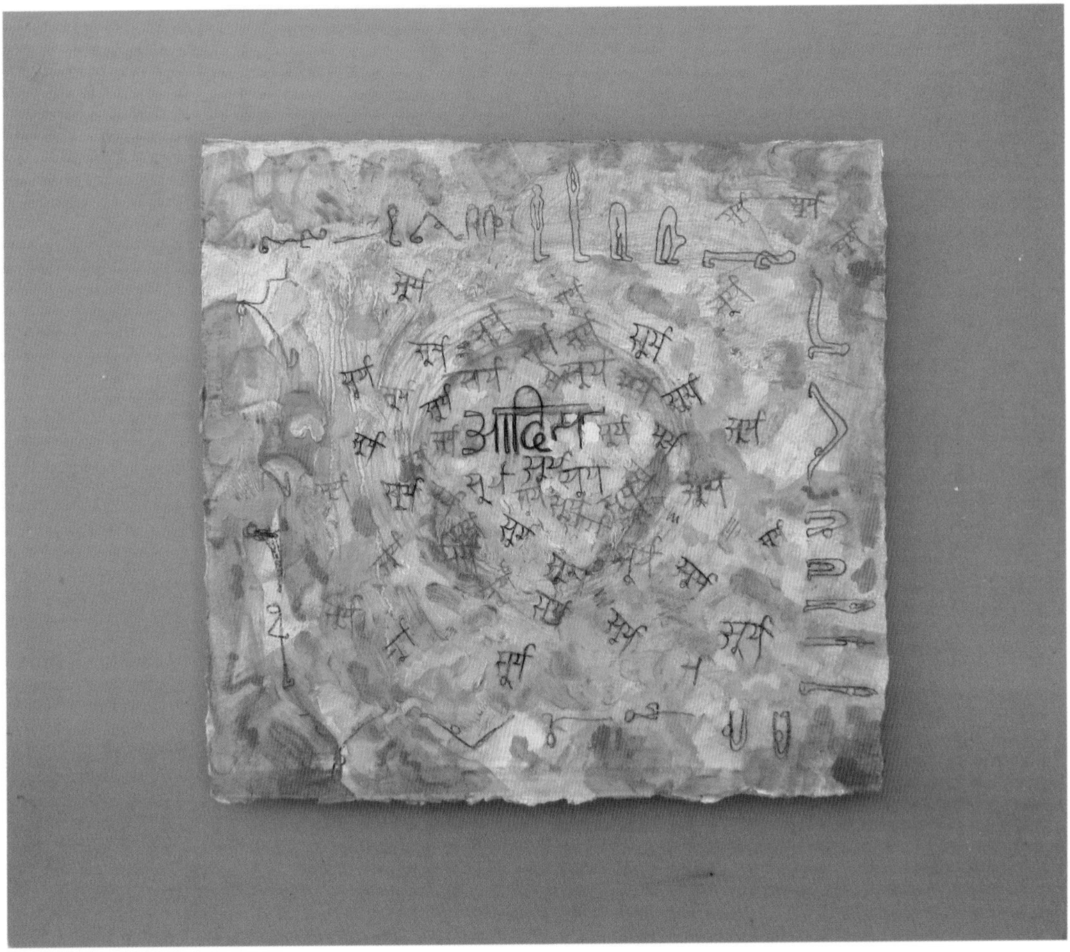

The *Ādityahṛdayam* is a hymn in praise of the Sun God, from the 107th chapter of the *Yuddha Kāṇḍa* (sixth book) of the *Rāmāyaṇa*. Rāma, the hero, has gone to rescue his beloved wife, Sītā, who has been kidnapped by Rāvaṇa; but just like Arjuna, he becomes paralyzed on the battlefield. The sage Agastya arrives and tells him to pray to the Sun God for strength and courage. This chant is said to convey all of the same benefits as *sūryanamaskāra* (sun salutations).

## Review Exercises

Contained within the *Śatapatha Brāhmaṇa*, the *Bṛhadāraṇyaka Upaniṣad*, "The Great Forest of Knowledge," is generally considered the oldest *upaniṣad*, dated to around the seventh or sixth century B.C.E. It is composed of three sections, the *Madhu-kāṇḍa* (the "Honey Section," named for its final portion), the *Yājñavalkya-kāṇḍa* (teachings of the sage Yājñavalkya), and the *Khila-kāṇḍa* (the "Supplementary Section").

Identify the underlined forms, translate, and memorize:

### I. *Bṛhadāraṇyakopaniṣat* 5.1.1

पूर्णमदः पूर्णमिदं पूर्णात्पूर्णमुदच्यते ।
पूर्णस्य पूर्णमादाय पूर्णमेवावशिष्यते ॥

Vocabulary

अदः that (n. nom. sg.)
इदम् this (n. nom. sg.)
उदच्यते it arises, comes forth (3rd p. sg. Ā उद्√अञ्च्)
पूर्णस्य note that the genitive here translates as "from the whole/full"
आदाय having taken (gerund आ√दा)
एव ind. only (governs the word which precedes it)
अवशिष्यते it remains (3rd p. sg. Ā अव√शिष्)

### J. *Maṅgala Mantra*

Translate the first line as one sentence—the subject is महीं महीशाः. The second line is two sentences.

स्वस्ति प्रजाभ्यः परिपालयन्तां न्यायेन मार्गेण महीं महीशाः ।
गोब्राह्मणेभ्यः शुभमस्तु नित्यं लोकाः समस्ताः सुखिनो भवन्तु ॥

Vocabulary

स्वस्ति well-being (n. acc. sg.)
प्रजाभ्यः for/of the people (f. dat. pl.)
परिपालयन्ताम् May they protect (3rd p. pl. Ā imperative परि√पा)
न्यायः m. justice, virtue
मार्गः m. path, right way, custom
महीम् the earth (f. acc. sg.)
महीशः m. ruler, king
गोब्राह्मणः m. cows and Brahmins (e.g., living beings)
शुभ mfn. good fortune, auspiciousness

अस्तु May there be (3rd p. sg. imperative √अस्)
नित्यम् ind. always

K. *Viṣṇu Mantra* I

Note that यथा in the second *pāda* goes with तोयम् in the first *pāda*.

आकाशात्पतितं तोयं यथा गच्छति सागरम् ।
सर्वदेवनमस्कारः केशवं प्रतिगच्छति ॥

This verse is the main refrain in the movie *Adi Shankaracharya*, the first and only movie ever made in Sanskrit, telling the beautiful story of Śaṅkarācārya's life and teachings.

Vocabulary
पतित mfn. fallen
यथा ind. in the same way as, just as
सागरः m. ocean
सर्वदेवनमस्कारः m. salutations to all the gods
केशवः m. Viṣṇu, Kṛṣṇa
प्रति√गम् 1P, to go toward, go back, return

# 4
# VERBS: PRESENT TENSE, *ĀTMANEPADA*, FIRST, FOURTH, SIXTH, AND TENTH CLASS; FEMININE NOUNS ENDING IN आ AND ई; *SANDHI* REVIEW

तदा द्रष्टुः स्वरूपेऽवस्थानम् ॥ १.३ ॥
**tadā draṣṭuḥ svarūpe 'vasthānam**
Then there is stability of the Seer in its own true nature.
॥ *Yogasūtra* 1.3 ॥

## PRESENT TENSE VERBS, *ĀTMANEPADA* CONJUGATIONS

All of the verbs we have learned so far have been in the present tense, परस्मैपद् voice. There is a parallel system of verbs, divided into the same ten *gaṇas* and conjugated in all of the same tenses, called the आत्मनेपद् voice. The word आत्मनेपद् literally means "word for oneself," indicating that unlike परस्मैपद् verbs, the action revolves around the agent, rather than a separate object. The आत्मनेपद् voice was originally used for self-reflexive verbs, such as to bathe/dress oneself, or intransitive verbs (verbs that take no object), such as to sit/stand.

The traditional example is the verb √यज्, "to sacrifice":

*Parasmaipada*: ब्राह्मणो यजति । The priest offers a sacrifice (for someone else's benefit).
*Ātmanepada*: नृपो यजते । The king offers a sacrifice (for his own benefit).

These distinctions are no longer readily apparent in classical Sanskrit; however, the two categories still remain. Most verbs will be cited as belonging to one of these two voices. Some verbs, उभयपद्, "word for both," can be seen with both sets of endings. Additionally, the आत्मनेपद् endings are used for all verbs in the passive construction, as we will see in Chapter 11.

## *Ātmanepada* Endings

| | Singular | Dual | Plural |
|---|---|---|---|
| 3rd person | -ते | -एते | -अन्ते |
| 2nd person | -से | -एथे | -ध्वे |
| 1st person | -ए | -वहे | -महे |

Just like in the परस्मैपद present tense conjugations, first, the verbal base is formed from the root. Then the specific *gaṇa* sign is added to create the verbal stem and the appropriate आत्मनेपद ending is suffixed to the end. As in the परस्मैपद conjugations, for first and sixth *gaṇa* verbs, the *gaṇa* sign अ is added before second- and third-person endings and आ is added before first-person endings. Fourth *gaṇa* verbs add the *gaṇa* sign य and या, respectively, and tenth class verbs add the *gaṇa* sign अय and अया. Note, however, that the final अ or आ of all of these *gaṇa* signs is lost before endings beginning with ए or अ.

**√मुद् (root) to rejoice, 1Ā ⇒ मोद् (base)**

| | Verbal Stem | | | | | | |
|---|---|---|---|---|---|---|---|
| | Base | | Gaṇa Sign | | Ending | | |
| 3rd person singular | मोद् | + | अ | + | ते | ⇒ | मोदते |
| 1st person singular | मोद् | + | आ | + | ए | ⇒ | मोदे |

| | Singular | Dual | Plural |
|---|---|---|---|
| 3rd person | मोदते<br>He/she rejoices | मोदेते<br>They both rejoice | मोदन्ते<br>They all rejoice |
| 2nd person | मोदसे<br>You rejoice | मोदेथे<br>You both rejoice | मोदध्वे<br>You all rejoice |
| 1st person | मोदे<br>I rejoice | मोदावहे<br>We both rejoice | मोदामहे<br>We all rejoice |

**√मन् (root) to think, 4Ā ⇒ मन् (base)**

| | Verbal Stem | | | | | | |
|---|---|---|---|---|---|---|---|
| | Base | | Gaṇa Sign | | Ending | | |
| 3rd person singular | मन् | + | य | + | ते | ⇒ | मन्यते |
| 1st person singular | मन् | + | या → य् | + | ए | ⇒ | मन्ये |

| | Singular | Dual | Plural |
|---|---|---|---|
| 3rd person | मन्यते | मन्येते | मन्यन्ते |
| 2nd person | मन्यसे | मन्येथे | मन्यध्वे |
| 1st person | मन्ये | मन्यावहे | मन्यामहे |

## Conjugate

| Root | | 3rd person singular |
|---|---|---|
| √ईक्ष् | to see (1Ā) | ईक्षते |
| √भाष् | to speak (1Ā) | भाषते |
| √लभ् | to obtain (1Ā) | लभते |
| √वन्द् | to honor, bow (1Ā) | वन्दते |
| √वृत् | to be, exist (1Ā) | *वर्तते |
| √जन् | to be born (4Ā) | *जायते |
| √मन्त्र् | to advise (10Ā) | मन्त्रयते |

You might know the word वन्दे, the first-person singular conjugation of √वन्द्, from the well-known invocation to Patañjali, the *Aṣṭāṅga Yoga Mantra*, वन्दे गुरूणां चरनारविन्दे, meaning "I bow to the two lotus feet of the gurus."

## Example: *Bhagavadgītā* 2.40

Kṛṣṇa is speaking to Arjuna about yoga practice. The subject of the second line is "one."

नेहाभिक्रमनाशोऽस्ति प्रत्यवायो न विद्यते ।
स्वल्पमप्यस्य धर्मस्य त्रायते महतो भयात् ॥

### Vocabulary

इह ind. here (i.e., in yoga practice)
अभिक्रमनाशः m. loss of effort, waste of an attempt
  अभिक्रमः m. undertaking, attempt, effort
  नाशः m. loss, disappearance
प्रत्यवायः m. contrary course, harm
√विद् 4Ā, to exist
स्वल्पः m. a little
अपि ind. even, also
अस्य of this (m. gen. sg.)
धर्मः m. practice, discipline
√त्रै 1Ā, to protect

*Sandhi* Rule: Two dissimilar vowels will coalesce only if the first vowel is अ / आ.

अ / आ + इ / ई ⇒ ए
अ / आ + उ / ऊ ⇒ ओ
अ / आ + ए / ऐ ⇒ ऐ
अ / आ + ओ / औ ⇒ औ
अ / आ + ऋ / ॠ ⇒ अर्

Example:
न + इह ⇒ नेह
च + एव ⇒ चैव

महतः from great (n. abl. sg.)
भयम् n. fear, danger

| न | इह | अभिक्रमनाशः | अस्ति | प्रत्यवायः | न | विद्यते । |
|---|---|---|---|---|---|---|
| no | here | loss of effort | there is | harm | no | exists |

| स्वल्पम् | अपि | अस्य | धर्मस्य | त्रायते | महतः | भयात् ॥ |
|---|---|---|---|---|---|---|
| a little | even | of this | of practice | protects | from great | from danger |

Here, [in yoga practice] (इह), there is (अस्ति) no (न) loss of effort (अभिक्रमनाशो),
Nor (न) does any harm (प्रत्यवायो) **exist** (विद्यते).
Even (अपि) a little (स्वल्पम्) of this (अस्य) practice (धर्मस्य)
**Protects** (त्रायते) [one] from great (महतो) danger (भयात्).

## NOTE ON COMPOUNDS

One of the richest but potentially most intimidating aspects of learning Sanskrit is the numerous compound words. In Chapters 11–14, we will learn how to break down these compound words and understand the relationship between the component parts. Some compounds consist of a list of two or more words that are considered together (a + b + c + . . .); some compounds consist of words related to each other through the case functions we have learned in Chapter 3, and other compounds describe some entity external to the compound. For now, when you see a compound word, try to distinguish the words that compose it (in most instances provided in the vocabulary list below the compound itself) and begin to pay attention to the relationship between them.

### Translate

#### A. *Kṛṣṇāṣṭakam*, "The Eight Verses to Kṛṣṇa," 1

Note that the main sentence is in the last *pāda*. The long compounds are all in the accusative case and describe Kṛṣṇa (in the fourth *pāda*).

वसुदेवसुतं देवं कंसचाणूरमर्दनम् ।
देवकीपरमानन्दं कृष्णं वन्दे जगद्गुरुम् ॥

Vocabulary

वसुदेवसुतः m. son of Vasudeva
  वसुदेवः m. father of Kṛṣṇa
  सुतः m. son
कंसचाणूरमर्दनः m. destroyer of Kaṃsa and Cāṇūra
  कंसः m. king of Mathurā, brother of Devakī
  चाणूरः m. a wrestler in Kaṃsa's service
  मर्दन mfn. destroying
देवकीपरमानन्दः m. the greatest joy (i.e., the son) of Devakī
  देवकी f. mother of Kṛṣṇa
  परम mfn. highest, best, greatest
  आनन्दः m. happiness, joy, delight
जगद्गुरुम् spiritual teacher of the universe (m. acc. sg.)
  जगत् n. the world, universe
  गुरुः m. teacher

> After the marriage of Devakī and Vasudeva, it was prophesied to Kaṃsa, Devakī's brother, that the eighth child of Devakī would kill him. Kaṃsa then threw them both in prison and killed their first six children. The seventh and eighth, Balarāma and Kṛṣṇa, were saved. Kṛṣṇa was raised by the cowherd couple Nanda and Yaśodā and grew up to fulfill the prophecy.

B. *Śivasaṃhitā* 4.17

The subject must be inferred as "the yogī" or simply "one." In trying to distinguish the words in this verse, note the repeated use of अभ्यासाद् / अभ्यासात्, "from practice," in each *pāda*. Each *pāda* is a separate sentence.

संवित्तिं लभतेऽभ्यासाद्योगोऽभ्यासात्प्रवर्तते ।
मन्त्राणां सिद्धिरभ्यासादभ्यासाद्वायुसाधनम् ॥

> The *Śivasaṃhitā* is a collection of verses on yoga, taught by Śiva to his wife, Pārvatī. It was written sometime between 1300 and 1500 C.E.

Vocabulary

संवित्तिम् knowledge, understanding (f. acc. sg.)
प्र√वृत् 1Ā, to occur, happen
मन्त्रः m. a sacred prayer
सिद्धिः fulfillment, accomplishment, success (f. nom. sg.)
वायुसाधनम् n. mastery of the breath
  वायुः m. wind, air, breath
  साधनम् n. accomplishment, attainment, mastery

> *Sandhi* Rule: In the case of a final ए before an initial अ, the अ is dropped and is replaced by an *avagraha* (ऽ).
>
> Example: लभते अभ्यासाद् ⇒ लभतेऽभ्यासाद्

## FEMININE NOUNS ENDING IN आ

**माला f. garland**

| | Singular | Dual | Plural |
|---|---|---|---|
| **Nominative** | माला<br>the garland (subject) | माले<br>the two garlands (subject) | मालाः<br>the garlands (subject) |
| **Accusative** | मालाम्<br>the garland (object) | माले<br>the two garlands (object) | मालाः<br>the garlands (object) |
| **Instrumental** | मालया<br>with the garland | मालाभ्याम्<br>with the two garlands | मालाभिः<br>with the garlands |
| **Dative** | मालायै<br>to/for the garland | मालाभ्याम्<br>to/for the two garlands | मालाभ्यः<br>to/for the garlands |
| **Ablative** | मालायाः<br>from garland | मालाभ्याम्<br>from the two garlands | मालाभ्यः<br>from the garlands |
| **Genitive** | मालायाः<br>of the garland | मालयोः<br>of the two garlands | मालानाम्<br>of the garlands |
| **Locative** | मालायाम्<br>in/on the garland | मालयोः<br>in/on the two garlands | मालासु<br>in/on the garlands |
| **Vocative** | माले<br>O garland | माले<br>O two garlands | मालाः<br>O garlands |

Vocabulary

अविद्या f. ignorance
अहिंसा f. nonviolence
कथा f. story
करुणा f. compassion
चेतना f. consciousness, understanding, intelligence
निद्रा f. sleep
प्रजा f. people, subjects, offspring
बाला f. girl
माया f. illusion
विद्या f. knowledge
श्रद्धा f. faith, confidence, trust

### Decline

अहिंसा, करुणा, विद्या, and श्रद्धा

## FEMININE NOUNS ENDING IN ई

**नदी f. river**

| | Singular | Dual | Plural |
|---|---|---|---|
| **Nominative** | नदी<br>the river (subject) | नद्यौ<br>the two rivers (subject) | नद्यः<br>the rivers (subject) |
| **Accusative** | नदीम्<br>the river (object) | नद्यौ<br>the two rivers (object) | नदीः<br>the rivers (object) |
| **Instrumental** | नद्या<br>by the river | नदीभ्याम्<br>by the two rivers | नदीभिः<br>by the rivers |
| **Dative** | नद्यै<br>to/for the river | नदीभ्याम्<br>to/for the two rivers | नदीभ्यः<br>to/for the rivers |
| **Ablative** | नद्याः<br>from the river | नदीभ्याम्<br>from the two rivers | नदीभ्यः<br>from the rivers |
| **Genitive** | नद्याः<br>of the river | नद्योः<br>of the two rivers | नदीनाम्<br>of the rivers |
| **Locative** | नद्याम्<br>in the river | नद्योः<br>in the two rivers | नदीषु<br>in the rivers |
| **Vocative** | नदि<br>O river | नद्यौ<br>O two rivers | नद्यः<br>O rivers |

Vocabulary

देवी f. goddess
नाडी f. subtle channel
नारी f. woman
मही f. earth
लक्ष्मी f. goddess of wealth
सरस्वती f. goddess of knowledge

## Decline

देवी, नाडी, मही, and सरस्वती

## Example: *Śivasaṃhitā* 2.24

The main noun is वाग्देवी in the third *pāda*, referenced by the pronoun सा in the first *pāda*. The other words ending in आ are feminine adjectives describing her.

जगत्संसृष्टिरूपा सा निर्माणे सततोद्यता ।
वाचामवाच्या वाग्देवी सदा दैवैर्नमस्कृता ॥

### Vocabulary

जगत्संसृष्टिरूप mfn. having the form of the creation of the world
निर्माणम् n. creating
सततोद्यत mfn. always active
वाचाम् of/by words (f. gen. pl.)
अवाच्य mfn. not to be expressed
वाग्देवी f. goddess of speech
सदा ind. always
नमस्कृत mfn. saluted, worshipped, adored

| जगत्संसृष्टिरूपा | सा | निर्माणे | सततोद्यता । |
|---|---|---|---|
| having the form of the creation of the world | she | in creating | always active |

| वाचाम् | अवाच्या | वाग्देवी | सदा | देवैर् | नमस्कृता ॥ |
|---|---|---|---|---|---|
| by words | not to be expressed | goddess of speech | always | by the gods | adored |

She (सा) **has the form of the creation of the world** (जगत्संसृष्टिरूपा),
**Always active** (सततोद्यता) in creating (निर्माणे).
**The goddess of speech** (वाग्देवी) **is inexpressible** (अवाच्या) by words (वाचाम्),
Always (सदा) adored (नमस्कृता) by the gods (देवैर्).

## C. Morning Mantra

करााग्रे वसते लक्ष्मी करमध्ये सरस्वती ।
करमूले स्थिता गौरी प्रभाते करदर्शनम् ॥

This chant is traditionally recited first thing in the morning.

Vocabulary

करराग्रम् n. tip of the hand
    करः m. hand, the doer
    अग्रम् n. tip
√वस् 1U, to live
करमध्यम् n. middle of the hand
    मध्य mfn. middle
करमूलम् n. root of the hand
    मूलम् n. root
स्थित mfn. situated
गौरी f. the goddess Parvatī
प्रभातम् n. daybreak, dawn, morning
करदर्शनम् n. looking at the hand
    दर्शनम् n. looking at, seeing

The word मूल occurs in the compound मूलबन्ध, "the lock at the root [of the body]."

**D. Bathing Mantra**

This chant is traditionally recited when taking a bath and evokes the presence of all of the sacred rivers of India. Accordingly, the subject implied in this verse is "I."

गङ्गे च यमुने चैव गोदावरि सरस्वति ।
नर्मदे सिन्धु कावेरि जलेऽस्मिन्सन्निधिं कुरु ॥

Vocabulary

गङ्गा f. the Ganges River
यमुना f. the Jumna/Jamuna River
गोदावरी f. a river in the south
सरस्वती f. legendary river, part of which dried up and another part that joins the Ganges and the Jumna at Allahabad
नर्मदा f. river
सिन्धु O Sindu River (f. voc. sg.)
कावेरी f. a river in the south
जलम् n. water
अस्मिन् in this (m. loc. sg.)
सन्निधिम् vicinity, presence (m. acc. sg.)
कुरु do, make, invoke (2nd p. sg. imperative √कृ)

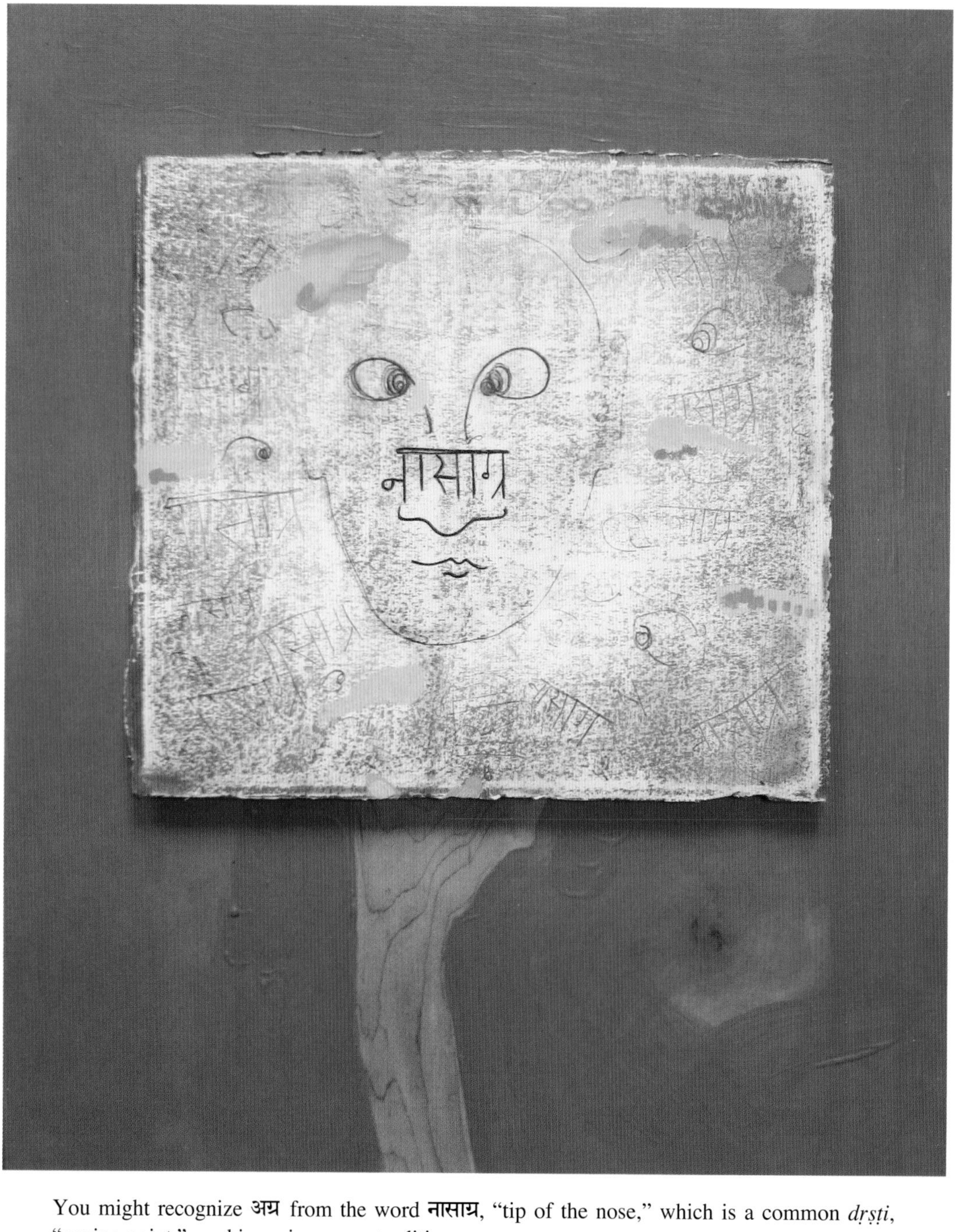


You might recognize अग्र from the word नासाग्र, “tip of the nose,” which is a common *dṛṣṭi*, “gazing point,” used in various yoga traditions.

### E. *Śivasaṃhitā* 2.23

Remember that adjectives can be masculine, feminine, or neuter, depending on their case ending. When you see an adjective ending in आ or ई, near a feminine noun, it will generally be a feminine adjective describing that noun. Here the main feminine noun is कुण्डली.

तत्र विद्युल्लताकारा कुण्डली परदेवता ।
सार्द्धत्रिकरा कुटिला सूक्ष्मा भुजगसंनिभा ॥

> *Sandhi* Rule: A final त् changes to ल् before an initial ल्.
>
> Example: विद्युत् लताकारा ⇒ विद्युल्लताकारा

Vocabulary

तत्र ind. there
विद्युल्लताकारा f. in the form of a creeping-vine of lightning, forked or zigzag lightning
- विद्युत् lightning (f.)
- लता f. creeper, creeping vine, winding plant
- आकारा f. form

कुण्डली f. Kuṇḍalinī
परदेवता f. highest deity
सार्द्धत्रिकर mfn. three and a half times
कुटिल mfn. curled, coiled
सूक्ष्म mfn. subtle
भुजगसंनिभ mfn. resembling a snake
- भुजगः m. snake
- संनिभ mfn. like, resembling

## *SANDHI* REVIEW

In addition to the rules given in the next few pages, you should go back and review the rules at the end of Chapter 2 at this point.

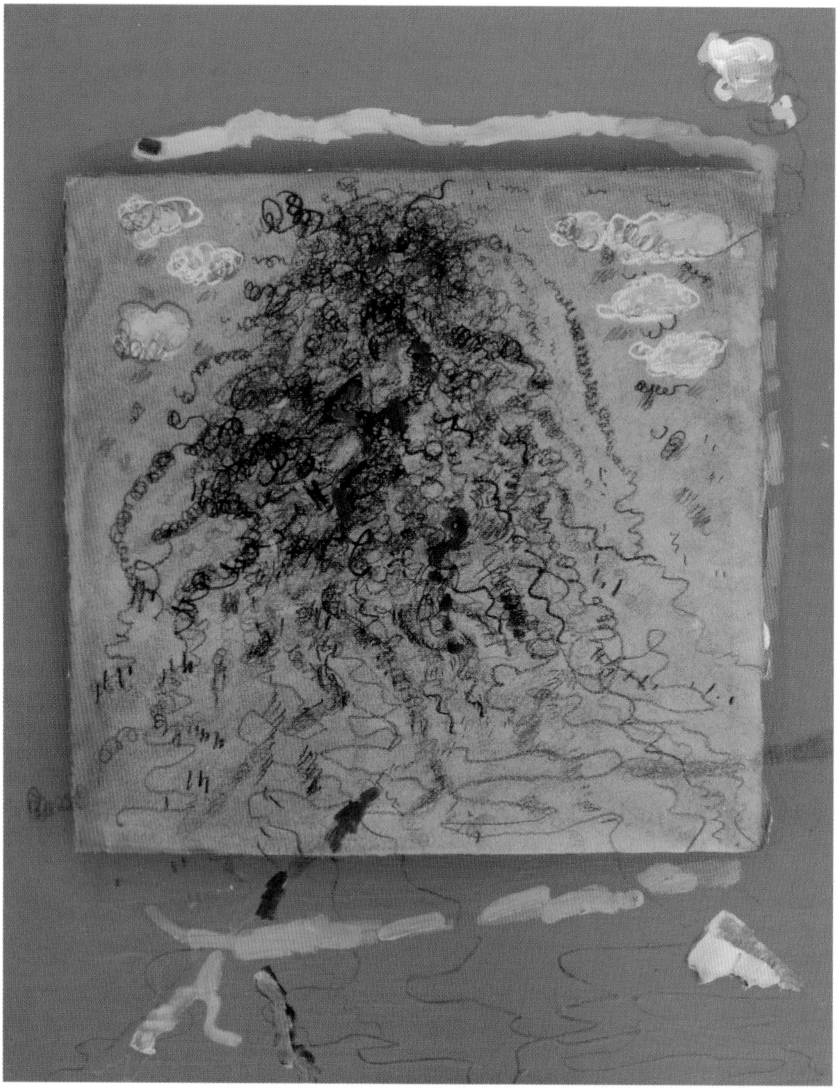

The Gaṅgā River is considered the most sacred of all the rivers in India. Originally residing in the sky, Gaṅgā was brought down to earth in response to the *tapas* (penance) performed by Bhagiratha to cleanse the souls of his ancestors, the sixty thousand sons of Sāgara, who had been burnt to ash when they offended the sage Kapila. Gaṅgā decided she would destroy the earth with the power of her waters; however, Lord Śiva intervened and broke her fall by trapping her in his matted locks of hair. He then let her cascade down to the earth, as well as to the netherworlds, in small streams. She is still thought to purify the souls of both the living and the dead with her waters.

## Vowel *Sandhi*

The main principle of vowel *sandhi*, both internal (within a word) and external (between two words), is that two vowels should generally not be directly next to each other. In order to avoid this juxtaposition, vowels coalesce in one of four ways: the two vowels become one, the first vowel becomes a consonant, one of the vowels disappears, or the first vowel changes to a different vowel to facilitate reading.

1. Two dissimilar vowels will coalesce only if the first vowel is अ / आ.

   अ / आ + इ / ई ⇒ ए
   अ / आ + उ / ऊ ⇒ ओ
   अ / आ + ए / ऐ ⇒ ऐ
   अ / आ + ओ / औ ⇒ औ
   अ / आ + ऋ / ॠ ⇒ अर्

**Example 1: *Yogasūtra* 2.55**

ततः परमा वश्यता इन्द्रियाणाम् ⇒ ततः परमा वश्यतेन्द्रियाणाम् ।

**Example 2: *Yogasūtra* 3.12**

ततः पुनः शान्त उदितौ तुल्यप्रत्ययौ चित्तस्य एकाग्रतापरिणामः ⇒ ततः पुनः शान्तोदितौ तुल्यप्रत्ययौ चित्तस्यैकाग्रतापरिणामः ।

**Example 3: *Yogasūtra* 4.1**

जन्म ओषधिमन्त्रतपःसमाधिजाः सिद्धयः ⇒ जन्मौषधिमन्त्रतपःसमाधिजाः सिद्धयः ।

2. In the case of a final ए before an initial अ, the अ is dropped and is replaced by an *avagraha* (ऽ).

**Example: *Yogasūtra* 1.3**

तदा द्रष्टुः स्वरूपे अवस्थानम् ⇒ तदा द्रष्टुः स्वरूपेऽवस्थानम् ।

3. When two dissimilar vowels are next to each other and the first vowel is a simple vowel other than अ / आ, the first vowel will change into its corresponding semivowel.

इ / ई ⇒ य्
उ / ऊ ⇒ व्
ऋ / ॠ ⇒ र्

**Example 1:** ***Yogasūtra* 2.13**

सति मूले तद्विपाको जाति अयुर्भोगाः ⇒ सति मूले तद्विपाको जात्ययुर्भोगाः ।

**Example 2:** ***Yogasūtra* 3.39**

उदानजयाज्जलपङ्ककण्टकादिषु असङ्ग उत्क्रान्तिश्च ⇒ उदानजयाज्जलपङ्ककण्टकादिष्वसङ्ग उत्क्रान्तिश्च ।

## *Visarga Sandhi*

4. If a *visarga* is preceded by अ and followed by a vowel other than अ, the *visarga* is dropped and the hiatus remains.

**Example:** ***Yogasūtra* 2.21**

तदर्थः एव दृश्यस्यात्मा ⇒ तदर्थ एव दृश्यस्यात्मा ।

5. If a *visarga* is preceded by आ and followed by a voiced consonant or vowel, the *visarga* is dropped and the hiatus remains.

**Example:** ***Yogasūtra* 1.46**

ताः एव सबीजः समाधिः ⇒ ता एव सबीजः समाधिः ।

6. A *visarga* before a च or छ becomes a श्.
   A *visarga* before a ट or ठ becomes a ष्.
   A *visarga* before a त or थ becomes a स्.

**Example 1:** ***Yogasūtra* 1.2**

योगः चित्तवृत्तिनिरोधः ⇒ योगश्चित्तवृत्तिनिरोधः ।

**Example 2:** ***Yogasūtra* 2.11**

ध्यानहेयाः तद्वृत्तयः ⇒ ध्यानहेयास्तद्वृत्तयः ।

7. If a *visarga* is preceded by a vowel other than अ / आ and followed by an unvoiced consonant, there is no change. If it is followed by a voiced consonant or vowel, it becomes र्.

**Example: *Yogasūtra* 2.23–24**

स्वस्वामिशक्त्योः स्वरूपोपलब्धिहेतुः संयोगः ⇒ स्वस्वामिशक्त्योः स्वरूपोपलब्धिहेतुः संयोगः ।
तस्य हेतुः अविद्या ⇒ तस्य हेतुरविद्या ।

## Consonant *Sandhi*

8. An unvoiced final consonant becomes the unaspirated voiced consonant of the same class, before an initial voiced consonant or vowel.

**Example: *Yogasūtra* 1.23**

ईश्वरप्रणिधानात् वा ⇒ ईश्वरप्रणिधानाद्वा

9. Exception to Rule 8: A final consonant before a word beginning with a nasal becomes the corresponding nasal.

   त् + न ⇒ न्न

**Example: *Yogasūtra* 1.12**

अभ्यासवैराग्याभ्यां तत् निरोधः ⇒ अभ्यासवैराग्याभ्यां तन्निरोधः ।

10. Before a retroflex or palatal consonant, त changes to the corresponding unaspirated consonant.

    त् + च ⇒ च्च
    त् + छ ⇒ च्छ
    त् + ज ⇒ ज्ज
    त् + ट ⇒ ट्ट

**Example 1:** ***Yogasūtra*** **1.28**

तत् जपस्तदर्थभावनम् ⇒ तज्जपस्तदर्थभावनम्।

**Example 2:** ***Yogasūtra*** **2.15**

परिणामतापसंस्कारदुःखैर्गुणवृत्तिविरोधात् च दुःखमेव सर्वं विवेकिनः ⇒
परिणामतापसंस्कारदुःखैर्गुणवृत्तिविरोधाच्च दुःखमेव सर्वं विवेकिनः।

**Example 3:** ***Yogasūtra*** **4.27**

तत् छिद्रेषु प्रत्ययान्तराणि संस्कारेभ्यः ⇒ तच्छिद्रेषु प्रत्ययान्तराणि संस्कारेभ्यः।

11. A final त् changes to ल् before an initial ल्.

**Example:** ***Yogasūtra*** **3.42**

कायाकाशयोः संबन्धसंयमात् लघुतूलसमापत्तेश्चाकाशगमनम् ⇒
कायाकाशयोः संबन्धसंयमाल्लघुतूलसमापत्तेश्चाकाशगमनम्।

## Internal *Sandhi*

12. Dental न् changes to retroflex ण् if, within the same word, it is preceded by र्, ऋ, or ष् and immediately followed by a vowel, semivowel, or nasal, if no palatal, retroflex, or dental consonant (except य्) intervenes.

**Example:** ***Yogasūtra*** **2.4**

अविद्याक्षेत्रमुत्तरेषां प्रसुप्ततनुविच्छिन्नोदाराणाम्।

### F. *Yogayājñavalkya* 1.46–49

Write with correct *sandhi* and translate. Yājñavalkya is speaking to his wife, Gārgī, enumerating the limbs of yoga and their respective components.

यमः च नियमः च एव आसनम् च तथा एव च ।
प्राणायामः तथा गार्गि प्रत्याहारः च धारणा ॥

ध्यानम् समाधिः एतानि योगाङ्गानि वरानने ।
यमः च नियमः च एव दशधा संप्रकीर्तितः ॥

आसनानि उत्तमानि अष्टौ त्रयम् तेषु उत्तमोत्तमम् ।
प्राणायामः त्रिधा प्रोक्तः प्रत्याहारः च पंचधा ॥

धारणा पंचधा प्रोक्ता ध्यानम् षोढा प्रकीर्तितम् ।
त्रयम् तेषु उत्तम् प्रोक्तम् समाधिः तु एकरूपकः ॥

The *Yogayājñavalkya* is a dialogue between the sage Yājñavalkya and his wife, Maitreyī, that takes place in front of an assembly of *ṛṣis*, or sages, in which he explains the path of *aṣṭāṅgayoga*. Written sometime between the thirteenth and fourteenth century C.E., it is one of the oldest texts on yoga and illustrates the historical importance of women as philosophers and practitioners of yoga.

Vocabulary

प्राणायामः m. breath control
तथा ind. in that way
गार्गी f. belonging to the Garga lineage, Yājñavalkya's wife
प्रत्याहारः m. sensory withdrawal
धारणा f. concentration
ध्यानम् n. meditation
समाधिः meditative absorption (m. nom. sg.)
एतानि these (n. nom. pl.)
योगाङ्गानि limbs/aspects of yoga (n. nom. pl.)
वरानना f. lovely-faced woman
दशधा ind. tenfold, in ten parts
संप्रकीर्तित mfn. mentioned, designated, called
उत्तम mfn. best, greatest, highest, end, ultimate stage
उत्तमोत्तम mfn. best of the best
अष्टौ eight (n. nom. sg.)
त्रय mfn. threefold
त्रिधा ind. threefold
प्रोक्त mfn. told, taught
पंचधा ind. fivefold
षोढा ind. in six ways, sixfold
प्रकीर्तित mfn. proclaimed, declared, said
एकरूपकः m. having [only] one form

## Review Exercises

### G. *Śivasaṃhitā* 2.25–26

Note that in both verses, the indeclinable verbal forms व्यवस्थिता, समाश्लिष्य, and गता all refer to the preceding word.

इडानाम्नी तु या नाडी वाममार्गे व्यवस्थिता ।
मध्यनाडीं समाश्लिष्य वामनासापुटे गता ॥

पिंगला नाम या नाडी दक्षमार्गे व्यवस्थिता ।
सुषुम्णां सा समाश्लिष्य दक्षनासापुटे गता ॥

Vocabulary

इडानाम्नी f. named Iḍā
या which (f. nom. sg.)
वाममार्गः m. the left-hand path
    वाम mfn. left, situated on the left side
व्यवस्थित mfn. situated
मध्यनाडी f. the central channel
समाश्लिष्य clinging to, attached to (gerund समा√श्लिष्)
वामनासापुटः m. left nostril
गत mfn. gone to, situated in, contained in, connected to
पिंगला f. name of the right-hand channel
नाम ind. by name, named
दक्षमार्गः m. right-hand path
    दक्ष mfn. right, situated on the right side
सुषुम्णा f. name of the central channel
दक्षनासापुटः m. right nostril

### H. *Bhagavadgītā* 2.65

The first two *pādas* should be read together as one sentence, with the main subject and verb in the second *pāda*; the third and fourth form a separate sentence with the subject and verb in the fourth *pāda*.

प्रसादे सर्वदुःखानां हानिरस्योपजायते ।
प्रसन्नचेतसो ह्याशु बुद्धिः पर्यवतिष्ठते ॥

Vocabulary

प्रसादः m. calmness, tranquillity
सर्वदुःखम् n. all suffering/sorrow
हानिर् cessation, disappearance (f. nom. sg.)
अस्य of him, his, of one's (m. gen. sg.)
उप√जन् 4Ā, to be born or produced, originate, arise
प्रसन्नचेतसः of one whose mind is tranquil (m. gen. sg)
हि ind. for, because
आशु ind. quickly, immediately
बुद्धिः understanding, discernment, wisdom, intellect (f. nom. sg.)
पर्यव√स्था 1Ā, to become firm or steady

I. *Gheraṇḍasaṃhitā* 2.43

The first three *pādas* list three separate results of the activity in the fourth *pāda*.

देहाग्निर्वर्धते नित्यं सर्वरोगविनाशनम् ।
जागर्ति भुजगी देवी भुजङ्गासनसाधनात् ॥

Vocabulary

देहाग्निर् fire in the body (m. nom. sg.)
  देह mn. the body
  अग्निः m. fire
√वृध् 1Ā, to grow, increase
नित्यम् ind. constantly, regularly, steadily
सर्वरोगविनाशनम् n. destruction of all diseases
  रोगः m. disease
  विनाशनम् n. removal, destruction
जागर्ति he/she/it awakens (3rd p. sg.)
भुजगी f. a female snake, serpent
भुजङ्गासनसाधनः m. the practice of *bhujaṅgāsana* (serpent pose)

# 5
# Masculine and Feminine Nouns Ending in इ and उ; Verbs: Imperative and Optative

वृत्तिसारूप्यमितरत्र ॥ १.४ ॥
**vṛtti-sārūpyam itaratra**
Otherwise, there is identification with the fluctuations of the mind.
॥ *Yogasūtra* 1.4 ॥

## MASCULINE NOUNS ENDING IN इ AND उ

Nouns ending in consonants other than अ differ slightly in their declensions; however, you will notice similar patterns and endings to the nouns we have learned so far. Masculine nouns ending in इ and उ have parallel declensions, with the following correspondences in the formation of the endings:

| Example | | Masc. Nouns in इ | Masc. Nouns in उ |
|---|---|---|---|
| Nom. sg. | इ ⇒ उ | मुनिः | गुरुः |
| Nom. du. | ई ⇒ ऊ | मुनी | गुरू |
| Nom. pl. | य ⇒ व | मुनयः | गुरवः |
| Voc. sg. | ए ⇒ ओ | मुने | गुरो |

### Masculine Nouns Ending in इ

**मुनिः m. sage**

| | Singular | Dual | Plural |
|---|---|---|---|
| **Nominative** (subject) | मुनिः | मुनी | मुनयः |
| **Accusative** (object) | मुनिम् | मुनी | मुनीन् |
| **Instrumental** (by/with) | मुनिना | मुनिभ्याम् | मुनिभिः |
| **Dative** (to/for) | मुनये | मुनिभ्याम् | मुनिभ्यः |
| **Ablative** (from) | मुनेः | मुनिभ्याम् | मुनिभ्यः |
| **Genitive** (of) | मुनेः | मुन्योः | मुनीनाम् |
| **Locative** (in/on) | मुनौ | मुन्योः | मुनिषु |
| **Vocative** (O) | मुने | मुनी | मुनयः |

## Masculine Nouns Ending in उ

**गुरुः m. teacher, heavy**

| | Singular | Dual | Plural |
|---|---|---|---|
| **Nominative** (subject) | गुरुः | गुरू | गुरवः |
| **Accusative** (object) | गुरुम् | गुरू | गुरून् |
| **Instrumental** (by/with) | गुरुणा | गुरुभ्याम् | गुरुभिः |
| **Dative** (to/for) | गुरवे | गुरुभ्याम् | गुरुभ्यः |
| **Ablative** (from) | गुरोः | गुरुभ्याम् | गुरुभ्यः |
| **Genitive** (of) | गुरोः | गुर्वोः | गुरूणाम् |
| **Locative** (in) | गुरौ | गुर्वोः | गुरुषु |
| **Vocative** (O) | गुरो | गुरू | गुरवः |

### Vocabulary

अथितिः m. guest
अरिः m. enemy
ऋषिः m. sage
कविः m. poet
रविः m. sun
समाधिः m. meditative absorption
इन्दुः m. moon
तरुः m. tree
बाहुः m. arm
वायुः m. wind, air, breath
शिशुः m. baby, child
साधुः m. holy man

There is a famous निर्वचनम् (saying) about the गुरुः (teacher) in the *Advayatārakopaniṣat*, V. 16:

गुशब्दस्त्वन्धकारः स्यात् रुशब्दस्तन्निरोधकः ।
अन्धकारनिरोधत्वात् गुरुरित्यभिधीयते ॥

The syllable "gu" denotes darkness,
The syllable "ru" denotes the dispeller of that.
Because of the ability to dispell darkness,
One is called a guru.

### Decline

ऋषिः, कविः, समाधिः, वायुः, and साधुः

*Sandhi* Rule: If a *visarga* is preceded by a letter other than अ / आ and followed by an unvoiced consonant, there is no change.

Example: गुरुः साक्षात् ⇒ गुरुः साक्षात्

If it is followed by a voiced consonant, it becomes र्.

Example: गुरुः ब्रह्मा ⇒ गुरुर्ब्रह्मा

## Translate and Memorize

### A. *Guru Stotram* I

गुरुर्ब्रह्मा गुरुर्विष्णुः गुरुर्देवो महेश्वरः ।
गुरुः साक्षात्परं ब्रह्म तस्मै श्रीगुरवे नमः ॥

Vocabulary

ब्रह्मा God of Creation (m. nom. sg. ब्रह्मन्)
विष्णुः m. God of Preservation
महेश्वरः m. Śiva, God of Destruction, "The Great Lord"
साक्षात् ind. clearly
पर mfn. highest, supreme
ब्रह्म the Supreme Spirit (n. nom. sg. ब्रह्मन्)
तस्मै to him (dative sg. तत्)
श्रीगुरुः m. sacred/revered teacher
श्री mfn. sacred, holy, revered
नमः m. a bow, salutations

Note the difference between the masc. ब्रह्मा, the God of Creation, mentioned in the first *pāda*, and the neuter ब्रह्म, the Supreme Spirit, mentioned in the third *pāda*.

## Translate

### B. *Ādityahṛdayam* 16

नमः पूर्वाय गिरये पश्चिमायाद्रये नमः ।
ज्योतिर्गणानां पतये दिनाधिपतये नमः ॥ १६ ॥

Vocabulary

पूर्व mfn. eastern
गिरिः m. mountain
पश्चिम mfn. western
अद्रिः m. mountain
ज्योतिर्गणः m. the heavenly bodies collectively
ज्योतिस् n. light
पतिः m. lord, master, ruler
दिनाधिपतिः m. lord of the day

### C. *Bhagavadgītā* 10.37

This verse comes in a series of verses in which Kṛṣṇa describes his many forms to Arjuna. Each *pāda* can be read as a separate sentence, explaining that, among various groups, he is the best of each group.

वृष्णीनां वासुदेवोऽस्मि पाण्डवानां धनंजयः ।
मुनीनामप्यहं व्यासः कवीनामुशना कविः ॥

Vocabulary

वृष्णिः m. family from which Kṛṣṇa is descended
वासुदेवः m. son of Vasudeva, name for Kṛṣṇa

पाण्डवः m. descendant of Pāṇḍu
धनंजयः m. name for Arjuna, "conqueror of wealth"
अपि ind. and, also, moreover
व्यासः m. "compiler, arranger" of the Vedas, author of the *Mahābhārata* and the *Purāṇas*
उशना name of an ancient sage (m. nom. sg.उशनस्)

Pāṇḍu, "the pale," is considered the father of Arjuna and his brothers. However, before their birth, when hunting in the forest, Pāṇḍu accidentally shot a sage and his wife in the act of love-making, mistaking them for deer. He was then cursed that if he were to make love with a woman, he would die in the act. So, he lived in celibacy with his two wives, Kuntī and Mādrī, in the forest. Pāṇḍu, wishing for a son, asked Kuntī to use a boon granted to her by the sage Durvāsas, which allowed her to call upon any God to give her a child. She prayed to Dharma, who gave her Yudhiṣṭhira, Vāyu, who gave her Bhīma, and Indra, who gave her Arjuna. She also allowed Mādrī to use the boon to call upon the Aśvins, who gave her Nakula and Sahadeva. Thus the five brothers were all partial incarnations of gods.

## Feminine Nouns Ending in इ and उ

Feminine nouns ending in इ and उ are identical to their masculine equivalents, with the exception of the accusative plural and instrumental singular forms. Additionally, the dative, ablative, genitive, and locative singular forms can take either the same endings as their masculine equivalents or the same endings as feminine nouns ending in ई and ऊ. One reason that multiple endings are permissible is to add to the tools at a poet's disposal. Sanskrit poems are categorized according to meter and each meter consists of a certain number of syllables per *pāda*, or quarter. Thus, the choice between वृत्त्यै and वृत्तये is a choice between two and three syllables.

## Feminine Nouns Ending in इ

**वृत्तिः f. fluctuating state**

| | Singular | Dual | Plural |
|---|---|---|---|
| **Nominative** (subject) | वृत्तिः | वृत्ती | वृत्तयः |
| **Accusative** (object) | वृत्तिम् | वृत्ती | वृत्तीः |
| **Instrumental** (by/with) | वृत्त्या | वृत्तिभ्याम् | वृत्तिभिः |
| **Dative** (to/for) | वृत्त्यै, वृत्तये | वृत्तिभ्याम् | वृत्तिभ्यः |
| **Ablative** (from) | वृत्त्याः, वृत्तेः | वृत्तिभ्याम् | वृत्तिभ्यः |
| **Genitive** (of) | वृत्त्याः, वृत्तेः | वृत्त्योः | वृत्तीनाम् |

| | | | |
|---|---|---|---|
| **Locative** (in/on) | वृत्त्याम्, वृत्तौ | वृत्त्योः | वृत्तिषु |
| **Vocative** (O) | वृत्ते | वृत्ती | वृत्तयः |

## Feminine Nouns Ending in उ

**तनुः f. body**

| | Singular | Dual | Plural |
|---|---|---|---|
| **Nominative** (subject) | तनुः | तनू | तनवः |
| **Accusative** (object) | तनुम् | तनू | तनूः |
| **Instrumental** (by/with) | तन्वा | तनुभ्याम् | तनुभिः |
| **Dative** (to/for) | तन्वै, तनवे | तनुभ्याम् | तनुभ्यः |
| **Ablative** (from) | तन्वाः, तनोः | तनुभ्याम् | तनुभ्यः |
| **Genitive** (of) | तन्वाः, तनोः | तन्वोः | तनूनाम् |
| **Locative** (in/on) | तन्वाम्, तनौ | तन्वोः | तनुषु |
| **Vocative** (O) | तनो | तनू | तनवः |

Vocabulary

दृष्टिः f. seeing, gaze
प्रकृतिः f. Nature
बुद्धिः f. understanding, discernment, wisdom, intelligence, intellect
भक्तिः f. devotion, love
भूमिः f. earth
मतिः f. thought, mind, intelligence
रात्रिः f. night
शक्तिः f. power
शान्तिः f. peace
स्थितिः f. stability
धेनुः f. cow
रज्जुः f. rope
रेणुः f. dust
हनुः f. jaw

The practice of दृष्टिः (*dṛṣṭi*), of a focused "gaze," which is used in yoga practice, is a means to a concentrated state of awareness; a bridge between the external world and the Soul. "Arjuna, what do you see?" asked Droṇa, the archery instructor in the *Mahābhārata*. "I see the head of a bird," Arjuna replied, and proceeded to cut off the bird's head with his arrow. Unlike his brothers and cousins, who had been distracted by the surrounding trees and sky, and were therefore certain to miss their target, Arjuna had a focused gaze and, thus, he instantly hit his mark. Studying Sanskrit requires a similar one-pointed concentration—each word, as well as the verse in its entirety, must be focused upon and understood in order to arrive at an understanding of the whole.

### Decline

भक्तिः, भूमिः, शान्तिः, धेनुः, and हनुः

हनुमान् (Hanumān), the famous monkey-god, who helped Rāma save Sītā from the demon Rāvaṇa, is so-called because he has large jaws.

## Translate

### D. *Bhagavadgītā* 2.66

Note that the genitives in this verse can be translated as "for" one who is X, rather than "of." The नास्ति, "there is no," in the first *pāda* is also implied by the न in the second and third *pādas*.

नास्ति बुद्धिरयुक्तस्य न चायुक्तस्य भावना ।
न चाभावयतः शान्तिरशान्तस्य कुतः सुखम् ॥

Vocabulary

अयुक्तः m. one who is not concentrated/yoked/attentive
भावना f. meditation, imagination, thought
अभावयतः of/for one who is not meditating/concentrating/perceiving (m. gen. sg.)
अशान्तः m. one who is unpeaceful
कुतः ind. from where? how can there be?

### E. *Haṭhapradīpikā* 1.32

In the second *pāda*, read together तत् शयनम्, "that act of rest," and then infer "is called."

उत्तानं शववद्भूमौ शयनं तच्छवासनम् ।
शवासनं श्रान्तिहरं चित्तविश्रान्तिकारकम् ॥

*Sandhi* Rule: A final त् before an initial श् together changes to च्छ्.
Example: तत् शवासनम् ⇒ तच्छवासनम्

Vocabulary

उत्तान mfn. stretched out, lying on the back
शववत् like a corpse (n. nom. sg.)
शयनम् n. act of lying down, rest, repose
शवासनम् n. corpse pose
श्रान्तिहरम् n. removing, taking away fatigue
चित्तविश्रान्तिकारकम् n. creating repose in the mind
  विश्रान्तिः f. rest, repose
  कारक mfn. making, doing, creating

F. *Yogasūtra* 1.5

वृत्तयः पञ्चतय्यः क्लिष्टाक्लिष्टाः ।

Vocabulary

पञ्चतय्य mfn. fivefold
क्लिष्टाक्लिष्टाः afflicted and unafflicted (f. nom. pl.)
  क्लिष्ट mfn. afflicted, distressed
  अक्लिष्ट mfn. unafflicted, untroubled

G. *Yogasūtra* 1.13

तत्र स्थितौ यत्नोऽभ्यासः ।

Vocabulary

तत्र ind. there, among those, with respect to that
यत्नः m. effort

The word तत्र has a locative sense. Here, it refers back to the previous *sūtra*, which states अभ्यासवैराग्याभ्यां तन्निरोधः ।. The stilling of those [fluctuations of the mind] is from अभ्यासः and वैराग्यम्, practice and dispassion. This *sūtra* defines the former.

## THE IMPERATIVE

The imperative mood is used for injunctions—to express a command, advice, instruction, or request. The imperative is also used to express a negative command when preceded by the particle मा. The endings (seen below) are added directly to the stem form. Because the imperative is mainly used for injunctions, the second-person forms are most common. Note that the second-person singular *parasmaipada* form is identical to the stem form. The third-person plural form is also frequently used to express a wish or blessing, in the sense of "may there be X . . ." or "may X happen."

**Imperative Endings**

| | Parasmaipada | | | Ātmanepada | | |
|---|---|---|---|---|---|---|
| | Singular | Dual | Plural | Singular | Dual | Plural |
| 3rd person | -तु | -ताम् | -अन्तु | -ताम् | -एताम् | -अन्ताम् |
| 2nd person | ∅ | -तम् | -त | -स्व | -एथाम् | -ध्वम् |
| 1st person | -आनि | -आव | -आम | -ऐ | -आवहै | -आमहै |

As in previous conjugations, note that the final अ / आ of the *gaṇa* sign is lost before endings beginning with a vowel.

**√भू (root) 1P, to be, to become ⇒ भव् (base)**

| | Verbal Stem | | | | | | |
|---|---|---|---|---|---|---|---|
| | Base | | Gaṇa Sign | | Ending | | |
| 3rd person singular | भव् | + | अ | + | तु | ⇒ | भवतु |
| 1st person singular | भव् | + | आ | + | आनि | ⇒ | भवानि |

| | Singular | Dual | Plural |
|---|---|---|---|
| 3rd person | भवतु<br>May he/she, it be | भवताम्<br>May they both be | भवन्तु<br>May they all be |
| 2nd person | भव<br>Be | भवतम्<br>May you both be | भवत<br>May you all be |
| 1st person | भवानि<br>May I be | भवाव<br>May we both be | भवाम<br>May we all be |

**√मुद् (root), 1Ā, to rejoice ⇒ मोद् (base)**

| | Verbal Stem | | | | | | |
|---|---|---|---|---|---|---|---|
| | Base | | Gaṇa Sign | | Ending | | |
| 3rd person singular | मोद् | + | अ | + | ताम् | ⇒ | मोदताम् |
| 1st person singular | मोद् | + | आ | + | ऐ | ⇒ | मोदै |

**√मुद् to rejoice (1Ā)**

| | Singular | Dual | Plural |
|---|---|---|---|
| 3rd person | मोदताम्<br>May he/she rejoice | मोदेताम्<br>May they both rejoice | मोदन्ताम्<br>May they all rejoice |
| 2nd person | मोदस्व<br>Rejoice | मोदेथाम्<br>May you both rejoice | मोदध्वम्<br>May you all rejoice |
| 1st person | मोदै<br>May I rejoice | मोदावहै<br>May we both rejoice | मोदामहै<br>May we all rejoice |

*Note the frequently used irregular imperative conjugations of the verb √अस् (to be):
3rd person singular: अस्तु May it be
3rd person plural: सन्तु May they be

## Conjugate in the Imperative

| Root | | 3rd person singular |
|---|---|---|
| √वद् | to speak (1P) | वदतु |
| √गम् | to go (1P) | गच्छतु |
| √नृत् | to dance (4P) | नृत्यतु |
| √चिन्त् | to contemplate (10P) | चिन्तयतु |
| √लभ् | to obtain (1Ā) | लभताम् |
| √मन् | to think (4Ā) | मन्यताम् |

## Example: *Dattātreyayogaśāstra* 8

The first line quotes Dattātreya speaking to Sāṃkṛti, marked by the first two words in the third *pāda*, इति पृष्टः, "thus asked."

सांकृते कथय त्वं मां किमुद्दिश्य इहागतः।
इति पृष्टस्तु स प्राह योगं ज्ञातुमिहागतः॥

### Vocabulary

मा्म् me (1st p. acc. sg.)
किम् ind. what, why
उद्दिश्य ind. with regard to, for the sake of
इह ind. here, to this place
आगत mfn. come, arrived
इति ind. thus (quotative particle)
पृष्ट mfn. asked
प्राह he said (3rd p. sg. perfect प्र√अह्)
ज्ञातुम् to learn (ind. infinitive √ज्ञा)

The *Dattātreyayogaśāstra* was composed in the twelfth to thirteenth century C.E., in the form of a teaching on yoga by the sage Dattātreya to Sāṃkṛti. It explains a traditional *aṣṭāṅgayoga* as taught by Yājñavalkya and others, and it is the earliest text to teach a systematized form of *haṭhayoga* as taught by seers such as Kapila, describing *mudrās*, *bandhas*, and *prāṇāyāma*.

| | | | | | | | |
|---|---|---|---|---|---|---|---|
| सांकृते | कथय | त्वं | मां | किम | उद्दिश्य | इह | आगतः । |
| O Sāṃkṛti | tell | you | me | what | with regard to | here | come |

| | | | | | | | | |
|---|---|---|---|---|---|---|---|---|
| इति | पृष्टस् | तु | स | प्राह | योगं | ज्ञातुम् | इह | आगतः ॥ |
| thus | asked | and | he | said | yoga | to learn | here | come |

"O Sāṃkṛti (सांकृते), **tell** (कथय) me (माम्),
With regard to (उद्दिश्य) what (किम्) have you (त्वम्) come (आगतः) here (इह)?"
And (तु) thus (इति) asked (पृष्टः), he (स) said (प्राह),
He had come (आगतः) here (इह) to learn (ज्ञातुम्) yoga (योगम्).

## Translate

### H. *Śānti Mantra* I

Note that अस्तु is implied in the second and third *pādas*.

काले वर्षतु पर्जन्यः पृथिवी सस्यशालिनी ।
देशोऽयं क्षोभरहितो ब्राह्मणाः सन्तु निर्भयाः ॥

#### Vocabulary

कालः m. proper time or season
√वृष् 1P, to rain down, shower down
पर्जन्यः m. rain-cloud, god of rain
पृथिवी f. earth
सस्यशालिनी f. full of crops
  सस्यम् n. crop
देशः m. place, country
अयम् this (m. nom. sg.)
क्षोभरहित mfn. free from disturbance
  क्षोभः m. agitation, disturbance
ब्राह्मणः m. Brahmin, one who has divine knowledge, a person belonging to the priestly class
निर्भय mfn. free from fear

### I. *Śānti Mantra* II

अपुत्राः पुत्रिणः सन्तु पुत्रिणः सन्तु पौत्रिणः ।
अधनाः सधनाः सन्तु जीवन्तु शरदां शतम् ॥

Vocabulary

अपुत्र mfn. sonless, childless
पुत्रिणः those possessing children, parents (m. nom. pl.)
पौत्रिणः those who have grandchildren, grandparents (m. nom. pl)
अधन mfn. poor, without wealth
  धनम् n. wealth, riches
सधन mfn. wealthy, with wealth
√जीव् 1P, to live
शरदाम् of, for autumns (f. gen. pl.)
शतम् n. a hundred

J. *Bhagavadgītā* 2.49

दूरेण ह्यवरं कर्म बुद्धियोगाद्धनंजय ।
बुद्धौ शरणमन्विच्छ कृपणाः फलहेतवः ॥

Vocabulary

दूरेण ind. by far
अवर mfn. inferior, below (goes with the ablative)
कर्म action (n. nom. sg.)
बुद्धियोगः m. the yoga of understanding/wisdom/discernment
शरणम् n. refuge
अन्व्√इष् 1P (अन्विच्छति), to desire, seek
कृपण mfn. pitiable, miserable, wretched
फलहेतवः those whose motives are the fruits [of action] (m. nom. pl.)

## THE OPTATIVE

The optative, or potential mood, is used to express a wish, possibility, instruction, or prescription. It is usually translated as "may," "might," "should," or "would." Note in particular the use of the third-person singular form without a specific subject, to express a duty, recommendation, or command, often translated as "one should . . ." The optative is marked by a special mode sign that is inserted between the verbal stem and the endings. For the *gaṇas* we have learned thus far (1, 4, 6, 10), this sign is ई. This ई joins with the preceding *gaṇa* sign ending in अ / आ to become ए. However, this ए cannot come into direct contact with an ending beginning with a vowel. To avoid this contact, for endings beginning with a vowel, a य् is inserted between the ए (*gaṇa* sign + mode sign) and the ending.

**Optative Endings**

| | Parasmaipada | | | Ātmanepada | | |
|---|---|---|---|---|---|---|
| | Singular | Dual | Plural | Singular | Dual | Plural |
| 3rd person | -त् | -ताम् | -उः | -त | -आताम् | -रन् |
| 2nd person | -ः | -तम् | -त | -थाः | -आथाम् | -ध्वम् |
| 1st person | -अम् | -व | -म | -अ | -वहि | -महि |

**√भू (root) 1P, to be, to become ⇒ भव् (base)**

| | Verbal Stem: Base | Gaṇa Sign | Mode Sign | Ending | | | | | | |
|---|---|---|---|---|---|---|---|---|---|---|
| 3rd person singular | भव् | + अ | + ई | + त् | ⇒ भव् | + ए | | + त् | ⇒ भवेत् |
| 1st person singular | भव् | + आ | + ई | + य् + अम् | ⇒ भव् | + ए | + य् | + अम् | ⇒ भवेयम् |

| | Singular | Dual | Plural |
|---|---|---|---|
| 3rd person | भवेत्<br>He/she, it may be | भवेताम्<br>They both may be | भवेयुः<br>They all may be |
| 2nd person | भवेः<br>You may be | भवेतम्<br>You both may be | भवेत<br>You all may be |
| 1st person | भवेयम्<br>I may be | भवेव<br>We both may be | भवेम<br>We all may be |

**√मुद् (root), 1Ā, to rejoice ⇒ मोद् (base)**

| | Verbal Stem: Base | Gaṇa Sign | Mode Sign | Ending | | | | | |
|---|---|---|---|---|---|---|---|---|---|
| 3rd person singular | मोद् | + अ | + ई | + त | ⇒ मोद् | + ए | | + त | ⇒ मोदेत |
| 1st person singular | मोद् | + आ | + ई | + य् + अ | ⇒ मोद् | + ए | + य् | + अ | ⇒ मोदेय |

| | Singular | Dual | Plural |
|---|---|---|---|
| 3rd person | मोदेत<br>He/she may rejoice | मोदेयाताम्<br>They both may rejoice | मोदेरन्<br>They all may rejoice |

| | | | |
|---|---|---|---|
| 2nd person | मोदेथाः<br>You may rejoice | मोदेयाथाम्<br>You both may rejoice | मोदेध्वम्<br>You all may rejoice |
| 1st person | मोदेय<br>I may rejoice | मोदेवहि<br>We both may rejoice | मोदेमहि<br>We all may rejoice |

## Conjugate in the Optative

| Root | | 3rd person singular |
|---|---|---|
| √वद् | to speak (1P) | वदेत् |
| √गम् | to go (1P) | गच्छेत् |
| √नृत् | to dance (4P) | नृत्येत् |
| √चिन्त् | to contemplate (10P) | चिन्तयेत् |
| √लभ् | to obtain (1Ā) | लभेत |
| √मन् | to think (4Ā) | मन्येत |

*Note the frequently used irregular optative conjugations of the verb √अस् (to be):

| | | |
|---|---|---|
| 3rd person singular: | स्यात् | It should/might be |
| 3rd person plural: | स्युः | They should/might be |

## Example: *Yogacūḍāmaṇyupaniṣat* 121

यथा तृतीयकाले तु रविः प्रत्याहरेत्प्रभाम् ।
तृतीयाङ्गस्थितो योगी विकारं मनसं हरेत् ॥

Vocabulary

**यथा** ind. just as
**तृतीयकालः** m. third quarter
**प्रत्या√हृ** 1U, to draw in or back
**प्रभा** f. light, splendor, radiance
**तृतीयाङ्गस्थित** mfn. established in the third limb (in this text, which describes a *sadaṅga*, or six-limbed yoga, the third limb is *pratyāhāra*, "sensory withdrawal")
**विकारः** m. disturbance

And (तु) just as (यथा) the sun (रविः), in the third quarter [of the day] (तृतीयकाले),
**Should draw back in** (प्रत्याहरेत्) its radiance (प्रभाम्),

[So,] the yogī (योगी), established in the third limb (तृतीयाङ्गस्थितो),
**Should subdue** (हरेत्) the disturbances (विकारम्) of the mind (मनसम्).

## Translate

### K. *Haṭhapradīpikā* 2.12–13

In the first verse, translate each *pāda* as a separate phrase, with the conclusion in the fourth *pāda*. In the second verse, translate each line as a separate phrase.

कनीयसि भवेत्स्वेदः कम्पो भवति मध्यमे ।
उत्तमे स्थानमाप्नोति ततो वायुं निबन्धयेत् ॥

जलेन श्रमजातेन गात्रमर्दनमाचरेत् ।
दृढता लघुता चैव तेन गात्रस्य जायते ॥

Vocabulary

कनीयसि at the beginning (m. loc. sg.)
स्वेदः m. sweat, perspiration
कम्पः m. trembling, shaking
मध्यम mfn. middle
उत्तम mfn. highest, end, ultimate stage
स्थानम् n. stability, place, state
आप्नोति one obtains (3rd p. sg. √आप्)
ततः ind. from that, therefore
निबन्धयेत् one should restrain, control (3rd p. sg. optative नि√बन्ध्)
जलम् n. water, that is, sweat
श्रमजात mfn. born from exertion
    श्रमः m. fatigue, exertion
    जात mfn. born
गात्रमर्दनम् n. rubbing of the limbs
आ√चर् 1P, to act, undertake, practice, perform
दृढता f. firmness, solidity, strength, steadiness
लघुता f. lightness
तेन by that (n. inst. sg.)
गात्रम् n. body, limbs

### L. *Haṭhapradīpikā* 2.15

यथा सिंहो गजो व्याघ्रो भवेद्वश्यः शनैः शनैः ।
तथैव सेवितो वायुरन्यथा हन्ति साधकम् ॥

Vocabulary

सिंहः m. lion
गजः m. elephant
व्याघ्रः m. tiger
वश्य mfn. subdued, tamed
शनैः शनैः ind. softly, gently, gradually
तथा ind. so, in that way
सेवित mfn. attended upon
अन्यथा ind. otherwise
हन्ति it kills/destroys (3rd p. sg. √हन्)
साधकः m. practitioner

### M. *Bhagavadgītā* 2.54

Arjuna is speaking to Kṛṣṇa.

स्थितप्रज्ञस्य का भाषा समाधिस्थस्य केशव ।
स्थितधीः किं प्रभाषेत किमासीत व्रजेत किम् ॥

Vocabulary

स्थितप्रज्ञः m. one whose wisdom is steady
    प्रज्ञा f. wisdom, knowledge, intelligence, discrimination
का what (f. nom. sg.)
भाषा f. description, language, speech
समाधिस्थः m. one who is situated/established in meditative absorption
स्थितधीः m. one who has a steady mind
प्र√भाष् 1Ā, to speak
आसीत he might/should sit (3rd p. sg. optative √आस्)
√व्रज् 1U, to go, wander, move

## Review Exercises

### N. *Haṭhapradīpikā* 1.65–66

क्रियायुक्तस्य सिद्धिः स्यादक्रियस्य कथं भवेत्।
न शास्त्रपाठमात्रेण योगसिद्धिः प्रजायते ॥

न वेषधारणं सिद्धेः कारणं न च तत्कथा।
क्रियैव कारणं सिद्धेः सत्यमेतन्न संशयः ॥

Vocabulary

क्रियायुक्तः m. engaged/absorbed in practice
  क्रिया f. action, practice
  युक्त mfn. yoked to, engaged in, absorbed in
सिद्धिः f. fulfillment, accomplishment, attainment, success
अक्रिय mfn. inactive, without practice
कथम् ind. how
शास्त्रपाठमात्रम् n. merely by reading sacred texts
योगसिद्धिः f. attainment of yoga, fulfillment in yoga
वेषधारण mfn. wearing [particular] clothes, assuming an appearance
  वेषः m. dress, clothing, assumed appearance
कारणम् n. cause (goes with सिद्धेः)
तत्कथा f. talking about it

### O. *Śānti Mantra* III

सर्वे भवन्तु सुखिनः। सर्वे सन्तु निरामयाः।
सर्वे भद्राणि पश्यन्तु। मा कश्चिद्दुःखभाग् भवेत् ॥

Vocabulary

सर्वे all (m. nom. pl.)
सुखिनः possessing happiness, happy (m. nom. pl.)
निरामयः m. freedom from disease, health
भद्रम् n. good fortune
मा कश्चित् ind. no one
दुःखभाग् m. bad luck

P. *Bhagavadgītā* 18.48

The subject in the first line is "one," which goes with the verb न त्यजेत्. The object is कर्म. The verbal form आवृताः goes with both the clause in the third *pāda* and in the fourth. Remember, इव means "like, as" and is used for comparison.

सहजं कर्म कौन्तेय सदोषमपि न त्यजेत् ।
सर्वारम्भा हि दोषेण धूमेनाग्निरिवावृताः ॥

Vocabulary
सहज mfn. inborn, natural, innate
कर्म action (n. acc. sg.)
कौन्तेयः m. son of Kuntī, Arjuna
सदोष mfn. having faults/deficiencies
सर्वारम्भः m. all undertakings
दोषः m. fault, deficiency
धूमः m. smoke
आवृत mfn. covered, surrounded, enveloped

# 6
# Familial and Agent Nouns Ending in ऋ; Past Imperfect Tense; Verbal Prefixes; Gerunds and Infinitives

मैत्रीकरुणामुदितोपेक्षाणां सुखदुःखपुण्यापुण्यविषयाणां भावनातश्चित्तप्रसादनम् ॥ १.३३ ॥
**maitrī-karuṇā-muditopekṣāṇāṃ sukha-duḥkha-puṇyāpuṇya-viṣayāṇāṃ bhāvanātaś citta-prasādanam**
From the cultivation of friendship toward the happy, compassion toward the suffering, joy toward the virtuous, and indifference toward the nonvirtuous, there is clarity of mind.
॥ *Yogasūtra* 1.33 ॥

## MASCULINE AND FEMININE NOUNS ENDING IN ऋ

There are two types of masculine nouns ending in ऋ. The first are agent nouns (verbal root + तृ) and the second are nouns expressing familial relationships. These declensions are similar, except in the nominative, accusative, and vocative cases.

**दातृ m. giver, donor, generous person**

| | Singular | Dual | Plural |
|---|---|---|---|
| **Nominative** | दाता | दातारौ | दातारः |
| **Accusative** | दातारम् | दातारौ | दातॄन् |
| **Instrumental** | दात्रा | दातृभ्याम् | दातृभिः |
| **Dative** | दात्रे | दातृभ्याम् | दातृभ्यः |
| **Ablative** | दातुः | दातृभ्याम् | दातृभ्यः |
| **Genitive** | दातुः | दात्रोः | दातॄणाम् |
| **Locative** | दातरि | दात्रोः | दातृषु |
| **Vocative** | दातर् | दातारौ | दातारः |

**पितृ m. father**

| | Singular | Dual | Plural |
|---|---|---|---|
| **Nominative** | पिता | पितरौ | पितरः |
| **Accusative** | पितरम् | पितरौ | पितॄन् |
| **Instrumental** | पित्रा | पितृभ्याम् | पितृभिः |
| **Dative** | पित्रे | पितृभ्याम् | पितृभ्यः |
| **Ablative** | पितुः | पितृभ्याम् | पितृभ्यः |
| **Genitive** | पितुः | पित्रोः | पितॄणाम् |
| **Locative** | पितरि | पित्रोः | पितृषु |
| **Vocative** | पितर् | पितरौ | पितरः |

Feminine nouns ending in ऋ express familial relationships and are identical to the masculine nouns of the same category, except in the accusative plural.

**मातृ f. mother**

| | Singular | Dual | Plural |
|---|---|---|---|
| **Nominative** | माता | मातरौ | मातरः |
| **Accusative** | मातरम् | मातरौ | मातॄः |
| **Instrumental** | मात्रा | मातृभ्याम् | मातृभिः |
| **Dative** | मात्रे | मातृभ्याम् | मातृभ्यः |
| **Ablative** | मातुः | मातृभ्याम् | मातृभ्यः |
| **Genitive** | मातुः | मात्रोः | मातॄणाम् |
| **Locative** | मातरि | मात्रोः | मातृषु |
| **Vocative** | मातर् | मातरौ | मातरः |

Vocabulary

कर्तृ m. doer, maker
दुहितृ f. daughter
द्रष्टृ m. seer, Soul
धातृ m. establisher, supporter
नेतृ m. leader
भर्तृ m. bearer, sustainer, preserver
भ्रातृ m. brother
वक्तृ m. eloquent speaker, orator
स्वसृ f. sister

## Decline

कर्तृ, भ्रातृ, वक्तृ, and स्वसृ

## Translate

### A. "You Alone"

Note that "my" is implied in all of the equations given.

त्वमेव माता च पिता त्वमेव त्वमेव बन्धुश्च सखा त्वमेव ।
त्वमेव विद्या द्रविणं त्वमेव त्वमेव सर्वं मम देव देव ॥

Vocabulary
बन्धुः m. relative
सखा friend (m. nom. sg. सखि)
द्रविणम् n. wealth
सर्वम् everything (n. nom. sg.)
मम to me (gen. sg.)

The word एव is used for emphasis and usually governs the word preceding it. It can mean "only," "alone," "exactly," "indeed," "truly." In this verse:

त्वम् एव = त्वमेव, means "You, alone."

### B. "Relatives"

Note the implied equivalency between all of the pairs in the first three *pādas* and the implied "my" in each pair (i.e., X is my Y).

सत्यं माता पिता ज्ञानं धर्मो भ्राता दया सखा ।
शान्तिः पत्नी क्षमा पुत्रः षडेते मम बान्धवाः ॥

Vocabulary
दया f. compassion
पत्नी f. wife
क्षमा f. patience
षड् m. six
एते these (m. nom. pl.)
मम of me, my (gen. sg.)
बान्धवः m. relative

### C. *Bhagavadgītā* 9.17

पिताहमस्य जगतो माता धाता पितामहः ।
वेद्यं पवित्रमोंकार ऋक्साम यजुरेव च ॥

Vocabulary

अस्य जगतः of this world (n. gen. sg.)
पितामहः m. grandfather
वेद्य mfn. to be learned or known
पवित्रम् n. a means of purification, the purifier
ओंकारः m. the sacred and mystical syllable *oṃ*

D. *Yogasūtra* 1.3

तदा द्रष्टुः स्वरूपेऽवस्थानम् ।

Vocabulary

तदा ind. then
स्वरूपम् n. one's own true nature
अवस्थानम् n. residing, dwelling, stability

## PAST IMPERFECT TENSE

The first past tense we will learn is the imperfect. The imperfect represents completed past action (e.g., he went). It can be formed by taking the present stem, adding the augment अ, and appending the past tense endings. (An augment is a prefixed vowel or a lengthening of the initial vowel, used to indicate the past tense.) Note the similarities between these endings and the optative endings we learned in Chapter 5. Also note that, as previously, the *gaṇa* sign अ / आ disappears before an ending beginning with अ.

Past Imperfect Endings

| | Parasmaipada | | | Ātmanepada | | |
|---|---|---|---|---|---|---|
| | Singular | Dual | Plural | Singular | Dual | Plural |
| 3rd person | -त् | -ताम् | -अन् | -त | -एताम् | -अन्त |
| 2nd person | -ः | -तम् | -त | -थाः | -एथाम् | -ध्वम् |
| 1st person | -अम् | -व | -म | -ए | -वहि | -महि |

**√भू (root) 1P, to be, to become ⇒ भव् (base)**

Verbal Stem

| | Augment | | Base | | Gaṇa Sign | | Ending | | |
|---|---|---|---|---|---|---|---|---|---|
| 3rd person singular | अ | + | भव् | + | अ | + | त् | ⇒ | अभवत् |
| 1st person singular | अ | + | भव् | + | आ | + | अम् | ⇒ | अभवम् |

| | Singular | Dual | Plural |
|---|---|---|---|
| 3rd person | अभवत्<br>He/she, it was | अभवताम्<br>They both were | अभवन्<br>They all were |
| 2nd person | अभवः<br>You were | अभवतम्<br>You both were | अभवत<br>You all were |
| 1st person | अभवम्<br>I was | अभवाव<br>We both were | अभवाम<br>We all were |

**√मुद् (root), 1Ā, to rejoice ⇒ मोद् (base)**

| | Verbal Stem | | | | | | | | | |
|---|---|---|---|---|---|---|---|---|---|---|
| | Augment | | Base | | Gaṇa Sign | | Ending | | | |
| 3rd person singular | अ | + | मोद् | + | अ | + | त | ⇒ | अमोदत |
| 1st person singular | अ | + | मोद् | + | आ | + | ए | ⇒ | अमोदे |

| | Singular | Dual | Plural |
|---|---|---|---|
| 3rd person | अमोदत<br>He/she rejoiced | अमोदेताम्<br>They both rejoiced | अमोदन्त<br>They all rejoiced |
| 2nd person | अमोदथाः<br>You rejoiced | अमोदेथाम्<br>You both rejoiced | अमोदध्वम्<br>You all rejoiced |
| 1st person | अमोदे<br>I rejoiced | अमोदावहि<br>We both rejoiced | अमोदामहि<br>We all rejoiced |

## Conjugate in the Imperfect

| Root | | 3rd person singular |
|---|---|---|
| √वद् | to speak (1P) | अवदत् |
| √गम् | to go (1P) | अगच्छत् |
| √नृत् | to dance (4P) | अनृत्यत् |
| √चिन्त् | to contemplate (10P) | अचिन्तयत् |
| √लभ् | to obtain (1Ā) | अलभत |
| √मन् | to think (4Ā) | अमन्यत |

## Translate

### E. *Bhagavadgītā* 1.13

ततः शङ्खाश्च भेर्यश्च पणवानकगोमुखाः ।
सहसैवाभ्यहन्यन्त स शब्दस्तुमुलोऽभवत् ॥

Vocabulary

ततः ind. then, after that
शङ्खः m. conch shell (used as a horn or trumpet in battle)
भेरी f. kettledrum
पणवानकगोमुखाः m. nom. pl. cymbals, drums, and trumpets
    पणवः m. small drum or cymbal
    आनकः m. drum
    गोमुखः m. trumpet, "cow-faced"
सहसा ind. suddenly, quickly, all at once
अभ्यहन्यन्त they were struck (3rd p. pl. imperfect, passive अभि√हन्)
शब्दः m. sound, noise
तुमुल mfn. tumultuous, noisy

### F. *Bhagavadgītā* 1.26

तत्रापश्यत्स्थितान्पार्थः पितॄनथ पितामहान् ।
आचार्यान्मातुलान्भ्रातॄन्पुत्रान्पौत्रान्सखींस्तथा ॥

Vocabulary

स्थितः m. standing, situated
पार्थः m. son of Pṛthā, matronymic name for Arjuna
अथ ind. then, also
आचार्यः m. teacher
मातुलः m. maternal uncle
पुत्रः m. son
पौत्रः m. grandson
सखीन् friends (m. acc. pl.)

## VERBAL PREFIXES, उपसर्ग

Verbal prefixes add nuance and depth of meaning to verbs and are an important part of the rich fabric of Sanskrit poetry. Becoming familiar with these prefixes will help you to break down and understand longer words and dramatically increase your vocabulary. These prefixes can be added to verbs to alter the meaning, either directly or idiomatically, or sometimes with no change in meaning, for metrical purposes. The standard meanings of these prefixes are given in the next two pages as well as some examples of their usage (idiomatic usages are starred). In most cases, the addition of verbal prefixes necessitates internal *sandhi* changes.

| Prefix | | Examples |
|---|---|---|
| अति beyond, surpassing | + | √क्रम् 1P, to step ⇒ अतिक्रामति he/she steps beyond, surpasses, oversteps, transgresses |
| अधि over and above | + | √गम् 1P, to go ⇒ अधिगच्छति he/she obtains, attains* |
| अनु after, alongside | + | √वद् 1P, to speak ⇒ अनुवदति he/she repeats |
| | + | √सृ 1P, to move, go toward ⇒ अनुसरति he/she follows |

You might know the verb अनु√सृ from the word अनुसार, meaning "in accordance with custom, established practice, and natural condition."

| | | |
|---|---|---|
| अन्तर् within, between | + | √भू 1P, to be ⇒ अन्तर्भवति he/she is contained, included in |
| अप away | + | √नी 1P, to lead ⇒ अपनयति he/she leads away |
| अभि to, toward | + | √गम् 1P, to go ⇒ अभिगच्छति he/she approaches sexually |
| अव down | + | √गम् 1P, to go ⇒ अवगच्छति he/she knows, understands* |
| | + | √तृ 1P, to cross ⇒ अवतरति he/she descends |

You might know the verb अव√तृ from the word अवतार, "a descent or incarnation of a deity on earth."

| | | |
|---|---|---|
| आ toward, back | + | √गम् 1P, to go ⇒ आगच्छति he/she comes |
| (reverses action) | + | √हृ 1P, to take ⇒ आहरति he/she brings, fetches |
| उद् up, upward | + | √स्था 1P, to stand ⇒ उत्तिष्ठति he/she stands up |
| | + | √भू 1P, to be ⇒ उद्भवति he/she arises, springs up |
| उप toward | + | √गम् 1P, to go ⇒ उपगच्छति he/she approaches |
| | + | √विश् 6P, to enter ⇒ उपविशति he/she sits down |

You might know the verb उप√विश् from the yoga posture उपविष्टकोणासन, "seated angle pose."

| | | |
|---|---|---|
| नि down, into | + | √वस् 1P, to dwell, live ⇒ निवसति he/she dwells in, inhabits |
| निः out of, away from | + | √वस् 1P, to dwell, live ⇒ निर्वसति he/she dwells abroad |
| परा away | + | √गम् 1P, to go ⇒ परागच्छति he/she returns |
| परि around, about | + | √ईक्ष् 1Ā, to see, look at ⇒ परीक्षते he/she examines |
| प्र forward, onward | + | √ईक्ष् 1Ā, to see, look at ⇒ प्रेक्षते he/she looks at, beholds |
| | + | √नम् 1P, to bow ⇒ प्रणमति he/she bows to |

> You might know the verb प्र√णम् from the word प्रणाम, "a bow or salutation."

| | | |
|---|---|---|
| | + | √भू 1P, to be ⇒ प्रभवति he/she arises, appears, is powerful, rules* |
| प्रति against, in opposition to | + | √गम् 1P, to go ⇒ प्रतिगच्छति he/she goes back, returns |
| वि division, opposition | + | √स्मृ 1P, to remember ⇒ विस्मरति he/she forgets |
| | + | √हृ 1P, to take ⇒ विहरति he/she amuses, takes pleasure* |
| सम् together | + | √गम् 1P, to go ⇒ संगच्छति he/she comes together with |
| | + | √कृ 8P, to do, make ⇒ संस्करोति he/she puts together well, refines, makes perfect |

> The word for the Sanskrit language, संस्कृत, means "refined or polished speech."

Sometimes, two or three prefixes may be simultaneously added to one verb:

सम् आ√गम् 1P, to come together with
उप आ√गम् 1P, to come near, approach

When forming the past tense of a verb with a verbal prefix, the augment अ is added after the verbal prefix but before the verbal root, often necessitating internal *sandhi* changes.

### Examples

| | Preverb | | Augment | | Base | | Gaṇa Sign | | Ending | | 3rd p. sg. |
|---|---|---|---|---|---|---|---|---|---|---|---|
| √गम् to go ⇒ | | | अ | + | गच्छ् | + | अ | + | त् | ⇒ | अगच्छत् |
| निर्√गम् to go out, come forth ⇒ | निर् | + | अ | + | गच्छ् | + | अ | + | त् | ⇒ | निरगच्छत् |
| अव√गम् to go down ⇒ | अव | + | अ | + | गच्छ् | + | अ | + | त् | ⇒ | अवागच्छत् |
| प्रति√गम् to go back, return ⇒ | प्रति | + | अ | + | गच्छ् | + | अ | + | त् | ⇒ | प्रत्यगच्छत् |
| अनु√गम् to go after, follow ⇒ | अनु | + | अ | + | गच्छ् | + | अ | + | त् | ⇒ | अन्वगच्छत् |

### Example: *Bhagavadgītā* 2.11

अशोच्यानन्वशोचस्त्वं प्रज्ञावादांश्च भाषसे ।
गतासूनगतासूंश्च नानुशोचन्ति पण्डिताः ॥

Vocabulary

अशोच्यान् those who are not to be mourned (m. acc. pl. gerundive अ√शुच्)
अनु√शुच् 1P, to mourn, lament
अन्वशोचः 2nd p. sg. past imperfect
प्रज्ञावादान् words of wisdom (idiomatic expression), i.e., words that appear to be wisdom but are not (m. acc. pl.)
गतासून् the dead, literally, those whose breaths are gone (m. acc. pl.)
अगतासून् the alive, literally, those whose breaths are not gone (m. acc. pl.)
पण्डितः m. wise person, scholar, philosopher

> *Sandhi* Rule: A final न् before an unvoiced palatal, retroflex, or dental stop ( च्, छ्, ट्, ठ्, त्, थ्) is replaced by an *anusvāra* plus the homorganic (articulated in the same place in the mouth) sibilant to the following stop.
>
> प्रज्ञावादान् च ⇒ प्रज्ञावादांश्च;
> अगतासून् च ⇒ अगतासूंश्च

You (त्वम्) **have mourned** (अन्वशोचः) those who are not to be mourned (अशोच्यान्),
And (च) you speak (भाषसे) words that appear to be wisdom but are not (प्रज्ञावादान्).
Those whose breaths are gone (गतासून्) and (च) whose breaths are not gone (अगतासून्),
The wise (पण्डिताः) do not (न) mourn (अनुशोचन्ति).

## GERUNDS (ABSOLUTIVES)

Gerunds are used to express multiple verbal actions in the same sentence. They are indeclinable and are derived from the verbal root. They express previous actions and concepts, translated as "having done X" or "doing X, Y happens." The gerund often refers to the preceding word.

There is no limit to how many gerunds can be used in a sentence; however, the final verb, although it may be expressed in any tense or mood, must be declined. Sometimes, in poetry, the final verb can be found in the following verse. The other restriction is that the agent of the gerund and the main verb must be the same.

There are two suffixes used to form gerunds: त्वा and य. These suffixes are added to the verbal root. त्वा is appended to a simple verb without a prefix, sometimes with the letter इ infixed between the root and the suffix; य is added to a verb with a prefix(es).

### Examples

√गम् ⇒ गत्वा, but आ√गम् ⇒ आगम्य / आगत्य
√त्यज् ⇒ त्यक्त्वा, but सं√त्यज् ⇒ संत्यज्य
√पत् ⇒ पतित्वा, but नि√पत् ⇒ निपत्य
√भू ⇒ भूत्वा, but सं√भू ⇒ संभूय

### Example: *Haṭhapradīpikā* 1.14

The previous verses describe the yogī's hut. Among other things, it should be secluded, have a small door, no holes or hollows, not too high, too low, or too long, completely smeared with cow dung, clean, and free from insects. The subject of this verse is the *haṭhayogī*.

एवंविधे मठे स्थित्वा सर्वचिन्ताविवर्जितः ।
गुरूपदिष्टमार्गेण योगमेव समभ्यसेत् ॥

#### Vocabulary

एवंविध mfn. of such a kind, in such a form or manner
मठ mn. a hut, cottage
सर्वचिन्ताविवर्जितः m. free from all anxieties
  चिन्ता f. thought, care, anxiety
गुरूपदिष्टमार्गः m. the path taught by the teacher
समभ्यू√अस् 4P, to practice

**Having settled** (स्थित्वा) in such (एवंविधे) a hut (मठे),
Free from all anxieties (सर्वचिन्ताविवर्जितः).
[One] should practice (समभ्यसेत्) yoga (योगम्), exactly (एव),
By means of the path taught by the guru (गुरूपदिष्टमार्गेण).

### G. *Ādityahṛdayam* 29–30

The subject is Rāma.

आदित्यं प्रेक्ष्य जप्त्वा तु परं हर्षमवाप्तवान् ।
त्रिराचम्य शुचिर्भूत्वा धनुरादाय वीर्यवान् ॥

रावणं प्रेक्ष्य हृष्टात्मा युद्धाय समुपागमत्।
सर्वयत्नेन महता वधे तस्य धृतोऽभवत्॥

Vocabulary
आदित्यः m. the sun
प्र√ईक्ष् = √प्रेक्ष् 1Ā, to look at, behold
√जप् 1P, to utter in a low voice, mutter, chant
हर्षः m. joy
अवाप्तवान् he attained (m. nom. sg. past active participle अव√आप्)
त्रिर् ind. three times, thrice
आ√चम् 1P, to sip water from the palm of the hand for purification
शुचि mfn. clear, pure, radiant, shining
धनुर् a bow (n. acc. sg.)
आदाय taking hold of (gerund, आ√दा)
वीर्यवान् powerful, mighty, valorous [hero] (m. nom. sg.)
हृष्टात्मा thrilled, delighted-minded [Rāma] (m. nom. sg.)
युद्धम् n. battle, fight, war
सम् उप√गम् 1P, to approach
सर्वयत्नः m. every effort
महता with great (m. inst. sg.)
वधः m. killing
तस्य of him (m. gen. sg.)
धृत mfn. resolved

## H. *Dattātreyayogaśāstra* 58

The previous verses describe the yogī's hut and how to create a seat covered with a fine cloth. The subsequent verses describe how to practice *prāṇāyāma*.

तत्रोपविश्य मेधावी पद्मासनसमन्वितः।
समकायः प्राञ्जलिश्च प्रणम्य स्वेष्टदेवताम्॥

Vocabulary
उप√विश् 6P, to sit
मेधावी wise [yogī] (m. nom. sg. मेधाविन्)
पद्मासनसमन्वितः taking the lotus posture (m. nom. sg.)
समकायः with a straight, upright body (m. nom. sg.)

प्राञ्जलि mfn. joining and holding out the hollowed open hands as a mark of respect and humility
प्र√णम् 1P, to bow
स्वेष्टदेवता f. favorite deity

## INFINITIVES

Just like the gerund, the infinitive is an indeclinable form used in conjunction with another verb, both of which share the same agent. Because it is indefinite, the role of the infinitive is "unbounded," as its name suggests, and it is translated as "to X" or "to do X." An infinitive can express an action that is subordinate to the main action, indicating a goal, purpose, or reason; or it can be used with an auxiliary or helping verb. One of the most common formations is with the verb √अर्ह्, which, by itself, means "to be worthy or capable," but often, as in Exercise J, in conjunction with an infinitive means "one should/ought to do X." It is also often used with the verb √शक्, "to be able," as in the example below. An infinitive can be used both with and without an object. Infinitives are formed from the verbal root + the ending -तुम्. In some cases, the letter इ is infixed between the two.

### Examples

√गम् ⇒ गन्तुम् to go
√त्यज् ⇒ त्यक्तुम् to abandon
√दृश् ⇒ द्रष्टुम् to see
√पत् ⇒ पतितुम् to fall
√भू ⇒ भवितुम् to be

### Example: *Śivasaṃhitā* 3.3

Note that the second *pāda* should be translated before the first, and the fourth before the third.

प्राणस्य वृत्तिभेदेन नामानि विविधानि च ।
वर्तन्ते तानि सर्वाणि कथितुं नैव शक्यते ॥

Vocabulary

वृत्तिभेदेन m. inst. sg. according to its different actions/functions
नामानि names (n. nom. pl.)
विविध mfn. of various sorts, manifold
तानि सर्वाणि all those (n. nom. pl.)
शक्यते it is possible (3rd p. sg. passive √शक्)

And [there are] various names (नामानि विविधानि) of *prāṇa* (प्राणस्य),
According to its different functions (वृत्तिभेदेन).
It is not (न) even (एव) possible (शक्यते) **to describe** (कथितुम्)
All (सर्वाणि) those (तानि) that exist (वर्तन्ते).

### I. *Bhagavadgītā* 1.30

Arjuna is speaking to Kṛṣṇa.

गाण्डीवं स्रंसते हस्तात्त्वक्चैव परिदह्यते ।
न च शक्नोम्यवस्थातुं भ्रमतीव च मे मनः ॥

Vocabulary

गाण्डीव mn. name of Arjuna's bow, given to him by Agni
√स्रंस् 1Ā, to fall down, drop
हस्तः m. hand
त्वक् skin (f. nom. sg.)
परिदह्यते it burns (3rd p. sg. pass. परि√दह्)
शक्नोमि I am able/capable (1st p. sg. √शक्)
अव√स्था 1P, to remain standing
√भ्रम् 1P, to wander about
मे my (gen. sg.)
मनः mind (n. nom. sg)

### J. *Bhagavadgītā* 2.27

Note that the genitives in the first and second *pādas* can be read as "for X" instead of "of X."

जातस्य हि ध्रुवो मृत्युर्ध्रुवं जन्म मृतस्य च ।
तस्मादपरिहार्येऽर्थे न त्वं शोचितुमर्हसि ॥

Vocabulary

जातः m. one who has been born
ध्रुव mfn. certain
मृत्युः m. death
जन्मम् n. birth
मृतम् n. one who has died
तस्मात् ind. from that, therefore
अपरिहार्य mfn. unavoidable, inevitable
अर्थः m. object, affair, concern
√शुच् 1P, to grieve (takes the locative)
√अर्ह् 1P, to be able, should, ought

## Review Exercises

### K. *Bhagavadgītā* 1.47

एवमुक्त्वार्जुनः संख्ये रथोपस्थ उपाविशत्।
विसृज्य सशरं चापं शोकसंविग्नमानसः ॥

> *Sandhi* Rule: A final ए or ओ before a vowel other than अ becomes अ and the hiatus between the vowels remains.
>
> रथोपस्थे उपाविशत् ⇒ रथोपस्थ उपाविशत्

Vocabulary

एवम् ind. thus
उक्त्वा having said/spoken (gerund √वच्)
संख्यम् n. battle, conflict
रथोपस्थः m. chariot seat
  रथः m. chariot
वि√सृज् 6P, to throw down, cast aside
सशर mfn. together with an arrow
  शरः m. an arrow
चाप mn. a bow
शोकसंविग्नमानसः m. with a mind/heart overcome by sorrow
  शोकः m. sorrow, grief
  संविग्न mfn. agitated, disturbed, overcome by
  मानसम् n. the mind, heart, soul

### L. *Ādityahṛdayam* 2

दैवतैश्च समागम्य द्रष्टुमभ्यागतो रणम्।
उपागम्याब्रवीद्राममगस्त्यो भगवानृषिः ॥

Vocabulary

दैवतम् n. deity, god
समा√गम् 1P, to come together with
अभ्यागत mfn. arrived, approaching, imminent
रणम् n. battle, conflict
उपा√गम् 1P, to come near, approach
अब्रवीद् he said (3rd p. sg. imperfect √ब्रू)
अगस्त्यः m. name of famous sage
भगवान् holy, blessed, venerable, divine (m. nom. sg. भगवत्)

## M. “A Generous Person”

शतेषु जायते शूरः सहस्रेषु च पण्डितः।
वक्ता दशसहस्रेषु दाता भवति वा न वा॥

Vocabulary

शूरः m. hero
सहस्रम् n. a thousand
दशसहस्रम् n. ten thousand
वा न वा ind. either X or not X

# 7
# Verbs: Future Tense; Pronouns, Relative and Correlative Pronouns; Pronominal Adjectives

हेयं दुःखमनागतम् ॥ २.१६ ॥
**heyaṃ duḥkham anāgatam**
Suffering that has not yet come is to be avoided.
॥ *Yogasūtra* 2.16 ॥

## FUTURE TENSE

There are two types of future tense—general and periphrastic. In this chapter, we will consider the general future, which is much more common. It is formed by adding the future tense marker स्य or इष्य directly to the **verbal root** (not the stem form) and then adding the present tense endings, either *parasmaipada* or *ātmanepada*. Some roots change slightly before conjugation. In most cases, स्य is used for roots ending in a vowel and इष्य for roots ending in a consonant. Just as in the present tense, the अ before first-person endings is lengthened to आ.

**√स्था (1P) to stand, stay**

| | Singular | Dual | Plural |
|---|---|---|---|
| 3rd person | स्थास्यति<br>He/she will stand | स्थास्यतः<br>They both will stand | स्थास्यन्ति<br>They all will stand |
| 2nd person | स्थास्यसि<br>You will stand | स्थास्यथः<br>You both will stand | स्थास्यथ<br>You all will stand |
| 1st person | स्थास्यामि<br>I will stand | स्थास्यावः<br>We both will stand | स्थास्यामः<br>We all will stand |

### √भू (1P) to be, to become

| | Singular | Dual | Plural |
|---|---|---|---|
| 3rd person | भविष्यति<br>He/she, it will be | भविष्यतः<br>They both will be | भविष्यन्ति<br>They all will be |
| 2nd person | भविष्यसि<br>You will be | भविष्यथः<br>You both will be | भविष्यथ<br>You all will be |
| 1st person | भविष्यामि<br>I will be | भविष्यावः<br>We both will be | भविष्यामः<br>We all will be |

### √मुद् to rejoice (1Ā)

| | Singular | Dual | Plural |
|---|---|---|---|
| 3rd person | मोदिष्यते<br>He/she will rejoice | मोदिष्येते<br>They both will rejoice | मोदिष्यन्ते<br>They all will rejoice |
| 2nd person | मोदिष्यसे<br>You will rejoice | मोदिष्येथे<br>You both will rejoice | मोदिष्यध्वे<br>You all will rejoice |
| 1st person | मोदिष्ये<br>I will rejoice | मोदिष्यावहे<br>We both will rejoice | मोदिष्यामहे<br>We all will rejoice |

## Conjugate in the Future Tense

Note that in some cases, other *sandhi* changes are necessitated.

| Root | | 3rd person singular |
|---|---|---|
| √गम् | to go (1P) | गमिष्यति |
| √वद् | to speak (1P) | वदिष्यति |
| √दृश् | to see (1P) | *द्रक्ष्यति |
| √नृत् | to dance (4P) | *नर्तिष्यति |
| √चिन्त् | to contemplate (10P) | चिन्तयिष्यति |
| √लभ् | to obtain (1Ā) | *लप्स्यते |
| √मन् | to think (4Ā) | *मंस्यते |

## Example: *Bhagavadgītā* 2.12

Kṛṣṇa is speaking to Arjuna. Note the double negatives in the first and third *pādas*.

न त्वेवाहं जातु नासं न त्वं नेमे जनाधिपाः ।
न चैव न भविष्यामः सर्वे वयमतः परम् ॥

Vocabulary
जातु ind. ever
आसम् I was, I existed (1st p. sg. imperfect √अस्)
इमे these (m. nom. pl.)
जनाधिपः m. "ruler of people," king
सर्वे all (m. nom. pl.)
अतः परम् ind. from this point forward, henceforth

Indeed (तु), there was never (न जातु) [a time] when I (अहम्) did not exist (न आसम्),
Nor (न) you (त्वम्) nor (न) these (इमे) rulers of people (जनाधिपाः).
And (च) there will not (न) even (एव) be [a time]
When we (वयम्) all (सर्वे) **will** not (न) **exist** (भविष्यामः), from this point forward (अतः परम्).

## Translate

### A. *Śivasaṃhitā* 3.10

The object of the main verb in the first *pāda* must be inferred (i.e., some rules/guidelines; the following).

अधुना कथयिष्यामि क्षिप्रं योगस्य सिद्धये ।
यज्ज्ञात्वा नावसीदन्ति योगिनो योगसाधने ॥

Vocabulary
अधुना ind. now, at this time
क्षिप्रम् ind. quickly
यत् which (n. nom. sg.)
ज्ञात्वा having known, knowing (gerund √ज्ञा)
अव√सद् 1P, to sink down, become disheartened
योगिनः yogīs (m. nom. pl.)
योगसाधनः m. practice of yoga

### B. *Ādityahṛdayam* 26

पूजयस्वैनमेकाग्रो देवदेवं जगत्पतिम् ।
एतत्त्रिगुणितं जप्त्वा युद्धेषु विजयिष्यसि ॥ २६ ॥

Vocabulary

√पूज् 10U, to worship, honor
एनम् this (m. acc. sg.)
एकाग्र mfn. one-pointed attention
देवदेवः m. the God of gods
जगत्पतिः m. the Lord of the universe
एतत् this [prayer] (n. acc. sg.)
त्रिगुणित mfn. three times
वि√जि 1P, to succeed, conquer

## PRONOUNS

We have already learned the personal pronouns in the nominative case, as well as seen pronouns with other case endings in many of the verses we have read so far. The pronouns are inflected in a similar manner to the nouns we have learned, except that there is no vocative case.

### Third Person

The third-person paradigms are largely similar to the declensions of nouns ending in अ. The neuter paradigm differs from the masculine only in the nominative and accusative cases.

**सः m. he**

| | Singular | Dual | Plural |
|---|---|---|---|
| **Nominative** | सः<br>he | तौ<br>they both | ते<br>they all |
| **Accusative** | तम्<br>him | तौ<br>them both | तान्<br>them all |
| **Instrumental** | तेन<br>by him | ताभ्याम्<br>by them both | तैः<br>by them all |

| | | | |
|---|---|---|---|
| **Dative** | तस्मै<br>to/for him | ताभ्याम्<br>to/for them both | तेभ्यः<br>to/for them all |
| **Ablative** | तस्मात्<br>from him | ताभ्याम्<br>from them both | तेभ्यः<br>from them all |
| **Genitive** | तस्य<br>of him | तयोः<br>of them both | तेषाम्<br>of them all |
| **Locative** | तस्मिन्<br>in him | तयोः<br>in them both | तेषु<br>in them all |

### तत् n. that

| | Singular | Dual | Plural |
|---|---|---|---|
| **Nom./Acc.** | तत्<br>that | ते<br>them both | तानि<br>them all |

### सा f. she

| | Singular | Dual | Plural |
|---|---|---|---|
| **Nominative** | सा<br>she | ते<br>they both (f.) | ताः<br>they all (f.) |
| **Accusative** | ताम्<br>her | ते<br>them both (f.) | ताः<br>they all (f.) |
| **Instrumental** | तया<br>by her | ताभ्याम्<br>by them both (f.) | ताभिः<br>by them all (f.) |
| **Dative** | तस्यै<br>to/for her | ताभ्याम्<br>to/for them both (f.) | ताभ्यः<br>to/for them all (f.) |
| **Ablative** | तस्याः<br>from her | ताभ्याम्<br>from them both (f.) | ताभ्यः<br>from them all (f.) |
| **Genitive** | तस्याः<br>of her | तयोः<br>of them both (f.) | तासाम्<br>of them all (f.) |
| **Locative** | तस्याम्<br>in her | तयोः<br>in them both (f.) | तासु<br>in them all (f.) |

## Proximal Pronouns

The proximal pronouns ("this" instead of "that") can be formed by adding ए to the beginning of each of the above paradigms. Note that *sandhi* rules cause स ⇒ ष, but the rest of the paradigm remains the same.

m. सः ⇒ एषः; n. तत् ⇒ एतत्; f. सा ⇒ एषा

## First and Second Person

In the first- and second-person paradigms given below, pay particular attention to the enclitic forms (monosyllabic unstressed forms that always follow and attach to another word), which are quite common, in the accusative, dative, and genitive cases.

**अस्मद् I**

| | Singular | Dual | Plural |
|---|---|---|---|
| **Nominative** | अहम्<br>I | आवाम्<br>We both | वयम्<br>We all |
| **Accusative** | माम्, मा<br>Me | आवाम्, नौ<br>Us both | अस्मान्, नः<br>Us all |
| **Instrumental** | मया<br>By me | आवाभ्याम्<br>By us both | अस्माभिः<br>By us all |
| **Dative** | मह्यम्, मे<br>To/for me | आवाभ्याम्, नौ<br>To/for us both | अस्मभ्यम्, नः<br>To/for us all |
| **Ablative** | मत् / मत्तः<br>From me | आवाभ्याम्<br>From us both | अस्मत् / अस्मत्तः<br>From us all |
| **Genitive** | मम, मे<br>Of me | आवयोः, नौ<br>Of us both | अस्माकम्, नः<br>Of us all |
| **Locative** | मयि<br>In me | आवयोः<br>In us both | अस्मासु<br>In us all |

**युष्मद् you**

| | Singular | Dual | Plural |
|---|---|---|---|
| **Nominative** | त्वम्<br>You | युवाम्<br>You both | यूयम्<br>You all |

| | | | |
|---|---|---|---|
| **Accusative** | त्वाम्, त्वा<br>You | युवाम्, वाम्<br>You both | युष्मान्, वः<br>You all |
| **Instrumental** | त्वया<br>By you | युवाभ्याम्<br>By you both | युष्माभिः<br>By you all |
| **Dative** | तुभ्यम्, ते<br>To/for you | युवाभ्याम्, वाम्<br>To/for you both | युष्मभ्यम्, वः<br>To/for you all |
| **Ablative** | त्वत् / त्वत्तः<br>From you | युवाभ्याम्<br>From you both | युष्मत् / युष्मत्तः<br>From you all |
| **Genitive** | तव, ते<br>Of you | युवयोः, वाम्<br>Of you both | युष्माकम्, वः<br>Of you all |
| **Locative** | त्वयि<br>In you | युवयोः<br>In you both | युष्मासु<br>In you all |

## Vedic Chanting

The next two chants are from the *Taittirīyopaniṣat* (*Taittirīya Upaniṣad*) and are considered Vedic chants. A distinctive feature of Vedic chanting is the use of pitch accents to mark correct pronunciation. These pitch accents are divided into three types—*udātta*, raised or high pitch (unmarked), *anudātta*, unraised or low pitch (_), and *svarita*, sounded or falling pitch ( ˈ ). There is also an elongated *svarita*, indicated by a double vertical line. Traditionally, these chants are considered to be ineffective if not recited with the proper cadences.

### C. *Taittirīyopaniṣat* 2.1

Note that in the first two *pādas,* the verb is in the third person, implying that the subject is either "it" (i.e., our study) or "he or she" (i.e., the Supreme God).

सह नाववतु । सह नौ भुनक्तु । सह वीर्यं करवावहै ।
तेजस्वि नावधीतमस्तु मा विद्विषावहै ॥
ॐ शान्तिः शान्तिः शान्तिः ॥

> This chant is often recited at the beginning of a joint study or venture, to bring together the best energies of the student(s) and teacher.

Vocabulary

सह ind. together, with
√अव् 1P, to protect

भुनक्तु may it nourish (3rd p. sg. imperative √भुज्)
वीर्यम् n. strength, energy, vigor, power
करवावहै may we work (1st p. du. imperative Ā √कृ)
तेजस्वि brilliant, energetic, powerful, illuminating (n. acc. sg.)
अधीत mfn. study
वि√द्विष् 1Ā, to be hostile, hate, argue

> *Sandhi* Reminder: **नाव् = नौ**

> Remember that the particle **मा**, together with an imperative is used to express negation.

**D. *Taittirīyopaniṣat* 1.1**

शं नो मित्रः शं वरुणः । शं नो भवत्वर्यमा ।
शं न इन्द्रो बृहस्पतिः । शं नो विष्णुरुरुक्रमः ।
नमो ब्रह्मणे । नमस्ते वायो । त्वमेव प्रत्यक्षं ब्रह्मासि ।
त्वामेव प्रत्यक्षं ब्रह्म वदिष्यामि । ऋतं वदिष्यामि । सत्यं वदिष्यामि ।
तन्मामवतु । तद्वक्तारमवतु । अवतु माम् । अवतु वक्तारम् ।
ॐ शान्तिः शान्तिः शान्तिः ॥

Note that the verb भवतु in the second *pāda* is implied in the first, third, and fourth *pādas* as well. Each phrase can be translated as "May God [grant] us happiness and well-being" or "May God be favorable to us."

Vocabulary

शम् ind. happiness and well-being, auspiciously
मित्रः m. Sun God
वरुणः m. god of the oceans
अर्यमा Aryaman, an Āditya, chief of the Manes, who presides over the Milky Way (m. nom. sg.)
इन्द्रः m. Vedic lord of the gods, god of rain, who wields a thunderbolt
बृहस्पतिः m. lord of prayer and devotion
विष्णुः m. the all-pervader, god of light and sun
उरुक्रमः m. far-stepping
वायुः m. god of the wind
प्रत्यक्ष mfn. present before the eyes, perceptible
ऋतम् n. divine law, custom

> The *Taittirīyopaniṣat*, from the *Taittirīya Āraṇyaka* and associated with the *Yajur Veda*, is one of the earlier prose *upaniṣads*, composed around the sixth to fifth century B.C.E. The most well-known verses center around the student-teacher relationship and the path toward the realization of *Brahman*.

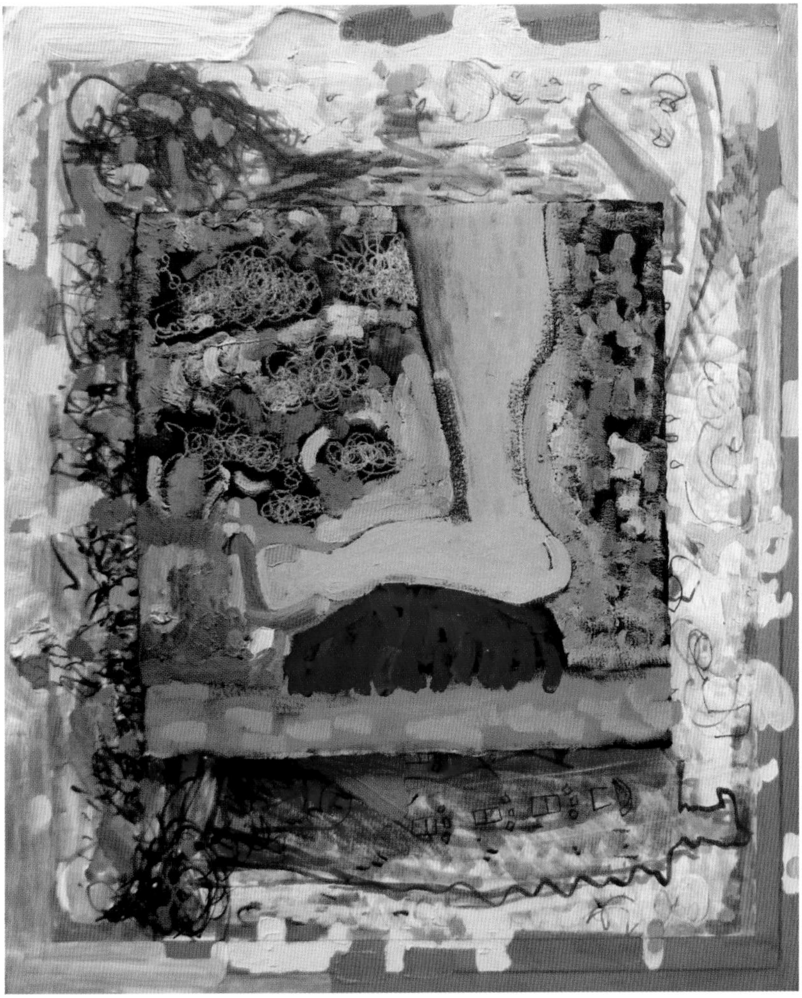

Viṣṇu is the god of preservation, most famous for his incarnations as Rāma and Kṛṣṇa. Here, the epithet *urukrama*, "far-stepping," refers to his incarnation as the dwarf Vāmana. A king named Bali had risen to power over the *asuras* (demons) and taken control of the earth and the heavens. The gods approached Viṣṇu for his help, and Viṣṇu, in the form of Vāmana, disguised as a Brahmin boy, approached Bali and asked for alms. Bali promised to grant him whatever he wished. In response, Vāmana asked for the amount of land he could cover with three steps, which Bali bemusedly agreed to grant. Vāmana then rose to great heights; with his first step he covered the entire earth, with his second step the heavens, and with his third step, since there was nothing left, Bali offered his head, which Vāmana stepped on, sending him down to the underworld. The yoga posture *trivikramāsana* is named for these three steps.

## Relative and Interrogative Pronouns

The relative pronoun यद्, "who, which," and the interrogative pronoun किम्, "what, how, why," are declined exactly like तद्, except for the latter in the neuter nominative and accusative singular forms. Relative pronouns usually occur in conjunction with a correlative pronoun (the third-person forms learned earlier).

**यः m. who, which**

| | Singular | Dual | Plural |
|---|---|---|---|
| **Nominative** | यः | यौ | ये |
| **Accusative** | यम् | यौ | यान् |
| **Instrumental** | येन | याभ्याम् | यैः |
| **Dative** | यस्मै | याभ्याम् | येभ्यः |
| **Ablative** | यस्मात् | याभ्याम् | येभ्यः |
| **Genitive** | यस्य | ययोः | येषाम् |
| **Locative** | यस्मिन् | ययोः | येषु |

**यत् n. which**

| | Singular | Dual | Plural |
|---|---|---|---|
| **Nom./Acc.** | यत् | ये | यानि |

**या f. who, which**

| | Singular | Dual | Plural |
|---|---|---|---|
| **Nominative** | या | ये | याः |
| **Accusative** | याम् | ये | याः |
| **Instrumental** | यया | याभ्याम् | याभिः |
| **Dative** | यस्यै | याभ्याम् | याभ्यः |
| **Ablative** | यस्याः | याभ्याम् | याभ्यः |
| **Genitive** | यस्याः | ययोः | यासाम् |
| **Locative** | यस्याम् | ययोः | यासु |

**कः m. what? why?**

| | Singular | Dual | Plural |
|---|---|---|---|
| **Nominative** | कः | कौ | के |
| **Accusative** | कम् | कौ | कान् |

| | | | |
|---|---|---|---|
| **Instrumental** | केन | काभ्याम् | कैः |
| **Dative** | कस्मै | काभ्याम् | केभ्यः |
| **Ablative** | कस्मात् | काभ्याम् | केभ्यः |
| **Genitive** | कस्य | कयोः | केषाम् |
| **Locative** | कस्मिन् | कयोः | केषु |

**किम् n. what? why?**

| | Singular | Dual | Plural |
|---|---|---|---|
| **Nom./Acc.** | किम् | के | कानि |

**का f. what? why?**

| | Singular | Dual | Plural |
|---|---|---|---|
| **Nominative** | का | के | काः |
| **Accusative** | काम् | के | काः |
| **Instrumental** | कया | काभ्याम् | काभिः |
| **Dative** | कस्यै | काभ्याम् | काभ्यः |
| **Ablative** | कस्याः | काभ्याम् | काभ्यः |
| **Genitive** | कस्याः | कयोः | कासाम् |
| **Locative** | कस्याम् | कयोः | कासु |

## Example: *Guru Stotram* II

Read the second line first. The words in the accusative case in the first line go with पदम् in the second.

अखण्डमण्डलाकारं व्याप्तं येन चराचरम् ।
तत्पदं दर्शितं येन तस्मै श्रीगुरवे नमः ॥

Vocabulary

अखण्डमण्डलाकारम् n. whose form is an unfragmented circle
 अखण्ड mfn. unfragmented
 मण्डलम् n. circle, globe, orb
 आकारः m. form, shape, appearance
व्याप्त mfn. pervaded
चराचरम् n. all created things, moving and unmoving, the whole world
पदम् n. state
दर्शित mfn. shown, revealed

[I] bow (नमः) to that (तस्मै) sacred guru (श्रीगुरवे),
**By whom** (येन) **that** (तत्) state (पदम्) was revealed (दर्शितम्),
Whose form is an unfragmented circle (अखण्डमण्डलाकारम्),
**By which** (येन) the whole universe—moving and unmoving (चराचरम्)—is pervaded (व्याप्तम्).

## Translate

### E. *Guru Stotram* III

As with the previous verse, translate the second line first.

अज्ञानतिमिरान्धस्य ज्ञानाञ्जनशलाकया ।
चक्षुरुन्मीलितं येन तस्मै श्रीगुरवे नमः ॥

Vocabulary

अज्ञानतिमिरान्धस्य of one who was blind because of the darkness of ignorance (m. gen. sg.)
 तिमिरम् n. darkness
 अन्ध mfn. blind
ज्ञानाञ्जनशलाका f. the collyrium pencil of knowledge
 अञ्जनम् n. collyrium, kohl, kajal, black pigment applied to eyelashes
 शलाका f. pencil
चक्षुः eye (n. nom. sg.)
उन्मीलित mfn. opened

### F. *Śivasaṃhitā* 5.213

The सः at the end of the second *pāda* refers to the yogī.

को बन्धः कस्य वा मोक्ष एकं पश्येत्सदा हि सः ।
एतत्करोति यो नित्यं स मुक्तो नात्र संशयः ।
स एव योगी मद्भक्तः सर्वलोकेषु पूजितः ॥

Vocabulary

बन्धः m. binding, bondage
एकम् n. unity
सदा ind. always
करोति to make, do (3rd p. sg. √कृ)

नित्यम् ind. constantly, continually, always
मुक्त mfn. liberated, set free
अत्र ind. here
संशयः m. doubt
मद्भक्त mfn. devoted to me
सर्वलोकः m. all the worlds
पूजित mfn. honored, worshipped, adored

Note also the following correspondences between interrogative, relative, and correlative pronouns.

| Interrogative | Relative | Correlative |
|---|---|---|
| कः who? | यः who, which | सः he, that |
| क्व / कुत्र where? | यत्र where | तत्र there |
| कुतः from what? who? | यतः from which, whence | ततः from that, thence |
| कदा when? | यदा when | तदा then |
| कथम् how? | यथा in which way, just as | तथा in that way, so |
| कीदृश् of what sort? | यादृश् of which sort | तादृश् of that sort |
| कीयन्त् how much? | यावन्त् as much | तावन्त् that much |
| | यावत् as long as | तावत् that long |
| | यदि / चेत् if | तर्हि / तत् then |
| | यद्यपि even if, although | तथापि even so |

## Example: *Śivasaṃhitā* 1.51

Translate the second *pāda* first. Note that the first line is the relative clause, the second is the correlative, and both lines have the same structure; the words are just in a slightly different order.

घटस्याभ्यन्तरे बाह्ये यथाकाशं प्रवर्तते ।
तथात्माभ्यन्तरे बाह्ये ब्रह्माण्डस्य प्रवर्तते ॥

Vocabulary
घटः m. pot, jar
अभ्यन्तर mfn. interior, inside
बाह्य mfn. exterior, outside
आत्मा the Soul (m. nom. sg.)
ब्रह्माण्डम् n. the universe, "Brahmā's egg"

**Just as** (यथा) space (आकाशम्) exists (प्रवर्तते),
On the inside (अभ्यन्तरे) [and] outside (बाह्ये) of a pot (घटस्य).
**So, in that way** (तथा), the Soul (आत्मा) exists (प्रवर्तते),
On the inside (अभ्यन्तरे) [and] outside (बाह्ये) of the universe (ब्रह्माण्डस्य).

### Translate

#### G. *Haṭhapradīpikā* 2.3

यावद्वायुः स्थितो देहे तावज्जीवनमुच्यते ।
मरणं तस्य निष्क्रान्तिस्ततो वायुं निरोधयेत् ॥

Vocabulary

स्थित mfn. standing, situated, abiding or remaining in
जीवनम् n. life
उच्यते it is said (3rd p. sg. pass. √वच्)
मरणम् n. death
निष्क्रान्तिः f. going out, departure
निरोधयेत् one should control (3rd p. sg. optative नि√रुध्)

#### H. *Haṭhapradīpikā* 3.2

सुप्ता गुरुप्रसादेन यदा जागर्ति कुण्डली ।
तदा सर्वाणि पद्मानि भिद्यन्ते ग्रन्थयोऽपि च ॥

Vocabulary

सुप्त mfn. sleeping
गुरुप्रसादः m. the grace of the teacher
जागर्ति is awakened (3rd p. sg. √जागृ)
सर्वाणि all (n. nom. pl.)
पद्म mn. lotus, here referring to the *cakras* (which appear like lotuses)
भिद्यन्ते are split open (3rd p. pl. passive √भिद्)
ग्रन्थिः m. knot

## PRONOMINAL ADJECTIVES

Certain adjectives are declined like the third-person pronoun as well.

अन्य mfn. other
अपर mfn. other, latter, lower

एक mfn. one
पर mfn. further, higher
पूर्व mfn. before, eastern
सर्व mfn. all, every

**सर्वः m. all**

| | Singular | Dual | Plural |
|---|---|---|---|
| **Nominative** | सर्वः | सर्वौ | सर्वे |
| **Accusative** | सर्वम् | सर्वौ | सर्वान् |
| **Instrumental** | सर्वेण | सर्वाभ्याम् | सर्वैः |
| **Dative** | सर्वस्मै | सर्वाभ्याम् | सर्वेभ्यः |
| **Ablative** | सर्वात् | सर्वाभ्याम् | सर्वेभ्यः |
| **Genitive** | सर्वस्य | सर्वयोः | सर्वेषाम् |
| **Locative** | सर्वस्मिन् | सर्वयोः | सर्वेषु |

**सर्वम् n. all**

| | Singular | Dual | Plural |
|---|---|---|---|
| **Nom./Acc.** | सर्वम् | सर्वे | सर्वाणि |

**सर्वा f. all**

| | Singular | Dual | Plural |
|---|---|---|---|
| **Nominative** | सर्वा | सर्वे | सर्वाः |
| **Accusative** | सर्वाम् | सर्वे | सर्वाः |
| **Instrumental** | सर्वया | सर्वाभ्याम् | सर्वाभिः |
| **Dative** | सर्वस्यै | सर्वाभ्याम् | सर्वाभ्यः |
| **Ablative** | सर्वस्याः | सर्वाभ्याम् | सर्वाभ्यः |
| **Genitive** | सर्वस्याः | सर्वयोः | सर्वासाम् |
| **Locative** | सर्वस्याम् | सर्वयोः | सर्वासु |

## Conjugate

अन्य, एक, पूर्व

## Translate

### I. *Śānti Mantra* IV

Note that the genitive सर्वेषाम् here translates as "for all."

सर्वेषां स्वस्तिर्भवतु । सर्वेषां शान्तिर्भवतु ।
सर्वेषां पूर्णं भवतु । सर्वेषां मङ्गलं भवतु ॥

Vocabulary
स्वस्तिः f. well-being, fortune
मङ्गलम् n. happiness, auspiciousness

### J. *Śivasaṃhitā* 1.4–5

These verses come in a series of verses explaining that there are many ways to liberation.

सत्यं केचित्प्रशंसन्ति तपः शौचं तथापरे ।
क्षमां केचित्प्रशंसन्ति तथैव शममार्जवम् ॥

केचिद्दानं प्रशंसन्ति पितृकर्म तथापरे ।
केचित्कर्म प्रशंसन्ति केचिद्वैराग्यमुत्तमम् ॥

Vocabulary
केचित् ind. some
प्र√शंस् 1P, proclaim, praise
तपः austerity, discipline (n. acc. sg.)
क्षमा f. patience
शमः m. tranquillity, equanimity
अर्जवम् n. honesty
पितृकर्म rites for the ancestors (n. acc. sg.)
कर्म action (n. acc. sg.)
केचित् . . . केचित् . . . ind. some . . . others . . .

### K. *Śivasaṃhitā* 1.15

This verse follows from the last one. एते refers to the methods just described.

एते चान्ये च मुनिभिः संज्ञाभेदाः पृथग्विधाः ।
शास्त्रेषु कथिता ह्येते लोकव्यामोहकारकाः ॥

Vocabulary

संज्ञाभेदः m. different conceptions/ideas
पृथग्विध mfn. of distinct kinds, manifold, various
शास्त्रम् n. an instrument of teaching, sacred text
कथित mfn. told, related, taught
लोकव्यामोहकारक mfn. creating confusion in people

## Review Exercises

### L. *Bhagavadgītā* 2.53

The subject of the first three *pādas* is ते बुद्धिः, found in the first and third *pādas*.

श्रुतिविप्रतिपन्ना ते यदा स्थास्यति निश्चला ।
समाधावचला बुद्धिस्तदा योगमवाप्स्यसि ॥

Vocabulary

श्रुतिविप्रतिपन्ना f. which is perplexed by hearing sacred texts (e.g., the Vedas) (describes बुद्धिः)

श्रुतिः f. a Vedic or sacred text

विप्रतिपन्न mfn. confused, bewildered, perplexed

निश्चल mfn. motionless, steady

अचल mfn. motionless, steady

अवाप्स्यसि you will attain (2nd p. sg. future अव√आप्)

### M. *Aparokṣānubhūti* 12

कोऽहं कथमिदं जातं को वै कर्तास्य विद्यते ।
उपादानं किमस्तीह विचारः सोऽयमीदृशः ॥

Vocabulary

इदम् this [world] (n. nom. sg.)

जात mfn. created

वै ind. indeed, truly (particle of emphasis)

उपादानम् n. material cause

इह ind. here, in this world

विचारः m. reflection, inquiry, consideration

अयम् this (m. nom. sg.)

ईदृश् mfn. endowed with such qualities, such

### N. *Bhagavadgītā* 8.7

तस्मात्सर्वेषु कालेषु मामनुस्मर युध्य च ।
मय्यर्पितमनोबुद्धिर्मामेवैष्यस्यसंशयम् ॥

Vocabulary

कालः m. time
अनु√स्मृ 1P, to remember
√युध् 4P, fight, engage in battle
अर्पितमनोबुद्धिः m. with mind and understanding fixed
    अर्पित mfn. fixed
एष्यसि you will come toward, attain (2nd p. sg. future √इ)
असंशयम् ind. without doubt, undoubtedly

O. *Bhagavadgītā* 2.46

अर्थ in the first *pāda*, is implied in the third *pāda* as well.

यावानर्थ उदपाने सर्वतः सम्प्लुतोदके ।
तावान्सर्वेषु वेदेषु ब्राह्मणस्य विजानतः ॥

Vocabulary

अर्थः m. value
उदपान mn. a well
सर्वतः ind. from all sides, in every direction, everywhere
सम्प्लुतोदके in which water is overflowing (n. loc. sg.)
    सम्प्लुत mfn. flooded over, overflowing
    उदकम् n. water
ब्राह्मणः m. Brahmin
विजानतः of/for one who is knowing, understanding (m. gen. sg.)

# *Sandhi* Review

The following charts illustrate all possible *sandhi* rules—vowel, *visarga*, and consonant. See each set of charts for examples of the rules that have not already been given. Review the *sandhi* rules at the end of Chapters 2 and 4 for rules that were explained previously. It may also be helpful at this point to review the meaning of the following words:

Stops or plosives: Sounds that block the flow of air within the vocal tract.

Voiced sounds: Sounds that use the vocal cords in pronunciation. In the chart of consonants, they constitute the last three columns of stops, the semivowels, and ह (which is guttural, aspirated, and voiced).

Unvoiced sounds: Sounds that do not use the vocal cords in pronunciation. In the chart of consonants, they constitute the first two columns of stops and the sibilants.

Unaspirated sounds: Sounds that do not create an explosion of breath as the sound is articulated. They constitute the first and third columns of stops.

Aspirated sounds: Sounds that create an explosion of breath as the sound is articulated. They constitute the second and fourth columns of stops.

Nasals: Voiced sounds that allow the air to pass through the nose, constituting the fifth column of stops.

Semivowels: Voiced sounds, considered somewhere between a consonant and a vowel, but treated as consonants.

Sibilants: Unvoiced sounds that make a hissing "sh" or "s" sound.

Homorganic: Articulated in the same place in the mouth.

Note: *Sandhi* may only be performed once at each juncture.
Do NOT perform *sandhi* upon *sandhi*!!!

## VOWEL *SANDHI*

| Final Letter of First Word | First Letter of Second Word: Vowels | | | | | | | | | | | |
|---|---|---|---|---|---|---|---|---|---|---|---|---|
| | अ | आ | इ | ई | उ | ऊ | ऋ | ॠ | ए | ऐ | ओ | औ |
| अ / आ | आ | आ | ए | ए | ओ | ओ | अर् | अर् | ऐ | ऐ | औ | औ |

| | | | | | | | | | | | | |
|---|---|---|---|---|---|---|---|---|---|---|---|---|
| इ / ई | य | या | ई | ई | यु | यू | यृ | यॄ | ये | यै | यो | यौ |
| उ / ऊ | व | वा | वि | वी | ऊ | ऊ | वृ | वॄ | वे | वै | वो | वौ |
| ऋ / ॠ | र | रा | रि | री | रु | रू | ऋ | ॠ | रे | रै | रो | रौ |
| ए | एऽ | अ_आ | अ_इ | अ_ई | अ_उ | अ_ऊ | अ_ऋ | अ_ॠ | अ_ए | अ_ऐ | अ_ओ | अ_औ |
| ऐ | आ_अ | आ_आ | आ_इ | आ_ई | आ_उ | आ_ऊ | आ_ऋ | आ_ॠ | आ_ए | आ_ऐ | आ_ओ | आ_औ |
| ओ | ओऽ | अ_आ | अ_इ | अ_ई | अ_उ | अ_ऊ | अ_ऋ | अ_ॠ | अ_ए | अ_ऐ | अ_ओ | अ_औ |
| औ | आव | आवा | आवि | आवी | आवु | आवू | आवृ | आवॄ | आवे | आवै | आवो | आवौ |

1. A final ए or ओ before a vowel other than अ becomes अ and the hiatus between the vowels remains.

### Example: *Bhagavadgītā* 1.47 ab

एवमुक्त्वार्जुन संख्ये रथोपस्थे उपाविशत् ⇒ एवमुक्त्वार्जुन संख्ये रथोपस्थ उपाविशत्।

2. A final ऐ before a vowel becomes आ and the hiatus between the vowels remains.

### Example: *Śivasaṃhitā* 4.59 ab

स्वप्राणैः सदृशो यस्तु तस्मै अपि न दीयते ⇒ स्वप्राणैः सदृशो यस्तु तस्मा अपि न दीयते।

3. A final औ before a vowel becomes आव्.

### Example: *Yogasūtra* 2.29

यमनियमासनप्राणायामप्रत्याहारधारणाध्यानसमाधयोऽष्टौ अङ्गानि ⇒
यमनियमासनप्राणायामप्रत्याहारधारणाध्यानसमाधयोऽष्टावङ्गानि।

## Exceptions to Vowel *Sandhi* Rules

Certain vowels, called प्रगृह्य vowels, do not follow normal *sandhi* rules.

4. The vowels ई, ऊ, and ए do not change if they occur at the end of dual forms of verbs or nouns.

### Example 1: *Yogayājñavalkya* 3.7 cd

उर्वोरुपरि विप्रेन्द्र कृत्वा पादतले उभे ⇒ उर्वोरुपरि विप्रेन्द्र कृत्वा पादतले उभे।

### Example 2: *Bhagavadgītā* 13.19 ab

प्रकृतिं पुरुषं चैव विद्ध्यनादी उभावपि ⇒ प्रकृतिं पुरुषं चैव विद्ध्यनादी उभावपि ।

5. The final vowels of particles or interjections (such as हे, आ, and अहो) do not change.
   Ex: अहो एषाम् ⇒ अहो एषाम्

## *VISARGA SANDHI*

The following charts illustrate all of the *visarga sandhi* rules. See the following page for examples of rules we have not encountered yet. *Visarga*, written in *devanāgarī* as ":" and transliterated as "ḥ," can derive from either of the two original sounds, "s" or "r," although the former is much more common.

**First Letter of Second Word: Unvoiced Consonants**

| Final Letter of First Word | क् / ख् | च् / छ् | ट् / ठ् | त् / थ् | प् / फ् | श् | ष् / स् |
|---|---|---|---|---|---|---|---|
| अः | अः | अश् | अष् | अस् | अः | अः | अः |
| आः | आः | आश् | आष् | आस् | आः | आः | आः |
| : * | : | श् | ष् | स् | : | : | : |

**First Letter of Second Word: Voiced Consonants**

| Final Letter of First Word | ग् / घ् | ज् / झ् | ड् / ढ् | द् / ध् | ब् / भ् | न् / म् |
|---|---|---|---|---|---|---|
| अः | ओ | ओ | ओ | ओ | ओ | ओ |
| आः | आ | आ | आ | आ | आ | आ |
| : * | र् | र् | र् | र् | र् | र् |

**First Letter of Second Word: Vowels, Semivowels**

| Final Letter of First Word | Vowels | य् | र् | ल् | व् | ह् |
|---|---|---|---|---|---|---|
| अः | अ** | ओ | ओ | ओ | ओ | ओ |
| आः | आ | आ | आ | आ | आ | आ |
| : * | र् | र् | _*** | र् | र् | र् |

* preceded by a vowel other than अ / आ
** except when followed by अ, where अः + अ = ओऽ
*** the final र् disappears and the preceding vowel is lengthened if possible (see the following page)

6. If a *visarga* or र् is preceded by a vowel other than अ and followed by an initial र्, the *visarga* or र् is dropped, and the final vowel is lengthened, if it is not already long.

**Example: *Chāndogyopaniṣat* 6.4.1**

यदग्नेः रोहितँ रूपं तेजसस्तद्रूपम् ⇒ यदग्ने रोहितँ रूपं तेजसस्तद्रूपम् ।

## CONSONANT *SANDHI*

In Sanskrit, words may end only in certain permitted finals: vowels, क्, ट्, त्, प्, ङ्, न्, or म्, in addition to *visarga* and र्, as described in the section on *visarga sandhi*. Note that if you encounter words ending in other consonants, it is due to *sandhi* changes. The letters in parentheses indicate a change in the initial vowel of the second word.

**First Letter of Second Word: Unvoiced Consonants**

| Final Letter of First Word | क् / ख् | च् / छ् | ट् / ठ् | त् / थ् | प् / फ् | श् | ष् / स् |
|---|---|---|---|---|---|---|---|
| क् | क् | क् | क् | क् | क् | क् | क् |
| ट् | ट् | ट् | ट् | ट् | ट् | ट् | ट् |
| त् | त् | च् | ट् | त् | त् | च(छ्) | त् |
| प् | प् | प् | प् | प् | प् | प् | प् |
| ङ् | ङ् | ङ् | ङ् | ङ् | ङ् | ङ् | ङ् |
| न् | न् | ंश् | ंष् | ंस् | न् | ञ(श्) / ञ(छ्) | न् |
| म् | ं(ṃ) | ं | ं | ं | ं | ं | ं |

**First Letter of Second Word: Voiced Consonants**

| Final Letter of First Word | ग् / घ् | ज् / झ् | ड् / द् | द् / ध् | ब् / भ् | न् / म् |
|---|---|---|---|---|---|---|
| क् | ग् | ग् | ग् | ग् | ग् | ङ् |
| ट् | ड् | ड् | ड् | ड् | ड् | ण् |
| त् | द् | ज् | ड | द् | द् | न् |
| प् | ब् | ब् | ब् | ब् | ब् | म् |
| ङ् | ङ् | ङ् | ङ् | ङ् | ङ् | ङ् |
| न् | न् | ञ् | ण् | न् | न् | न् |
| म् | ं | ं | ं | ं | ं | ं |

**First Letter of Second Word: Vowels, Semivowels**

| Final Letter of First Word | Vowels | य् | र् | ल् | व् | ह् |
|---|---|---|---|---|---|---|
| क् | ग् | ग् | ग् | ग् | ग् | ग (घ्) |
| ट् | ड् | ड् | ड् | ड् | ड् | ड् (ढ्) |
| त् | द् | द् | द् | ल् | द् | द् (ध्) |
| प् | ब् | ब् | ब् | ब् | ब् | ब (भ्) |
| ङ् | ङ् / ङ्ङ् | ङ् | ङ् | ङ् | ङ् | ङ् |
| न् | न् / न्न् | न् | न् | लँ् | न् | न् |
| म् | म् | ं | ं | ं | ं | ं |

7. A final consonant + an initial ह is replaced by a conjunct consonant consisting of a voiced unaspirated consonant + a voiced aspirated consonant, both with the same place of articulation as the original final consonant.

द् / ध् + ह ⇒ द्ध
ब् / प् + ह ⇒ ब्भ
क् / ग् + ह ⇒ ग्घ

**Example:** ***Yogayājñavalkya* 3.7ab**

अङ्गुष्ठौ च निबध्नीयाद् हस्ताभ्यां व्युत्क्रमेण तु ⇒ अङ्गुष्ठौ च निबध्नीयाद्धस्ताभ्यां व्युत्क्रमेण तु ।

8. A final त् before an initial श् changes to च्छ्.

**Example:** ***Bhāgavatapurāṇa* 11.28.43cd**

तत् श्रद्धध्यान्न मतिमान्योगमुत्सृज्य मत्परः ⇒ तच्छ्रद्धध्यान्न मतिमान्योगमुत्सृज्य मत्परः ।

9. A final न् before an unvoiced palatal, retroflex, or dental stop (च्, छ्, ट्, ठ्, त्, थ्) is replaced by *anusvāra*, plus the homorganic (articulated in the same place in the mouth) sibilant to the following stop.

**Example:** ***Bhagavadgītā* 13.19cd**

विकारान् च गुणान् चैव विद्धि प्रकृतिसंभवान् ⇒ विकारांश्च गुणांश्चैव विद्धि प्रकृतिसंभवान् ।

10. A final न् before an initial ल् changes to ल् and *candrabindu* (ँ), the special mark of nasalization, is added.

You will probably recognize the *candrabindu*, "moon-drop," from the word ॐ.

**Example:** ***Bhagavadgītā*** **18.71**

सोऽपि मुक्तः शुभान् लोकोन्प्राप्नुयात्पुण्यकर्मणाम् ⇒
सोऽपि मुक्तः शुभाँल्लोकान्प्राप्नुयात्पुण्यकर्मणाम् ।

11. A final न् , ण् , or ङ् is doubled after a short vowel, before any initial vowel.

**Example:** ***Aparokṣānubhūti*** **112ab**

सुखेनैव भवेद्यस्मिन् अजस्रं ब्रह्मचिन्तनम् ⇒ सुखेनैव भवेद्यस्मिन्नजस्रं ब्रह्मचिन्तनम् ।

## INTERNAL *SANDHI*

12. The letter स् changes to ष् if immediately preceded by a vowel other than अ or आ or the consonants क् or र्. This rule holds as long as स् is not at the end of a word or followed by र्.

Ex.: उप नि√सद् ⇒उपनिषद्

# Part I Review: *Gurvaṣṭakam*

## Write with Correct *Sandhi*, Translate, and Memorize (as Much as Possible)

गुर्वष्टकम् = गुरु + अष्टकम्

Written by Ādi Śaṅkarācārya, a teacher of *Advaita Vedānta* (nondualism), these are the eight verses to the guru. *Aṣṭaka* means consisting of eight parts (like *aṣṭāṅgayoga*—the yoga with eight limbs). There is a ninth verse that is a colophon, a concluding verse, which is not included in the count. The vocabulary for these nine verses is listed together after the colophon.

शरीरम् सुरूपम् तथा वा कलत्रम् यशः चारु चित्रम् धनम् मेरुतुल्यम् ।
मनस् चेत् न लग्नम् गुरोः अङ्घ्रिपद्मे ततः किम् ततः किम् ततः किम् ततः किम् ॥ १ ॥

कलत्रम् धनम् पुत्रपौत्रादि सर्वम् गृहम् बान्धवाः सर्वम् एतद् हि जातम् ।
मनस् चेत् न लग्नम् गुरोः अङ्घ्रिपद्मे ततः किम् ततः किम् ततः किम् ततः किम् ॥ २ ॥

षडङ्गादिवेदः मुखे शास्त्रविद्या कवित्वादि गद्यम् सुपद्यम् करोति ।
मनस् चेत् न लग्नम् गुरोः अङ्घ्रिपद्मे ततः किम् ततः किम् ततः किम् ततः किम् ॥ ३ ॥

विदेशेषु मान्यः स्वदेशेषु धन्यः सदाचारवृत्तेषु मत्तः न च अन्यः ।
मनस् चेत् न लग्नम् गुरोः अङ्घ्रिपद्मे ततः किम् ततः किम् ततः किम् ततः किम् ॥ ४ ॥

क्षमामण्डले भूपभूपालवृन्दैः सदा सेवितम् यस्य पादारविन्दम् ।
मनस् चेत् न लग्नम् गुरोः अङ्घ्रिपद्मे ततः किम् ततः किम् ततः किम् ततः किम् ॥ ५ ॥

यशः मे गतम् दिक्षु दानप्रतापात् जगद्वस्तु सर्वम् करे यत्प्रसादात् ।
मनस् चेत् न लग्नम् गुरोः अङ्घ्रिपद्मे ततः किम् ततः किम् ततः किम् ततः किम् ॥ ६ ॥

न भोगे न योगे न वा वाजिराजौ न कान्तामुखे नैव वित्तेषु चित्तम् ।
मनस् चेत् न लग्नम् गुरोः अङ्घ्रिपद्मे ततः किम् ततः किम् ततः किम् ततः किम् ॥ ७ ॥

अरण्ये न वा स्वस्य गेहे न कार्ये न देहे मनः वर्तते मे तु अनर्घ्ये ।
मनस् चेत् न लग्नम् गुरोः अङ्घ्रिपद्मे ततः किम् ततः किम् ततः किम् ततः किम् ॥ ८ ॥

गुरोः अष्टकम् यः पठेत् पुण्यदेही यतिः भूपतिः ब्रह्मचारी च गेही ।
लभेद् वाञ्छितार्थम् पदम् ब्रह्मसंज्ञम् गुरोः उक्तवाक्ये मनः यस्य लग्नम् ॥ ९ ॥

Vocabulary

Note that the vocabulary words are listed in Sanskrit alphabetical order. Remember that any vocabulary not listed is in the glossary, at the end of the book.

अङ्घ्रिपद्मे lotus feet (n. acc. du.)
अनर्घ्य mfn. priceless, invaluable
अरण्यम् n. a forest
उक्तवाक्यम् n. sayings
करोति to make, do, compose (3rd p. sg. √कृ)
कलत्रम् n. wife
कवित्वादि poetic skill, etc. (m. nom. sg.)
कान्तामुखम् n. the face of the beloved
  कान्त mfn. desired, loved, dear
कार्य mfn. to be done
क्ष्मामण्डलम् n. the whole earth
  क्ष्मा f. the earth
गत mfn. gone, spread
गद्यम् n. prose
गृहः m. a house, home
गेहम् n. a house
गेही householder (m. nom. sg. गेहिन्)
चारु mfn. pleasing, lovely, beautiful
चित्र mfn. excellent, manifold
चेत् ind. if
जगद्वस्तु things of the world (n. acc. sg.)
जात mfn. present, existent
दानप्रतापः m. generosity and prowess
  दानम् n. the act of giving, generosity
  प्रतापः m. prowess, splendor, brilliancy, majesty
दिक्षु in [all] the directions (f. loc. pl. दिश्)

धन्य mfn. fortunate, wealthy
न च अन्यः ind. there is no other
पादारविन्दम् n. lotus feet
पुण्यदेही virtuous person (m. nom sg. पुण्यदेहिन्)
पुत्रपौत्रादि children, grandchildren, etc. (m. nom. sg.)
ब्रह्मचारी student (m. nom. sg. ब्रह्मचारिन्)
ब्रह्मसंज्ञम् n. which is called *Brahman* (Spirit)
भूपतिः m. king
भूपभूपालवृन्दम् n. multitudes of princes and kings
भोगः m. enjoyment, pleasure
मनस् mind (n. nom. sg.)
मान्य mfn. to be respected or honored
मेरुतुल्य mfn. equal to Mt. Meru
    तुल्य mfn. equal to
यतिः m. ascetic
यत्प्रसादात् from whose (i.e., the guru's) favor (m. abl. sg.)
    प्रसादः m. graciousness, kindness, favor
यशस् fame (n. nom. sg.)
लग्न mfn. attached to
वाजिराजः m. the king's horses
वाञ्छितार्थः m. desired goal
    वाञ्छित mfn. wished, desired
वित्तम् n. wealth
विदेशः m. another country, abroad
√वृत् 1Ā, to exist, live, dwell
शास्त्रविद्या f. knowledge of sciences
षडङ्गादिवेदः m. the Vedas with their six limbs
सदाचारवृत्तम् n. ways of virtuous conduct
    सदाचारः m. virtuous conduct, good manners
सुपद्यम् n. beautiful poetry
सुरूप mfn. well formed, beautiful
    रूपम् n. form, shape
सेवित mfn. served
स्वदेशः m. one's own country
स्वस्य of oneself (m. gen. sg.)

# *Viṣkambha*: Interlude

## विष्कम्भ

*Viṣkambha*: "An interlude between the acts of a drama and performed by one or more characters, middling or inferior, who connect the story of the drama and the subdivisions of the plot by briefly explaining to the audience what has occurred in the intervals of the acts or what is likely to happen later on." Also "a particular posture practised by Yogins," according to Monier Williams.

In Part I, we have learned most of the basic grammatical structures of the Sanskrit language. Before you continue on to Part II, it is a good idea to review the verses we have read in Part I. As you revisit these verses, you will see that much of the grammar that was obscure the first time around has now become clear. *Svādhyāya*, the fourth *niyama* ("observance," the second limb of *aṣṭāṅgayoga*), as well as the second component of *kriyāyoga*, "the yoga of action," literally means "self-study," but has been translated by many teachers as going over your lessons!

Part II continues in a similar manner to Part I, introducing slightly more complex and interesting grammatical structures such as compounds and participles. We will learn the other six verbal *gaṇas* and their various conjugations, as well as declensions for nouns ending in consonants.

At this juncture, I would recommend getting a dictionary, if you haven't already. I am partial to Vaman Shivaram Apte's *The Practical Sanskrit-English Dictionary*, which lists meanings in order of the frequency of use. It also comes in a compact version for easy travel. If you use Monier Williams's dictionary, note that entries are listed chronologically, which means that, often, Vedic definitions will be given first. You should look for the definitions that are found in classical texts, for example, the *Mahābhārata*. Although all necessary vocabulary will still be provided with each example, it is a good idea to begin to get familiar with how to use a dictionary. All entries are listed in Sanskrit alphabetical order; often, nouns follow the verb they derive from. Have patience; it takes time to get comfortable with the way in which words are listed. But a dictionary will open up a world of possibility—every word has multiple meanings beyond what is provided in the vocabulary lists. As you get comfortable with the dictionary, you can put a little dot next to every word you look up. If you find that you look a word up multiple times—three or four dots—it is a good idea to memorize that word. Online dictionaries exist now, as well; however, I would encourage you to wait to explore them until you are thoroughly familiar with using the hard-bound ones.

# PART II

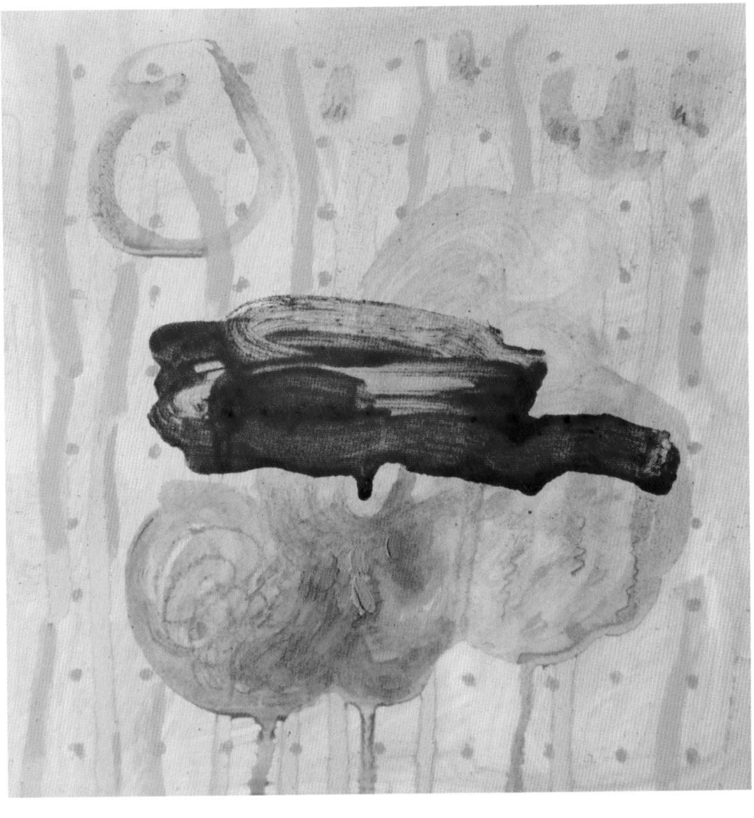

# 8
# Nouns Ending in Simple Consonants; Vowel Strength; Verb Conjugations: Second and Third Class

**तीव्रसंवेगानामासन्नः ॥ १.२१ ॥**
**tīvra-saṃvegānām āsannaḥ**
The attainment of *samādhi* is near for those who apply themselves intensely.
॥ *Yogasūtra* 1.21 ॥

## NOUNS ENDING IN CONSONANTS

All nouns ending in consonants have a distinctive set of endings, differing from those for the nouns ending in vowels that we have learned thus far. The masculine and feminine paradigms are identical, and in the neuter, they differ only in the nominative, accusative, and vocative forms, which are all equivalent. The stems remain unchanged before endings beginning with vowels, but undergo *sandhi* changes before endings beginning with consonants, as well as in the nominative and vocative singular. When you learn a new consonant-ending verb, take note of both the stem form and the nominative singular form. In this transition, the final letter changes according to the following rules:

क् ख् ग् घ् च् ज् श् ह् ⇒ क्
ट् ठ् ड् ढ् छ् ज् झ् श् ष् ह् ⇒ ट्
त् थ् द् ध् ह् ⇒ त्
प् फ् ब् भ् ⇒ प्
ङ् ञ् ⇒ ङ्
न् म् ⇒ remain unchanged
स् ⇒ *visarga*
र् ⇒ remains unchanged
ण् य् ल् व् ⇒ do not occur

Note that some consonants (ज्, श्, ह्) have two options.

This same ending used in the nominative and vocative singular forms is also used in the locative plural, with *sandhi* changes as necessary. Before all other endings beginning with a consonant (instrumental, dative, ablative dual, and plural) the final consonant is changed to the voiced equivalent of the nominative singular ending.

**सुहृद् m. friend, "good-hearted"**

| | Singular | Dual | Plural |
|---|---|---|---|
| **Nominative** | सुहृत् | सुहृदौ | सुहृदः |
| **Accusative** | सुहृदम् | सुहृदौ | सुहृदः |
| **Instrumental** | सुहृदा | सुहृद्भ्याम् | सुहृद्भिः |
| **Dative** | सुहृदे | सुहृद्भ्याम् | सुहृद्भ्यः |
| **Ablative** | सुहृदः | सुहृद्भ्याम् | सुहृद्भ्यः |
| **Genitive** | सुहृदः | सुहृदोः | सुहृदाम् |
| **Locative** | सुहृदि | सुहृदोः | सुहृत्सु |
| **Vocative** | सुहृत् | सुहृदौ | सुहृदः |

**जगत् n. world**

| | Singular | Dual | Plural |
|---|---|---|---|
| **Nominative** | जगत् | जगती | जगन्ति |
| **Accusative** | जगत् | जगती | जगन्ति |
| **Instrumental** | जगता | जगद्भ्याम् | जगद्भिः |
| **Dative** | जगते | जगद्भ्याम् | जगद्भ्यः |
| **Ablative** | जगतः | जगद्भ्याम् | जगद्भ्यः |
| **Genitive** | जगतः | जगतोः | जगताम् |
| **Locative** | जगति | जगतोः | जगत्सु |
| **Vocative** | जगत् | जगती | जगन्ति |

**वाच् f. speech**

| | Singular | Dual | Plural |
|---|---|---|---|
| **Nominative** | वाक् | वाचौ | वाचः |
| **Accusative** | वाचम् | वाचौ | वाचः |
| **Instrumental** | वाचा | वाग्भ्याम् | वाग्भिः |
| **Dative** | वाचे | वाग्भ्याम् | वाग्भ्यः |
| **Ablative** | वाचः | वाग्भ्याम् | वाग्भ्यः |
| **Genitive** | वाचः | वाचोः | वाचाम् |
| **Locative** | वाचि | वाचोः | वाक्षु |
| **Vocative** | वाक् | वाचौ | वाचः |

| Vocabulary | Nominative Singular |
| --- | --- |
| ऋत्विज् m. priest | ऋत्विक् |
| त्वच् f. skin | त्वक् |
| दिश् f. direction | दिक् |
| परिव्राज् m. wandering mendicant | परिव्राट् |
| मरुत् m. wind | मरुत् |
| शरद् f. autumn | शरत् |
| शुच् f. grief | शुक् |
| सम्राज् m. king, emperor | सम्राट् |
| सरित् f. river | सरित् |

## Decline

दिश्, शरद्, सम्राज्

## Translate

### A. *Gheraṇḍasaṃhitā* 5.9

वसन्ते शरदि प्रोक्तं योगारम्भं समाचरेत्।
तदा योगो भवेत्सिद्धो रोगान्मुक्तो भवेद् ध्रुवम्॥

Vocabulary
वसन्तः m. spring
प्रोक्त mfn. declared, said, taught
योगारम्भः m. beginning of yoga practice
आरम्भः m. undertaking, beginning, commencement
समा√चर् 1P, to act, practice
सिद्ध mfn. attained
रोगः m. disease
मुक्त mfn. liberated, freed (takes the ablative)
ध्रुवम् ind. certainly, surely

### B. *Bhagavadgītā* 16.5

In the first *pāda* infer "leads to."

दैवी संपद्विमोक्षाय निबन्धायासुरी मता ।
मा शुचः संपदं दैवीमभिजातोऽसि पाण्डव ॥

Vocabulary
दैवी f. divine
संपद् f. fate, destiny
विमोक्षः m. liberation
निबन्धः m. chain, fetter, bondage
असुरी f. demonic
मत mfn. thought, believed
मा शुचः don't grieve (2nd p. sg. injunctive aorist)
अभिजात mfn. born

## C. *Amaruśataka* 105

This verse can be translated as a series of short phrases, beginning with प्रासादे सा.

प्रासादे सा दिशि दिशि च सा पृष्ठतः सा पुरः सा
पर्यङ्के सा पथि पथि च सा तद्वियोगातुरस्य ।
हा हा चेतः प्रकृतिरपरा नास्ति मे कापि सा सा
सा सा सा सा जगति सकले कोऽयमद्वैतवादः ॥

The *Amaruśataka*, or "Hundred Verses of Amaru," is a collection of poems by Amaru from around the seventh to eighth century C.E. They are all verses about love in its various forms, although mainly about love in separation.

Vocabulary
प्रासादः m. palace
पृष्ठतः ind. behind
पुरः ind. in front
पर्यङ्कः m. bed, couch, sofa
पथि पथि on every path (m. loc. sg.)
    पथि on the path (m. loc. sg.)
तद्वियोगातुरस्य of/for one who is tortured by separation from her (m. gen. sg.)
    वियोगः m. disjunction, separation
    आतुर mfn. suffering, diseased or pained by
हा हा चेतः ind. Oh! My heart!
प्रकृतिः f. woman
कापि ind. someone
सकल mfn. with parts, whole, entire

अयम् this (m. nom. sg.)
अद्वैतवादः m. talk of nonduality
अद्वैतम् n. nonduality
वादः m. speech, discourse, talk

## VOWEL STRENGTH

An important distinction related to the vowel *sandhi* rules is vowel strength. The two degrees of strength are called गुण and वृद्धि. They are applied only to the simple vowels, increasing their strength by one or two degrees, respectively. As we will see, this vowel strengthening explains many of the internal *sandhi* changes that occur during conjugations, both those we have learned so far and those to come.

| | अ / आ | इ / ई | उ / ऊ | ऋ / ॠ |
|---|---|---|---|---|
| गुण | *अ / आ | ए | ओ | अर् |
| वृद्धि | आ | ऐ | औ | आर् |

*Note that the letter अ is unchanged by गुण (i.e., the गुण of अ is अ).

## OTHER VERB CONJUGATIONS

The verbs we have learned thus far belong to the thematic *gaṇas* (1, 4, 6, and 10) and are all conjugated in a similar way, adding *gaṇa* signs that end in "a," which are invariable before all endings. The remaining athematic verbs (belonging to the *gaṇas* 2, 3, 5, 7, 8, and 9) differ in that the *gaṇa* signs added do NOT end in "a." Because of this, the internal *sandhi* changes necessitated during conjugation are more complex, depending on which ending they are prefixed to. The endings are similar to those we learned in Part I; however, the verbal stems can take two forms—strong or weak—depending on the ending they precede. The strong forms are the first-, second-, and third-person singular forms of the present and past imperfect *parasmaipada* tenses, and all of the first-person forms of the imperative, both *parasmaipada* and *ātmanepada*, as well as the third-person singular imperative *parasmaipada* form. The chart below gives the final endings for these conjugations, with the strong forms emphasized in red.

### Parasmaipada

| | Present Tense | | | Past Imperfect | | |
|---|---|---|---|---|---|---|
| | Singular | Dual | Plural | Singular | Dual | Plural |
| 3 | -ति | -तः | -अन्ति | -त् | -ताम् | -अन् |
| 2 | -सि | -थः | -थ | -स् | -तम् | -त |
| 1 | -मि | -वः | -मः | -अम् | -व | -म |

| | Imperative | | | Optative | | |
|---|---|---|---|---|---|---|
| | Singular | Dual | Plural | Singular | Dual | Plural |
| 3 | -तु | -ताम् | -अन्तु | -यात् | -याताम् | -युः |
| 2 | -धि / -हि | -तम् | -त | -याः | -यातम् | -यात |
| 1 | -आनि | -आव | -आम | -याम् | -याव | -याम |

### Ātmanepada

| | Present Tense | | | Past Imperfect | | |
|---|---|---|---|---|---|---|
| | Singular | Dual | Plural | Singular | Dual | Plural |
| 3 | -ते | -आते | -अते | -त | -आताम् | -अत |
| 2 | -से | -आथे | -ध्वे | -थाः | -आथाम् | -ध्वम् |
| 1 | -ए | -वहे | -महे | -इ | -वहि | -महि |

| | Imperative | | | Optative | | |
|---|---|---|---|---|---|---|
| | Singular | Dual | Plural | Singular | Dual | Plural |
| 3 | -ताम् | -आताम् | -अताम् | -ईत | -ईयाताम् | -ईरन् |
| 2 | -स्व | -आथाम् | -ध्वम् | -ईथाः | -ईयाथाम् | -ईध्वम् |
| 1 | -ऐ | -आवहै | -आमहै | -ईय | -ईवहि | -ईमहि |

## SECOND CLASS VERBS

The second *gaṇa* is named after the root अद्, "to eat." It is also often known as the root class, because its present tense stem is exactly the same as the root. Because the root joins directly with the verbal endings, some complex internal *sandhi* changes can arise. Additionally, the root vowel takes गुण in strong forms. There is no need to memorize all of the paradigms, just try to learn to recognize and understand the different forms.

### √पा 2P, to protect

| | Present Tense | | | Past Imperfect | | |
|---|---|---|---|---|---|---|
| | Singular | Dual | Plural | Singular | Dual | Plural |
| 3 | पाति | पातः | पान्ति | अपात् | अपाताम् | अपान् |
| 2 | पासि | पाथः | पाथ | अपाः | अपातम् | अपात |
| 1 | पामि | पावः | पामः | अपाम् | अपाव | अपाम |

| | Imperative | | | Optative | | |
|---|---|---|---|---|---|---|
| | Singular | Dual | Plural | Singular | Dual | Plural |
| 3 | पातु | पाताम् | पान्तु | पायात् | पायाताम् | पायुः |
| 2 | पाहि | पातम् | पात | पायाः | पायातम् | पायात |
| 1 | पानि | पाव | पाम | पायाम् | पायाव | पायाम |

### √विद् 2P, to know, feel, consider

| | Present Tense | | | Past Imperfect | | |
|---|---|---|---|---|---|---|
| | Singular | Dual | Plural | Singular | Dual | Plural |
| 3 | वेत्ति | वित्तः | विदन्ति | अवेत् | अवित्ताम् | अविदन् / अविदुः |
| 2 | वेत्सि | वित्थः | वित्थ | अवेः / अवेत् | अवित्तम् | अवित्त |
| 1 | वेद्मि | विद्वः | विद्मः | अवेदम् | अविद्व | अविद्म |

| | Imperative | | | Optative | | |
|---|---|---|---|---|---|---|
| | Singular | Dual | Plural | Singular | Dual | Plural |
| 3 | वेत्तु | वित्ताम् | विदन्तु | विद्यात् | विद्याताम् | विद्युः |
| 2 | विद्धि | वित्तम् | वित्त | विद्याः | विद्यातम् | विद्यात |
| 1 | वेदानि | वेदाव | वेदाम | विद्याम् | विद्याव | विद्याम |

### √इ 2P, to go

| | Present Tense | | | Past Imperfect | | |
|---|---|---|---|---|---|---|
| | Singular | Dual | Plural | Singular | Dual | Plural |
| 3 | एति | इतः | यन्ति | ऐत् | ऐताम् | आयन् |
| 2 | एषि | इथः | इथ | ऐः | ऐतम् | ऐत |
| 1 | एमि | इवः | इमः | आयम् | ऐव | ऐम |

| | Imperative | | | Optative | | |
|---|---|---|---|---|---|---|
| | Singular | Dual | Plural | Singular | Dual | Plural |
| 3 | एतु | इताम् | यन्तु | इयात् | इयाताम् | इयुः |
| 2 | इहि | इतम् | इत | इयाः | इयातम् | इयात |
| 1 | अयानि | अयाव | अयाम | इयाम् | इयाव | इयाम |

**√आस् 2Ā, to sit**

| | Present Tense | | | Past Imperfect | | |
|---|---|---|---|---|---|---|
| | Singular | Dual | Plural | Singular | Dual | Plural |
| 3 | आस्ते | आसाते | आसते | आस्त | आसाताम् | आसत |
| 2 | आस्से | आसाथे | आद्ध्वे | आस्थाः | आसाथाम् | आस्ध्वम् |
| 1 | आसे | आस्वहे | आस्महे | आसि | आस्वहि | आस्महि |

| | Imperative | | | Optative | | |
|---|---|---|---|---|---|---|
| | Singular | Dual | Plural | Singular | Dual | Plural |
| 3 | आस्ताम् | आसाताम् | आसताम् | आसीत | आसीयाताम् | आसीरन् |
| 2 | आस्स्व | आसाथाम् | आस्ध्वम् | आसीथाः | आसीयाथाम् | आसीध्वम् |
| 1 | आसै | आसावहै | आसामहै | आसीय | आसीवहि | आसीमहि |

## Second Class Verbs

Difficult conjugations are given in parentheses in the present tense.

√अद् P, to eat (अत्ति अत्तः अदन्ति; अत्सि अत्थः अत्थ; अद्मि अद्वः अद्मः)
√ख्या P, to tell, narrate
√जागृ P, to be awake (जागर्ति जागृतः जाग्रति; जागर्षि जागृथः जागृथ; जागर्मि जागृवः जागृमः)
√द्विष् U, to hate (P: द्वेष्टि द्विष्टः द्विषन्ति; द्वेक्षि द्विष्ठः द्विष्ठ; द्वेष्मि द्विष्वः द्विष्मः)
√ब्रू U, to speak (P: ब्रवीति ब्रूतः ब्रुवन्ति; ब्रवीषि ब्रूथः ब्रुथ; ब्रवीमि ब्रूवः ब्रूमः)
√भा P, to shine
√या P, to go, move, proceed
√वच् P, to speak (वक्ति वक्तः वचन्ति; वक्षि वक्थः वक्थ; वच्मि वच्वः वच्मः)
√शास् P, to teach (शास्ति शिष्टः शासति; शाःसि शिष्ठः शिष्ठ; शास्मि शिष्वः शिष्मः)
√शी Ā, to lie, sleep (शेते शयाते शेरते; शेषे शयाथे शेध्वे; शये शेवहे शेमहे)
√श्वस् P, to breathe (श्वसिति श्वसितः श्वसन्ति; श्वसिषि श्वसिथः श्वसिथ; श्वसिमि श्वसिवः श्वसिमः)
√स्तु U, to praise (P: स्तौति स्तुतः स्तुवन्ति; स्तौषि स्तुथः स्तुथ; स्तौमि स्तुवः स्तुमः)
√स्ना P, to bathe
√स्वप् P, to sleep (स्वपिति स्वपितः स्वपन्ति; स्वपिषि स्वपिथः स्वपिथ; स्वपिमि स्वपिवः स्वपिमः)
√हन् P, to kill (हन्ति हतः घ्नन्ति; हंसि हथः हथ; हन्मि हन्वः हन्मः)

## Conjugate

√भा

## Translate

### D. "Truth"

सत्यं ब्रूयात्प्रियं ब्रूयान्न ब्रूयात्सत्यमप्रियम् ।
प्रियञ्च नानृतं ब्रूयातेष धर्मः सनातनः ॥

Vocabulary

प्रिय mfn. pleasant, agreeable
अप्रिय mfn. disagreeable, unkind
अनृतम् n. falsehood, lie
धर्मः m. law
सनातन mfn. eternal, ancient

### E. *Bhagavadgītā* 2.19

Note that both वेत्ति and मन्यते take two accusatives.

य एनं वेत्ति हन्तारं यश्चैनं मन्यते हतम् ।
उभौ तौ न विजानीतो नायं हन्ति न हन्यते ॥

Vocabulary

एनम् this [Soul] (m. acc. sg.)
हन्तृ mfn. a killer, slayer
हत mfn. slain, killed
उभ mfn. both
विजानीतः they both understand (3rd p. du. वि√जन्)
अयम् this [Soul] (m. nom. sg.)
हन्यते is killed, slain (3rd p. sg. passive √हन्)

### F. *Bhāgavatapurāṇa* 3.28.1

Having decided to teach his mother, Yaṣoda, yoga, Kṛṣṇa says . . .

योगस्य लक्षणं वक्ष्ये सबीजस्य नृपात्मजे ।
मनो येनैव विधिना प्रसन्नं याति सत्पथम् ॥

The *Bhāgavatapurāṇa*, or *Śrīmad Bhāgavatam*, written sometime between 500 and 1000 C.E., is a collection of stories and teachings attributed to Vyāsa that centers around *bhakti* or devotion to Lord Viṣṇu, particularly in his incarnation as Kṛṣṇa.

Vocabulary

लक्षणम् n. mark, sign, characteristic, attribute

सबीजः m. type of *samādhi* or meditative absorption in which some *samskāras* (past impressions) still exist, "with seed"

नृपात्मजा f. daughter of the king

नृपः m. king

मनः the mind (n. nom. sg.)

विधिः m. practice, method [of yoga]

प्रसन्न mfn. pure, bright, pleased, delighted

सत्पथम् the path of truth (m. acc. sg.)

G. *Bhagavadgītā* 2.69

या निशा सर्वभूतानां तस्यां जागर्ति संयमी ।
यस्यां जाग्रति भूतानि सा निशा पश्यतो मुनेः ॥

Vocabulary

निशा f. night

सर्वभूतानाम् of, for all beings (n. gen. pl.)

संयमी one who is absorbed in *saṃyama*, self-controlled (m. nom. sg.)

पश्यतः of, for the one [i.e., the sage] who sees (m. gen. sg.)

## THIRD CLASS VERBS

The third *gaṇa* of verbs is known as the reduplicative class. It is named after the root √हु, to sacrifice/offer. Like the second class, there is no *gaṇa* sign added between the root and the ending; however, the beginning of the root is repeated (exactly or with slight changes) in conjugation. Here, too, the root vowel takes गुण in strong forms. However, in all forms, in the reduplicated syllable, the root vowel appears in its short form. Note that in all third-person plural forms, the न् disappears.

## GENERAL RULES OF REDUPLICATION (ABHYĀSA)

The rules of reduplication given on the following page apply in all other instances of reduplication too—the perfect and the reduplicated aorist—which will be elaborated on in Part III.

The word *abhyāsa*, used for reduplication, literally means "repetition." It is the same word used for "practice" in yoga texts.

1. Only the first part of the root, ending with the root vowel, is reduplicated.
   √युज् ⇒ युयुज्

2. If the original root vowel is long, it is shortened in the reduplicating syllable.
   √दा ⇒ ददा

3. An initial aspirated consonant is reduplicated by its corresponding nonaspirated consonant.
   √धा ⇒ दधा
   √भी ⇒ बिभी

4. The vowel ऋ changes to इ in reduplication.
   √भृ ⇒ बिभृ

5. Roots beginning with ह् change to ज् in reduplication.
   √हु ⇒ जुहु

**√दा 3U, to give**

**Parasmaipada**

| | Present Tense | | | Past Imperfect | | |
|---|---|---|---|---|---|---|
| | Singular | Dual | Plural | Singular | Dual | Plural |
| 3 | ददाति | दत्तः | ददति | अददात् | अदत्ताम् | अददुः |
| 2 | ददासि | दत्थः | दत्थ | अददाः | अदत्तम् | अदत्त |
| 1 | ददामि | दद्वः | दद्मः | अददाम् | अदद्व | अदद्म |

| | Imperative | | | Optative | | |
|---|---|---|---|---|---|---|
| | Singular | Dual | Plural | Singular | Dual | Plural |
| 3 | ददातु | दत्ताम् | ददतु | दद्यात् | दद्याताम् | दद्युः |
| 2 | देहि | दत्तम् | दत्त | दद्याः | दद्यातम् | दद्यात |
| 1 | ददानि | ददाव | ददाम | दद्याम् | दद्याव | दद्याम |

**Ātmanepada**

| | Present Tense | | | Past Imperfect | | |
|---|---|---|---|---|---|---|
| | Singular | Dual | Plural | Singular | Dual | Plural |
| 3 | दत्ते | ददाते | ददते | अदत्त | अददाताम् | अददत |
| 2 | दत्से | ददाथे | दद्ध्वे | अदत्थाः | अददाथाम् | अदद्ध्वम् |
| 1 | ददे | दद्वहे | दद्महे | अददि | अदद्वहि | अदद्महि |

| | Imperative | | | Optative | | |
|---|---|---|---|---|---|---|
| | Singular | Dual | Plural | Singular | Dual | Plural |
| 3 | दत्ताम् | ददाताम् | ददताम् | ददीत | ददीयाताम् | ददीरन् |
| 2 | दत्स्व | ददाथाम् | दद्ध्वम् | ददीथाः | ददीयाथाम् | ददीध्वम् |
| 1 | ददै | ददावहै | ददामहै | ददीय | ददीवहि | ददीमहि |

## √भृ 3U, to support, hold

### Parasmaipada

| | Present Tense | | | Past Imperfect | | |
|---|---|---|---|---|---|---|
| | Singular | Dual | Plural | Singular | Dual | Plural |
| 3 | बिभर्ति | बिभृतः | बिभ्रति | *अबिभः | अबिभृताम् | अबिभरुः |
| 2 | बिभर्षि | बिभृथः | बिभृथ | *अबिभः | अबिभृतम् | अबिभृत |
| 1 | बिभर्मि | बिभृवः | बिभृमः | अबिभरम् | अबिभृव | अबिभृम |

*The final त् and स् become र् which becomes *visarga*.

| | Imperative | | | Optative | | |
|---|---|---|---|---|---|---|
| | Singular | Dual | Plural | Singular | Dual | Plural |
| 3 | बिभर्तु | बिभृताम् | बिभ्रतु | बिभृयात् | बिभृयाताम् | बिभृयुः |
| 2 | बिभृहि | बिभृतम् | बिभृत | बिभृयाः | बिभृयातम् | बिभृयात |
| 1 | बिभराणि | बिभराव | बिभराम | बिभृयाम् | बिभृयाव | बिभृयाम |

### Ātmanepada

| | Present Tense | | | Past Imperfect | | |
|---|---|---|---|---|---|---|
| | Singular | Dual | Plural | Singular | Dual | Plural |
| 3 | बिभृते | बिभ्राते | बिभ्रते | अबिभृत | अबिभ्राताम् | अबिभ्रत |
| 2 | बिभृषे | बिभ्राथे | बिभृध्वे | अबिभृथाः | अबिभ्राथाम् | अबिभृध्वम् |
| 1 | बिभ्रे | बिभृवहे | बिभृमहे | अबिभ्रि | अबिभृवहि | अबिभृमहि |

| | Imperative | | | Optative | | |
|---|---|---|---|---|---|---|
| | Singular | Dual | Plural | Singular | Dual | Plural |
| 3 | बिभृताम् | बिभ्राताम् | बिभ्रताम् | बिभ्रीत | बिभ्रीयाताम् | बिभ्रीरन् |
| 2 | बिभृष्व | बिभ्राथाम् | बिभृध्वम् | बिभ्रीथाः | बिभ्रीयाथाम् | बिभ्रीध्वम् |
| 1 | बिभरै | बिभरावहै | बिभरामहै | बिभ्रीय | बिभ्रीवहि | बिभ्रीमहि |

### √हु 3P, to sacrifice, to offer an oblation

| | Present Tense | | | Past Imperfect | | |
|---|---|---|---|---|---|---|
| | Singular | Dual | Plural | Singular | Dual | Plural |
| 3 | जुहोति | जुहुतः | जुह्वति | अजुहोत् | अजुहुताम् | अजुहवुः |
| 2 | जुहोषि | जुहुथः | जुहुथ | अजुहोः | अजुहुतम् | अजुहुत |
| 1 | जुहोमि | जुहुवः | जुहुमः | अजुहवम् | अजुहुव | अजुहुम |

| | Imperative | | | Optative | | |
|---|---|---|---|---|---|---|
| | Singular | Dual | Plural | Singular | Dual | Plural |
| 3 | जुहोतु | जुहुताम् | जुहवतु | जुहुयात् | जुहुयाताम् | जुहुयुः |
| 2 | जुहुधि | जुहुतम् | जुहुत | जुहुयाः | जुहुयातम् | जुहुयात |
| 1 | जुहवानि | जुहवाव | जुहवाम | जुहुयाम् | जुहुयाव | जुहुयाम |

## Third Class Verbs

√धा U, to put, place, create, make, compose
√भी P, to fear, be afraid of
√मा Ā, to measure
√हा U, to leave, abandon

## Conjugate

√धा, √भी

## Translate

### H. *Bhagavadgītā* 4.29

This verse comes in a sequence of verses explaining different kinds of sacrifices performed by yogīs. The subject is in the second *pāda*.

अपाने <u>जुह्वति</u> प्राणं प्राणेऽपानं तथापरे ।
प्राणापानगती रुद्ध्वा प्राणायामपरायणाः ॥

Vocabulary

अपानः m. exhalation
प्राणः m. inhalation
प्राणापानगती the movement of the inhalation and exhalation (f. acc. du.)
रुद्ध्वा restraining, stopping (gerund √रुध्)
प्राणायामपरायणः m. intent upon/completely focused on control of the breath

### I. *Bhagavadgītā* 11.8

Arjuna has just asked Kṛṣṇa to see his divine form. Kṛṣṇa tells him to look at his manifold forms.

न तु मां शक्यसे द्रष्टुमनेनैव स्वचक्षुषा ।
दिव्यं ददामि ते चक्षुः पश्य मे योगमैश्वरम् ॥

Vocabulary

शक्यसे you are able (2nd p. sg. passive √शक्)
अनेन with this (n. inst. sg.)
स्वचक्षुषा with your own eye (n. inst. sg.)
चक्षुः eye, sight (n. acc.sg.)
दिव्य mfn. divine
ऐश्वर mfn. powerful, majestic

### J. *Bhagavadgītā* 2.50

बुद्धियुक्तो जहातीह उभे सुकृतदुष्कृते ।
तस्माद्योगाय युज्यस्व योगः कर्मसु कौशलम् ॥

Vocabulary

बुद्धियुक्त mfn. one who is absorbed in understanding, yoked to wisdom/discernment
सुकृतदुष्कृते good and evil actions (n. acc. du.)
युज्यस्व Yoke yourself to! Unite yourself with! Absorb yourself in! (takes the dative) (2nd p. passive imperative √युज्)
कर्मसु in action (n. loc. sg.)
कौशलम् n. skillfulness, ease

### K. *Haṭhapradīpikā* 1.3

भ्रान्त्या बहुमतध्वान्ते राजयोगमजानताम् ।
हठप्रदीपिकां धत्ते स्वात्मरामः कृपाकरः ॥

Vocabulary

भ्रान्तिः f. wandering or roaming about
बहुमतध्वान्तम् n. the darkness of too many different opinions
    बहु mfn. much, many
    मतम् n. thought, opinion, belief
    ध्वान्तम् n. darkness
अजानताम् of/for those who do not know, are unaware (m. gen. sg.)
हठप्रदीपिका f. light/lamp on *haṭhayoga*
कृपाकरः m. very compassionate

## Review Exercises

### L. *Śivasaṃhitā* 1.61

बाह्यानि सर्वभूतानि विनाशं यान्ति कालतः।
यतो वाचो निवर्तन्ते आत्मा द्वैतविवर्जितः॥

#### Vocabulary

बाह्य mfn. outer part, exterior
सर्वभूतम् n. all beings
  भूतम् n. living being
विनाशः m. destruction, death
कालतः ind. in the course of time
यतः ind. from which, wherefore, for which reason, but
नि√वृत् 1Ā, to disappear, be ineffective, vanish, not exist
आत्मा the Soul (m. nom. sg.)
द्वैतविवर्जितः m. free from duality
  द्वैतम् n. duality
  विवर्जित mfn. free from

### M. *Vivekamārtaṇḍa* 112

आसनेन रुजो हन्ति प्राणायामेन पातकम्।
विकारं मानसं योगी प्रत्याहारेण मुञ्चति॥

#### Vocabulary

रुज् mfn. pain, illness, disease
पातकम् n. sin, crime, vice
विकारः m. disturbances, diseases
मानस mfn. pertaining to the mind, mental, spiritual
योगी the yogī (m. nom. sg.)
√मुच् 6U, to let go, free oneself of

The *Vivekamārtaṇḍa*, composed around the twelfth to thirteenth century C.E., teaches a *ṣaḍaṅga* or six-limbed yoga, which omits *yama* and *niyama*. Drawing from tantric Śaiva traditions, it refers to various *mudrās*, *bandhas*, *āsanas*, and *prāṇāyāmas*.

N. *Śivasaṃhitā* 3.34

अथ वर्ज्यं प्रवक्ष्यामि योगविघ्नकरं परम्।
येन संसारदुःखाब्धिं तीर्त्वा यास्यन्ति योगिनः॥

Vocabulary
अथ ind. now (a particle used at the beginning, mostly as a sign of auspiciousness)
वर्ज्य mfn. to be avoided
योगविघ्नकर mfn. obstacles to yoga
परम् ind. highest, supreme
संसारदुःखाब्धिः m. the ocean of the suffering of cyclic existence
  संसारः m. cyclic existence
  अब्धिः m. ocean, receptacle of water
√तॄ 1P, to cross over
योगिनः yogīs (m. nom. pl.)

# 9
# Nouns Ending in अन्; Verb Conjugations: Fifth and Eighth Class; Quotations and the Particle इति

**मृदुमध्याधिमात्रत्वात्ततोऽपि विशेषः ॥ १.२२ ॥**
**mṛdu-madhyādhimātratvāt tato 'pi viśeṣaḥ**
Therefore, even among those who apply themselves intensely, there is differentiation between mild, medium, and intense.
॥ *Yogasūtra* 1.22 ॥

## NOUNS ENDING IN अन्

Some nouns ending in consonants can have a strong, weak, and middle stem, depending on which ending follows. All nouns ending in -अन् are either masculine or neuter. The strong stem usually ends in -आन्, although the न् is dropped in the nominative singular and the stem is preserved intact in the vocative singular. The middle stem ends in -अ and precedes endings beginning with vowels. The weak stem ends in -न् or -अन् if the second consonant is part of a conjunct.

**Masculine Nouns—strong forms:**

Nominative—singular, dual, and plural
Accusative—singular and dual
Vocative—singular, dual, and plural

**Neuter Nouns—strong forms:**

Nominative—plural
Accusative—plural
Vocative—plural

Note below that strong forms are in red, weak stems in blue, and middle stems in black.

**आत्मन् m. the Soul, individual Soul, Self**

| | Singular | Dual | Plural |
|---|---|---|---|
| **Nominative** | आत्मा | आत्मानौ | आत्मानः |
| **Accusative** | आत्मानम् | आत्मानौ | आत्मनः |
| **Instrumental** | आत्मना | आत्मभ्याम् | आत्मभिः |
| **Dative** | आत्मने | आत्मभ्याम् | आत्मभ्यः |

| | | | |
|---|---|---|---|
| **Ablative** | आत्मनः | आत्मभ्याम् | आत्मभ्यः |
| **Genitive** | आत्मनः | आत्मनोः | आत्मनाम् |
| **Locative** | आत्मनि | आत्मनोः | आत्मसु |
| **Vocative** | आत्मन् | आत्मानौ | आत्मानः |

**राजन् m. king**

| | Singular | Dual | Plural |
|---|---|---|---|
| **Nominative** | राजा | राजानौ | राजानः |
| **Accusative** | राजानम् | राजानौ | राज्ञः |
| **Instrumental** | राज्ञा | राजभ्याम् | राजभिः |
| **Dative** | राज्ञे | राजभ्याम् | राजभ्यः |
| **Ablative** | राज्ञः | राजभ्याम् | राजभ्यः |
| **Genitive** | राज्ञः | राज्ञोः | राज्ञाम् |
| **Locative** | राज्ञि / राजनि | राज्ञोः | राजसु |
| **Vocative** | राजन् | राजानौ | राजानः |

**कर्मन् n. action**

| | Singular | Dual | Plural |
|---|---|---|---|
| **Nominative** | कर्म | कर्मणी | कर्माणि |
| **Accusative** | कर्म | कर्मणी | कर्माणि |
| **Instrumental** | कर्मणा | कर्मभ्याम् | कर्मभिः |
| **Dative** | कर्मणे | कर्मभ्याम् | कर्मभ्यः |
| **Ablative** | कर्मणः | कर्मभ्याम् | कर्मभ्यः |
| **Genitive** | कर्मणः | कर्मणोः | कर्मणाम् |
| **Locative** | कर्मणि | कर्मणोः | कर्मसु |
| **Vocative** | कर्मन् / कर्म | कर्मणी | कर्माणि |

Vocabulary

**नामन्** n. name
**ब्रह्मन्** n. universal Spirit
**मूर्धन्** m. head
**वार्त्मन्** n. path

## Decline

**ब्रह्मन्, मूर्धन्**

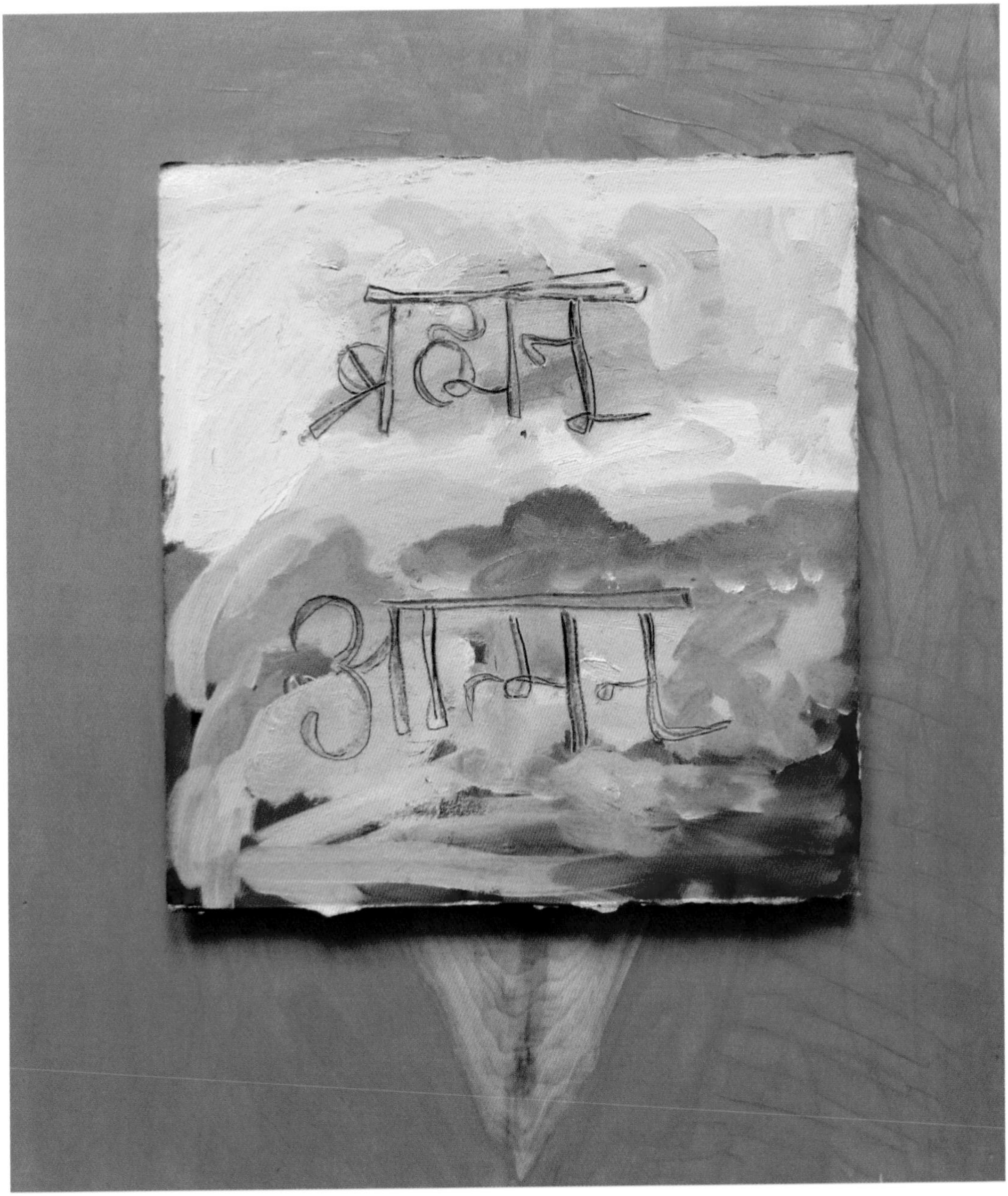


The equation of आत्मन् and ब्रह्मन्, between the individual, worldly, earthy, embodied Soul and the universal, transcendent Spirit, is at the heart of all of the *Upaniṣads*.

## Translate

### A. *Bhagavadgītā* 2.47

कर्मण्येवाधिकारस्ते मा फलेषु कदाचन ।
मा कर्मफलहेतुर्भूर्मा ते सङ्गोऽस्त्वकर्मणि ॥

Vocabulary
अधिकारः m. authority, right
मा ind. not
फलम् n. fruit
कदाचन ind. at any time
कर्मफलहेतुः m. the motive of fruits of action
  हेतुः m. motive, cause
मा भूः never should it be/arise (3rd p. sg. injunctive aorist)
सङ्गः m. association, attachment, desire
अकर्मन् m. inaction

### B. *Bhagavadgītā* 6.5

उद्धरेदात्मनात्मानं नात्मानमवसादयेत् ।
आत्मैव ह्यात्मनो बन्धुरात्मैव रिपुरात्मनः ॥

Vocabulary
उद्√धृ 1P, to raise up, uplift
अवसादयेत् one should cause to sink down/become disheartened (3rd p. sg. caus. optative अव√सद्)
बन्धुः m. friend
रिपुः m. enemy

### C. *Bhagavadgītā* 4.24

This prayer is often recited before eating a meal. It compares the eating of a meal to the Vedic fire sacrifice, analogizing between the eater and the priest, the act of eating and the act of sacrifice, the eaten and the sacrifice, and the digestive fire and the sacrificial fire.

ब्रह्मार्पणं ब्रह्म हविर्ब्रह्माग्नौ ब्रह्मणा हुतम् ।
ब्रह्मैव तेन गन्तव्यं ब्रह्मकर्मसमाधिना ॥

Vocabulary

अर्पणम् n. offering, the act of offering, entrusting
हविस् n. oblation, burnt offering
ब्रह्माग्निः m. the fire of *Brahman*/Spirit
हुत mfn. offered, poured out into the fire
गन्तव्य mfn. to be attained
ब्रह्मकर्मसमाधिना by one who is absorbed in the action of *Brahman*/Spirit (m. inst. sg.)

## FIFTH CLASS VERBS

The fifth *gaṇa* is named for the root √सु, "to press out." Fifth *gaṇa* verbs add नु as a suffix to the root. In strong forms, this suffix takes गुण and नु becomes नो. Before an ending beginning with a vowel, उ becomes व् or उव् and नो becomes नव्.

**√आप् 5P, to get, obtain**

| | Present Tense | | | Past Imperfect | | |
|---|---|---|---|---|---|---|
| | Singular | Dual | Plural | Singular | Dual | Plural |
| 3 | आप्नोति | आप्नुतः | आप्नुवन्ति | आप्नोत् | आप्नुताम् | आप्नुवन् |
| 2 | आप्नोषि | आप्नुथः | आप्नुथ | आप्नोः | आप्नुतम् | आप्नुत |
| 1 | आप्नोमि | आप्नुवः | आप्नुमः | आप्नवम् | आप्नुव | आप्नुम |

| | Imperative | | | Optative | | |
|---|---|---|---|---|---|---|
| | Singular | Dual | Plural | Singular | Dual | Plural |
| 3 | आप्नोतु | आप्नुताम् | आप्नुवन्तु | आप्नुयात् | आप्नुयाताम् | आप्नुयुः |
| 2 | आप्नुहि | आप्नुतम् | आप्नुत | आप्नुयाः | आप्नुयातम् | आप्नुयात |
| 1 | आप्नवानि | आप्नवाव | आप्नवाम | आप्नुयाम् | आप्नुयाव | आप्नुयाम |

**√अश् 5Ā, to eat, enjoy, obtain**

| | Present Tense | | | Past Imperfect | | |
|---|---|---|---|---|---|---|
| | Singular | Dual | Plural | Singular | Dual | Plural |
| 3 | अश्नुते | अश्नुवाते | अश्नुवते | आश्नुत | आश्नुवाताम् | आश्नुवत |
| 2 | अश्नुषे | अश्नुवाथे | अश्नुध्वे | आश्नुथाः | आश्नुवाथाम् | आश्नुध्वम् |
| 1 | अश्नुवे | अश्नुवहे | अश्नुमहे | आश्नुवि | आश्नुवहि | आश्नुमहि |

| | Imperative | | | Optative | | |
|---|---|---|---|---|---|---|
| | Singular | Dual | Plural | Singular | Dual | Plural |
| 3 | अश्नुताम् | अश्नुवाताम् | अश्नुवताम् | अश्नुवीत | अश्नुवीयाताम् | अश्नुवीरन् |
| 2 | अश्नुष्व | अश्नुवाथाम् | अश्नुध्वम् | अश्नुवीथाः | अश्नुवीयाथाम् | अश्नुवीध्वम् |
| 1 | अश्नवै | अश्नवावहै | अश्नवामहै | अश्नुवीय | अश्नुवीवहि | अश्नुवीमहि |

## Fifth Class Verbs

√शक् P, to be able or capable
√श्रु P, to hear, listen
√सु U, to press out, extract

## Conjugate

√शक्

## Translate

### D. *Haṭhapradīpikā* 1.64

युवा वृद्धोऽतिवृद्धो वा व्याधितो दुर्बलोऽपि वा।
अभ्यासात्सिद्धिमाप्नोति सर्वयोगेष्वतन्द्रितः॥

Vocabulary
युवन् m. youth, young
वृद्ध mfn. old
अतिवृद्ध mfn. very old
व्याधित mfn. sick, afflicted with disease
दुर्बल mfn. weak
सर्वयोग m. all yoga
अतन्द्रित mfn. free from lassitude, unwearied, vigilant, alert, not lazy

### E. *Bhagavadgītā* 3.4

न कर्मणामनारम्भान्नैष्कर्म्यं पुरुषोऽश्नुते।
न च संन्यसनादेव सिद्धिं समधिगच्छति॥

Vocabulary
अनारम्भः m. noncommencement, not undertaking
नैष्कर्म्यम् n. inactivity, exemption from acts and their consequences

संन्यसनम् n. renunciation
समधि√गम् 1P, go toward, approach

F. *Dattātreyayogaśāstra* 41–2ab

The construction "*vā* . . . *vā* . . ." means "whether a . . . or . . . or . . ."

ब्राह्मणः श्रमणो वापि बौद्धो वाप्यार्हतोऽथवा ।
कापालिको वा चार्वाकः श्रद्धया सहितः सुधीः ॥
योगाभ्यासरतो नित्यं सर्वसिद्धिमवाप्नुयात् ।

Vocabulary
श्रमणः m. ascetic, devotee
बौद्धः m. Buddhist
अर्हत् m. Jain
कापालिकः m. follower of a particular Śaiva sect that carries skulls
चार्वाकः m. follower of Cārvāka, a philosopher who propounded materialism
सहित mfn. possessed of, accompanied by
सुधीः wise person (m. nom. sg.)
योगाभ्यासरतः m. delighting in/intent upon/devoted to the practice of yoga
सर्वसिद्धिः f. complete fulfillment/attainment/perfection

## EIGHTH CLASS VERBS

The eighth *gaṇa* is named for the root √तन्, "to stretch," and is conjugated similarly to the fifth *gaṇa*. The eighth *gaṇa* adds उ as a suffix to the root. In strong forms, this suffix takes गुण and उ becomes ओ. Before an ending beginning with a vowel, उ becomes व् and ओ becomes अव्.

√कृ is one of the most commonly encountered roots and is slightly irregular.

**√कृ 8U, to do, make**

| | Parasmaipada | | | | | |
|---|---|---|---|---|---|---|
| | Present Tense | | | Past Imperfect | | |
| | Singular | Dual | Plural | Singular | Dual | Plural |
| 3 | करोति | कुरुतः | कुर्वन्ति | अकरोत् | अकुरुताम् | अकुर्वन् |
| 2 | करोषि | कुरुथः | कुरुथ | अकरोः | अकुरुतम् | अकुरुत |
| 1 | करोमि | कुर्वः | कुर्मः | अकरवम् | अकुर्व | अकुर्म |

| | Imperative | | | Optative | | |
|---|---|---|---|---|---|---|
| | Singular | Dual | Plural | Singular | Dual | Plural |
| 3 | करोतु | कुरुताम् | कुर्वन्तु | कुर्यात् | कुर्याताम् | कुर्युः |
| 2 | कुरु | कुरुतम् | कुरुत | कुर्याः | कुर्यातम् | कुर्यात |
| 1 | करवाणि | करवाव | करवाम | कुर्याम् | कुर्याव | कुर्याम |

Ātmanepada

| | Present Tense | | | Past Imperfect | | |
|---|---|---|---|---|---|---|
| | Singular | Dual | Plural | Singular | Dual | Plural |
| 3 | कुरुते | कुर्वाते | कुर्वते | अकुरुत | अकुर्वाताम् | अकुर्वत |
| 2 | कुरुषे | कुर्वाथे | कुरुध्वे | अकुरुथाः | अकुर्वाथाम् | अकुरुध्वम् |
| 1 | कुर्वे | कुर्वहे | कुर्महे | अकुर्वि | अकुर्वहि | अकुर्महि |

| | Imperative | | | Optative | | |
|---|---|---|---|---|---|---|
| | Singular | Dual | Plural | Singular | Dual | Plural |
| 3 | कुरुताम् | कुर्वाताम् | कुर्वताम् | कुर्वीत | कुर्वीयाताम् | कुर्वीरन् |
| 2 | कुरुष्व | कुर्वाथाम् | कुरुध्वम् | कुर्वीथाः | कुर्वीयाथाम् | कुर्वीध्वम् |
| 1 | करवै | करवावहै | करवामहै | कुर्वीय | कर्वीवहि | कुर्वीमहि |

## EIGHTH CLASS VERBS

√तन् U, to extend, stretch
√मन् Ā, to think, consider

### Conjugate

√तन्

### Translate

#### G. *Bhagavadgītā* 9.27

यत्करोषि यदश्नासि यज्जुहोषि ददासि यत्।
यत्तपस्यसि कौन्तेय तत्कुरुष्व मदपर्णम्॥

Vocabulary

यद् n. acc. sg. whatever
√तपस्य 10P, to undergo religious austerities
मदपर्णम् n. an offering to me

### H. *Gheraṇḍasaṃhitā* 5.3

दूरदेशे तथारण्ये राजधान्यां जनान्तिके ।
योगारम्भं न कुर्वीत कृतश्चेत्सिद्धिहा भवेत् ॥

> The yogī should practice in a place that is isolated and away from people and disturbances, but not so remote that necessities such as food and water are difficult to obtain.

Vocabulary

दूरदेशः m. remote place
  दूर mfn. distant, remote
राजधानी f. the king's residence, the capital, metropolis
  धानी f. receptacle, seat, home
जनान्तिकम् n. near people, in the vicinity of people
  अन्तिकम् n. vicinity, proximity, near
योगारम्भः m. beginning of yoga practice
  आरम्भः m. beginning, commencement, undertaking
कृत mfn. done
सिद्धिहा f. devoid of fulfillment

## THE QUOTATIVE PARTICLE इति

To illustrate a quotation, rather than punctuation marks, the particle इति is used at the end of the quote in order to set off a separate sentence—the quotation—within a longer sentence. It is often followed by some version of the verb √वच्, "to say," or √मन्, "to think." It can also be used to mean "thus" or to mark a cause.

> The *Kaṭhopaniṣat*, also known as the *Kāṭhaka Upaniṣad*, was probably composed in the last few centuries B.C.E. and is one of the oldest texts that speak of yoga. Written in verse form, it tells the story of Naciketas's encounter with Death. By fearlessly interacting with and questioning Death, Naciketas moves beyond the fear of death and thus is able to know his true self.

### Example: *Kaṭhopaniṣat* 6.11

तां योगमिति मन्यन्ते स्थिरामिन्द्रियधारणाम् ।
अप्रमत्तस्तदा भवति योगो हि प्रभवाप्ययौ ॥

Vocabulary

इन्द्रियधारणा f. restraint of the senses
अप्रमत्त mfn. not careless or inattentive, careful, attentive
प्रभवाप्ययौ origin and dissolution (m. nom. du.)
  प्रभवः m. origin, birth
  अप्ययः m. entering into, vanishing, absorption, dissolution

"That (ताम्) is yoga (योगम्)," (इति) [people] think (मन्यन्ते),
When the restraint of the senses (इन्द्रियधारणाम्) is steady (स्थिराम्).
[One] then (तदा) becomes (भवति) attentive (अप्रमत्तः),
For (हि) yoga (योगः) is both the origin and the dissolution (प्रभवाप्ययौ).

## Translate

### I. *Bhagavadgītā* 3.28

The previous verse speaks of those who are attached to their actions. The subject is "[one] who knows the truth."

तत्त्ववित्तु महाबाहो गुणकर्मविभागयोः ।
गुणा गुणेषु वर्तन्त इति मत्वा न सज्जते ॥

Vocabulary

तत्त्ववित् mfn. knowing the true nature/truth
तत्त्वम् n. real truth, true nature
गुणकर्मविभागयोः of the role of the three qualities and their actions (m. gen. du., read with तत्त्ववित्)
विभागः m. share, division, role
√सञ्ज् 1U, to be attached

### J. *Bhagavadgītā* 15.20

इति गुह्यतमं शास्त्रमिदमुक्तं मयानघ ।
एतद्बुद्ध्वा बुद्धिमान्स्यात्कृतकृत्यश्च भारत ॥

Vocabulary

गुह्यतमम् n. most hidden, secret
इदम् this (n. nom. sg.)
उक्त mfn. spoken, taught
अनघः m. faultless, sinless
बुद्धिमान् endowed with understanding, wise (m. nom. sg.)
कृतकृत्य mfn. one who has done his duties, one who has attained any object or purpose

इति is also the first half of the word इतिहास, literally meaning "so, indeed, it was." It is used to denote history or legend, and is implicitly acknowledged as subjective, since, by definition, it is quoted by someone.

## Review Exercises

K. *Yogatattvopaniṣat* 71

जिह्वया यद्रसं ह्यत्ति तत्तदात्मेति भावयेत्।
त्वचा यद्यत्स्पृशेद्योगी तत्तदात्मेति भावयेत्॥

This verse is speaking of what happens in the state of *pratyāhāra*, sensory withdrawal. Whatever object or person one looks at, one sees the same divine essence.

Vocabulary

जिह्वा f. tongue
भावयेत् may one consider (3rd p. sg. causative optative √भू)
योगी the yogī (m. nom. sg.)

L. *Haṭhapradīpikā* 1.29

The previous verse describes how to practice *paścimatānāsana*.

इति पश्चिमतानमासनाग्र्यं पवनं पश्चिमवाहिनं करोति।
उदयं जठरानलस्य कुर्यादुदरे कार्श्यमरोगतां च पुंसाम्॥

Vocabulary

पश्चिमतानः m. *paścimatānāsana*, stretch of the western part of the body (i.e., the back)
आसनाग्र्य mfn. the foremost among postures
    अग्र्य mfn. foremost
पवनः m. vital air, breath
पश्चिमवाहिन mfn. causing to flow in the back of the body
उदयः m. rise up, increase
जठरानलः m. abdominal fire
    जठरम् n. stomach, belly, abdomen
    अनलः m. fire
उदरम् n. belly, stomach
कार्श्यम् n. thinness
अरोगता f. health, the state of being disease-free
पुंसाम् for man, for human beings (m. gen. sg.)

पश्चिमतानासन (*Paścimatānāsana*) is often considered to have its name because traditionally, one practices yoga facing the rising sun in the east. When one bends forward in this posture, one's back, or western side, is brought to face the sun.

M. *Haṭhapradīpikā* 2.37

This verse provides an alternative view to the previous fifteen verses, which describe and advocate practicing the *ṣaṭkarman.*

प्राणायामैरेव सर्वे प्रशुष्यन्ति मला इति ।
आचार्याणां तु केषाञ्चिदन्यत्कर्म न संमतम् ॥

Vocabulary
प्र√शुष् 4P, to dry up, be extinguished, eliminated
केषाञ्चिद् ind. of some
संमत mfn. agreed or consented to, approved of

अन्यत्कर्म here refers to the *ṣaṭkarman*, or six cleansing rituals. These rituals (to be learned only from a teacher!) are *dhauti* (swallowing a cloth and drawing it back out in order to cleanse the digestive tract), *vasti/basti* (enema), *neti* (cleansing the nasal passages with a thread), *nauli* (revolving the stomach), *trāṭaka* (fixing the eyes on one point or candle flame), and *kapālabhāti* ("shining skull" breath, consisting of short, forceful exhalations).

N. *Mahābhārata* 12.289.12

In the last two *pādas*, the subject is "[those practicing] the yogas, i.e., the yogīs."

यथा चानिमिषाः स्थूला जालं छित्त्वा पुनर्जलम् ।
प्राप्नुवन्ति तथा योगास्तत्पदं वीतकल्मषाः ॥

Vocabulary
अनिमिषः m. a fish
स्थूल mfn. large, big
जालम् n. a net
पुनर् ind. again
तत्पदम् n. that state [of liberation]
वीतकल्मषाः whose impurities are gone, freed from sins (m. nom. pl.)
कल्मषम् n. stain, dirt, impurity, sin

The *Mahābhārata* contains more than 100,000 verses in its longest recension and is approximately ten times the length of the *Iliad* and the *Odyssey* put together. Originating somewhere around the ninth to eighth century B.C.E., it most likely reached its final form around the fourth century C.E. It is said that Vyāsa dictated the entire text to Gaṇeśa, who acted as scribe, under the condition that Vyāsa narrate the entire text without pause. Vyāsa agreed, with his own condition that Gaṇeśa understand everything before writing it down.

# 10
# Nouns Ending in स्; Verb Conjugations: Seventh and Ninth Class; Causative Verbs

प्रकाशक्रियास्थितिशीलं भूतेन्द्रियात्मकं भोगापवर्गार्थं दृश्यम् ॥ २.१८ ॥
**prakāśa-kriyā-sthiti-śīlaṃ bhūtendriyātmakaṃ bhogāpavargārthaṃ dṛśyam**
That which is seen is characterized by illumination, activity, and stability and consists of the elements and the senses. Its purpose is experience and liberation.
|| *Yogasūtra* 2.18 ||

## NOUNS ENDING IN स्

The masculine and feminine paradigms for nouns ending in स् are identical; the neuter differs only in the nominative, accusative, and vocative forms. In the masculine and feminine, the stem vowel is lengthened in the nominative singular and the final स् becomes a *visarga* before consonant endings, leading to internal *sandhi* changes.

**वेधस् m. creator**

| | Singular | Dual | Plural |
|---|---|---|---|
| **Nominative** | वेधाः | वेधसौ | वेधसः |
| **Accusative** | वेधसम् | वेधसौ | वेधसः |
| **Instrumental** | वेधसा | वेधोभ्याम् | वेधोभिः |
| **Dative** | वेधसे | वेधोभ्याम् | वेधोभ्यः |
| **Ablative** | वेधसः | वेधोभ्याम् | वेधोभ्यः |
| **Genitive** | वेधसः | वेधसोः | वेधसाम् |
| **Locative** | वेधसि | वेधसोः | वेधःसु |
| **Vocative** | वेधः | वेधसौ | वेधसः |

**तपस् n. burning devotion, austerity, discipline**

| | Singular | Dual | Plural |
|---|---|---|---|
| **Nominative** | तपः | तपसी | तपांसि |
| **Accusative** | तपः | तपसी | तपांसि |
| **Instrumental** | तपसा | तपोभ्याम् | तपोभिः |
| **Dative** | तपसे | तपोभ्याम् | तपोभ्यः |
| **Ablative** | तपसः | तपोभ्याम् | तपोभ्यः |
| **Genitive** | तपसः | तपसोः | तपसाम् |
| **Locative** | तपसि | तपसोः | तपःसु |
| **Vocative** | तपः | तपसी | तपांसि |

**आयुस् n. life**

| | Singular | Dual | Plural |
|---|---|---|---|
| **Nominative** | आयुः | आयुषी | आयूंषि |
| **Accusative** | आयुः | आयुषी | आयूंषि |
| **Instrumental** | आयुषा | आयुर्भ्याम् | आयुर्भिः |
| **Dative** | आयुषे | आयुर्भ्याम् | आयुर्भ्यः |
| **Ablative** | आयुषः | आयुर्भ्याम् | आयुर्भ्यः |
| **Genitive** | आयुषः | आयुषोः | आयुषाम् |
| **Locative** | आयुषि | आयुषोः | आयुःषु |
| **Vocative** | आयुः | आयुषी | आयूंषि |

आयुस् is the root of the word आयुर्वेद, the traditional Indian medical system, literally "the science of life."

Vocabulary

अप्सरस् f. nymph
ओजस् n. vitality, energy, strength
चक्षुस् n. eye, seeing
चेतस् n. mind
ज्योतिस् n. light, star
तमस् n. inertia (one of the three *guṇas* or qualities of mind)
तेजस् n. splendor, brilliance
धनुस् m. bow
मनस् n. mind
यशस् n. fame
रजस् n. activity (one of the three *guṇas* or qualities of mind)
हविस् n. oblation

## Decline

धनुस्, मनस्, रजस्

## Translate

### A. *Bhagavadgītā* 5.11

कायेन मनसा बुद्ध्या केवलैरिन्द्रियैरपि ।
योगिनः कर्म कुर्वन्ति सङ्गं त्यक्त्वात्मशुद्धये ॥

Vocabulary
कायः m. body
केवल mfn. only, merely, solely
इन्द्रियम् n. faculty of sense, sense, sense organ
योगिनः yogīs (m. nom. pl.)
आत्मशुद्धिः f. purification of the self, true knowledge of Soul
शुद्धिः f. purification, true knowledge

### B. *Praśnopaniṣat* 2.12

This verse comes in a series of verses that form a hymn to *prāṇa*, "the life force," or "breath." ते, "your," refers to *prāṇa*. The word तनूः is implied with each repetition of the word या in the second and third *pādas*.

या ते तनूर्वाचि प्रतिष्ठिता या श्रोत्रे या च चक्षुषि ।
या च मनसि सन्तता शिवां तां कुरु मोत्क्रमीः ॥

Vocabulary
तनूः f. form, body, self, manifestation
प्रतिष्ठित mfn. is situated, resides in
श्रोत्रम् n. ear, act of hearing
सन्तत mfn. extended, stretched
शिव mfn. auspicious, favorable, benevolent
मा उत्क्रमीः Don't go away! (second p. sg. inj. aorist उत्√क्रम्)

The *Praśnopaniṣat* is among the latest of the early prose *upaniṣads*, composed around the beginning of the Common Era, and is associated with the *Atharva Veda*. It consists of six *praśnas* or questions asked by six different Brahmins and the sage Pippalāda's answers to them, revolving around themes such as the origins of the universe, *prāṇa*, and *Brahman*.

### C. *Yogavāsiṣṭha* 2.16.10

यः स्नातः शीतसितया साधुसंगतिगङ्गया ।
किं तस्य दानैः किं तीर्थैः किं तपोभिः किमध्वरैः ॥

Vocabulary

स्नात mfn. bathed
शीतसिता f. cool and bright
  शीत mfn. cold, cool
  सित mfn. bright
साधुसंगतिगङ्गा f. the river *Gaṅgā*, meeting place of sages
  साधुः m. sage, seer
  संगतिः f. meeting
दानम् n. donation
तीर्थम् n. pilgrimage, bathing place
अध्वरः m. sacrifice

Written and expanded from the tenth to fourteenth century C.E., the *Yogavāsiṣṭha* is an *Advaita Vedantin* text of epic length, attributed to the sage Vālmīki. It precedes the story of the *Rāmāyaṇa*, recounting a dialogue lasting many days between the sage Vāsiṣṭha and the young prince Rāma. Rāma, feeling disillusioned upon seeing the state of the world, is consoled by Vāsiṣṭha, who answers his many questions, tells him stories, and discusses the true nature of reality, explaining to him that his feeling of detachment is a necessary step on the path to liberation.

## SEVENTH CLASS VERBS

The seventh *gaṇa* is named for the root √रुध्, "to obstruct." The roots of the seventh *gaṇa* all end in consonants. Rather than added to the end of the verbal root, the *gaṇa* sign is placed inside the root after the vowel. In strong forms this *gaṇa* sign is न and in weak forms it is न्.

The word किम् is used with a word in the instrumental case to mean "What is the use of, what is the need for, what good is it?"

For example, किं तीर्थैः

"What is the use of pilgrimage?"

**√युज् 7U, to join, yoke, unite, engage**

√युज् is the root of the word योग.

Parasmaipaida

| | Present Tense | | | Past Imperfect | | |
|---|---|---|---|---|---|---|
| | Singular | Dual | Plural | Singular | Dual | Plural |
| 3 | युनक्ति | युङ्क्तः | युञ्जन्ति | अयुनक् | अयुङ्क्ताम् | अयुञ्जन् |
| 2 | युनक्षि | युङ्क्थः | युङ्क्थ | अयुनक् | अयुङ्क्तम् | अयुङ्क्त |
| 1 | युनज्मि | युञ्ज्वः | युञ्ज्मः | अयुनजम् | अयुञ्ज्व | अयुञ्ज्म |

| | Imperative | | | Optative | | |
|---|---|---|---|---|---|---|
| | Singular | Dual | Plural | Singular | Dual | Plural |
| 3 | युनक्तु | युङ्क्ताम् | युञ्जन्तु | युञ्ज्यात् | युञ्ज्याताम् | युञ्ज्युः |
| 2 | युङ्ग्धि | युङ्क्तम् | युङ्क्त | युञ्ज्याः | युञ्ज्यातम् | युञ्ज्यात |
| 1 | युनजानि | युनजाव | युनजाम | युञ्ज्याम् | युञ्ज्याव | युञ्ज्याम |

### Ātmanepada

| | Present Tense | | | Past Imperfect | | |
|---|---|---|---|---|---|---|
| | Singular | Dual | Plural | Singular | Dual | Plural |
| 3 | युङ्क्ते | युञ्जाते | युञ्जते | अयुङ्क्त | अयुञ्जाताम् | अयुञ्जत |
| 2 | यङ्क्षे | युञ्जाथे | युङ्ग्ध्वे | अयुङ्क्थाः | अयुञ्जाथाम् | अयुङ्ग्ध्वम् |
| 1 | युञ्जे | युञ्ज्वहे | युञ्ज्महे | अयुञ्जि | अयुञ्ज्वहि | अयुञ्ज्महि |

| | Imperative | | | Optative | | |
|---|---|---|---|---|---|---|
| | Singular | Dual | Plural | Singular | Dual | Plural |
| 3 | युङ्क्ताम् | युञ्जाताम् | युञ्जताम् | युञ्जीत | युञ्जीयाताम् | युञ्जीरन् |
| 2 | युङ्क्ष्व | युञ्जाथाम् | युङ्ग्ध्वम् | युञ्जीथाः | युञ्जीयाथाम् | युञ्जीध्वम् |
| 1 | युनजै | युनजावहै | युनजामहै | युञ्जीय | युञ्जीवहि | युञ्जीमहि |

## Seventh Class Verbs

√छिद् U, to cut
√भिद् P, to split, break
√भुज् U, to eat, enjoy, experience
√रुध् U, to obstruct, restrain

## Conjugate

√भुज्

## Translate

### D. *Śivasaṃhitā* 2.41

This verse continues the discussion of the previous two verses on how the *jīva*, the embodied soul, is bound by *karma*.

यद्यत्संदृश्यते लोके सर्वं तत्कर्मसंभवम् ।
सर्वकर्मानुसारेण जन्तुर्भोगान्भुनक्ति वै ॥

Vocabulary

यद्यत् ind. whatever
संदृश्यते is seen (3rd p. sg. passive)
कर्मसंभव mfn. arises from actions
सर्वकर्मानुसारेण according to all of its actions (m. inst. sg.)
जन्तुः m. person
भोगः m. fruition, rewards, results

### E. *Bhāgavatapurāṇa* 11.28.41

This verse comes in a series of verses explaining that although one may attain physical benefits through the practice of yoga, this is not the goal, and can actually be a hindrance on the path to *samādhi*. Note that विधाय in the third *pāda* goes with the words in the second *pāda*. सिद्धिः refers to physical perfections or supernatural powers, and the implied object of the verb √युज् is yoga.

केचिद्देहमिमं धीराः सुकल्पं वयसि स्थिरम् ।
विधाय विविधोपयैरथ युञ्जन्ति सिद्धये ॥

Vocabulary

केचिद् ind. some [yogīs]
इमम् this (m. acc. sg.)
धीर mfn. strong-minded, persevering, resolute
सुकल्प mfn. very qualified or skilled
वयस् n. energy, strength, youth
वि√धा 3P, to make, render
विविधोपयः m. various means
    उपायः m. means, expedient

### F. *Vivekamārtaṇḍa* 55

सुस्निग्धं मधुराहारं चतुर्थांशविवर्जितम् ।
भुञ्जते सुरसं प्रीत्यै मिताहारी स उच्यते ॥

Vocabulary

सुस्निग्ध mfn. very oily/rich
मधुराहारः m. sweet food
  मधुर mfn. sweet, pleasant, charming
  आहारः m. food
चतुर्थांशविवर्जित mfn. excepting the fourth quarter, leaving the fourth quarter empty
  चतुर्थ mfn. the fourth
  अंशः m. a share, portion
सुरस mfn. well flavored, good tasting
  रसः m. taste
प्रीतिः f. pleasure, satisfaction
मिताहारी one who eats a moderate diet (m. nom .sg.)
उच्यते it is said (3rd p. sg. passive √वच्)

## NINTH CLASS VERBS

The ninth *gaṇa* is named for the root, √क्री, "to buy." Verbs of the ninth *gaṇa* add ना as a suffix to the root in strong forms. In weak forms, नी is added to the root before an ending beginning with a consonant, and न् is added before an ending beginning with a vowel.

**√ज्ञा 9U, to know (√ज्ञा ⇒ जा)**

Parasmaipada

| | Present Tense | | | Past Imperfect | | |
|---|---|---|---|---|---|---|
| | Singular | Dual | Plural | Singular | Dual | Plural |
| 3 | जानाति | जानीतः | जानन्ति | अजानात् | अजानीताम् | अजानन् |
| 2 | जानासि | जानीथः | जानीथ | अजानाः | अजानीतम् | अजानीत |
| 1 | जानामि | जानीवः | जानीमः | अजानाम् | अजानीव | अजानीम |

| | Imperative | | | Optative | | |
|---|---|---|---|---|---|---|
| | Singular | Dual | Plural | Singular | Dual | Plural |
| 3 | जानातु | जानीताम् | जानन्तु | जानीयात् | जानीयाताम् | जानीयुः |
| 2 | जानीहि | जानीतम् | जानीत | जानीयाः | जानीयातम् | जानीयात |
| 1 | जानानि | जानाव | जानाम | जानीयाम् | जानीयाव | जानीयाम |

### Ātmanepada

| | Present Tense | | | Past Imperfect | | |
|---|---|---|---|---|---|---|
| | Singular | Dual | Plural | Singular | Dual | Plural |
| 3 | जानीते | जानाते | जानते | अजानीत | अजानाताम् | अजानत |
| 2 | जानीषे | जानाथे | जानीध्वे | अजानीथाः | अजानाथाम् | अजानीध्वम् |
| 1 | जाने | जानीवहे | जानीमहे | अजानि | अजानीवहि | अजानीमहि |

| | Imperative | | | Optative | | |
|---|---|---|---|---|---|---|
| | Singular | Dual | Plural | Singular | Dual | Plural |
| 3 | जानीताम् | जानाताम् | जानताम् | जानीत | जानीयाताम् | जानीरन् |
| 2 | जानीष्व | जानाथाम् | जानीध्वम् | जानीथाः | जानीयाथाम् | जानीध्वम् |
| 1 | जानै | जानावहै | जानामहै | जानीय | जानीवहि | जानीमहि |

## Ninth Class Verbs

√क्री U, to buy
√ग्रह् U, to grasp (√ग्रह् ⇒ गृह्)
√पू U, to purify, sanctify (√पू ⇒ पु)
√बन्ध् P, to bind (√बन्ध् ⇒ बध्)
√मन्थ् P, to churn, agitate (√मन्थ् ⇒ मथ्)
√वृ U, to choose

## Conjugate

√ग्रह्, √बन्ध्

## Translate

### G. *Vivekamārtaṇḍa* 8

आसनानि च तावन्ति यावन्त्यो जीवजातयः।
एतेषामखिलान्भेदान्विजानाति महेश्वरः॥

Vocabulary
तावन्ति there are as many . . . (n. nom. pl. तावत्)
यावन्त्यः as . . . (f. nom. pl यावत्)
जीवजातिः f. species of living beings

जीवः m. life, living being
जातिः f. species, type, kind
अखिल mfn. without a gap, complete, whole, all
भेदः m. distinction, variety, difference

### H. *Bhagavadgītā* 9.19

The "I" in this verse is Kṛṣṇa.

तपाम्यहमहं वर्षं निगृह्णाम्युत्सृजामि च ।
अमृतं चैव मृत्युश्च सदसच्चाहमर्जुन ॥

Vocabulary
√तप् 1P, to give out heat, shine
वर्षः m. rain
नि√ग्रह् 9P, to hold back
उत्√सृज् 6P, to let loose, pour forth
अमृतम् n. immortality
सत् n. existence
असत् n. nonexistence

### I. *Bhagavadgītā* 14.5–8

Note that these verses are all speaking of the different ways in which the Soul is bound to the body by the three *guṇas*.

सत्त्वं रजस्तम इति गुणाः प्रकृतिसम्भवाः ।
निबध्नन्ति महाबाहो देहे देहिनमव्ययम् ॥

तत्र सत्त्वं निर्मलत्वात्प्रकाशकमनामयम् ।
सुखसङ्गेन बध्नाति ज्ञानसङ्गेन चानघ ॥

रजो रागात्मकं विद्धि तृष्णासङ्गसमुद्भवम् ।
तन्निबध्नाति कौन्तेय कर्मसङ्गेन देहिनम् ॥

तमस्त्वज्ञानजं विद्धि मोहनं सर्वदेहिनाम् ।
प्रमादालस्यनिद्राभिस्तन्निबध्नाति भारत ॥

Vocabulary

सत्त्वम् n. equilibrium, luminosity
प्रकृतिसम्भवः m. whose origins are in nature
सम्भवः m. origin, source
देह mn. the body
देहिनम् the embodied Soul (m. acc. sg.)
निर्मलत्वम् n. stainlessness, clearness, purity
प्रकाशक mfn. clear, bright, shining, illuminating
अनामय mfn. free from disease
सुखसङ्गः m. attachment to happiness
ज्ञानसङ्गः m. attachment to knowledge
ज्ञानम् n. knowledge
रागात्मक mfn. whose nature is passion
रागः m. passion
तृष्णासङ्गसमुद्भवः m. arising from thirst and attachment
तृष्णा f. thirst
कर्मसङ्गः m. attachment to action
अज्ञानज mfn. born from ignorance
अज्ञानम् n. ignorance
मोहनम् n. confusing, deluding
सर्वदेहिनाम् of all embodied beings (m. gen. sg.)
प्रमादालस्यनिद्रा f. intoxication, laziness, and sleepiness
प्रमादः m. intoxication, madness
आलस्यम् n. laziness, idleness

The three *guṇas*, as described in Sāṃkhya philosophy, are considered to be the fundamental constituents of *prakṛti* (Nature), and it is through a disturbance in their equilibrium that the transformation (*pariṇāma*) from unmanifest to manifest nature occurs. The word *guṇa* has multiple technical meanings; however, in this context, it means "a characteristic, a quality, an attribute," or literally, "a thread." Each person is born with different proportions of these three psychophysical components, and this determines his or her individual personality. As detailed in the *Sāṃkhyakārikā*, *rajas* (activity or energy), *tamas* (inertia or stability), and *sattva* (equilibrium, balance, or luminescence) are associated respectively with the psychological qualities of aversion or pain (*aprīti*), depression or despair (*viṣāda*), and pleasure or joy (*prīti*), and the physical qualities of inciting and fluctuating (*upaṣṭambhaka* and *cala*), heavy and enveloping (*guru* and *varaṇaka*), and light and shining (*laghu* and *prakāśa*). As explained in the *Bhagavadgītā*, the *guṇas* can be influenced and balanced by what a person takes into his or her body and mind, analogously to the three *doṣas* in Āyurvedic theory. Over time, yoga practice is meant to lead to a decrease of *rajas* and *tamas* and an increase of *sattva*, and eventually, to a state that is beyond the three *guṇas*.

## CAUSATIVE VERBS

A verb from any of the ten *gaṇas* can be turned into a causative verb by adding the suffix अय to the verbal root and conjugating it as a tenth class verb. Although most commonly used in the present tense, these causative verbs can be conjugated in any mood and tense.

1. In most cases, the first vowel takes *guṇa* strengthening.

   √गम् to go ⇒ गच्छति he/she goes ⇒ गमयति he/she causes to go
   √बुध् to be awake ⇒ बोधति he/she is awake ⇒ बोधयति he/she causes to be awake
   √शुष् to be dry ⇒ शुष्यति he/she is dry ⇒ शोषयति he/she causes to be dry

2. If *guṇa* does not produce a heavy syllable, as in the case of अ, it is upgraded to *vṛddhi* and becomes आ.

   √कृ to do ⇒ करोति he/she does ⇒ कारयति he/she causes to do
   √पत् to fall ⇒ पतति he/she falls ⇒ पातयति he/she causes to fall
   √भू to become ⇒ भवति he/she becomes ⇒ भावयति he/she causes to become

3. In some roots ending in आ, a प् is added before the infix अय.

   √ज्ञा to know ⇒ जानाति he/she knows ⇒ ज्ञापयति he/she causes to know
   √दा to give ⇒ ददाति he/she gives ⇒ दापयति he/she causes to give
   √स्था to stand ⇒ तिष्ठति he/she stands ⇒ स्थापयति he/she causes to stand

4. The absolutive/gerund of a causative with no preverb is formed by replacing अय with अयित्वा. With a preverb, अय is replaced with य.

   √स्था to stand ⇒ स्थापयति he/she causes to stand ⇒ स्थापयित्वा having caused to stand
   प्रति√ष्ठा to stand firm ⇒ प्रतिष्ठापयति he/she establishes ⇒ प्रतिष्ठाप्य having established

### Translate

#### J. *Bhagavadgītā* 2.23

नैनं छिन्दन्ति शस्त्राणि नैनं दहति पावकः ।
न चैनं क्लेदयन्त्यापो न शोषयति मारुतः ॥

Vocabulary
एनम् this [Soul] (m. acc. sg.)
शस्त्रम् n. weapon
√दह् 1P, to burn
पावकः m. fire

√क्लिद् 4P, to be wet
आपः water (f. nom. pl.)
√शुष् 4P, to be dry
मारुतः m. wind

### K. *Yogāñjalisāram* 32

बन्धय वायुं नन्दय जीवं
धारय चित्तं दहरे परमे ।
इति तिरुमल कृष्णो योगी
प्रदिशति वाचं सन्देशाख्याम् ॥

Vocabulary
√नन्द् 1P, to rejoice, delight, be pleased
दहरः m. the heart
तिरुमल कृष्णो योगी the yogī Tirumalai Krishnamacharya (m. nom. sg.)
प्र√दिश् 3P, to point out, indicate, teach
सन्देशः m. message
आख्य mfn. named, called (at the end of compounds)

*Yogāñjalisāram* is a poem, composed of thirty-two verses, written by Śrī Tirumalai Krishnamacharya. Krishnamacharya, often considered the grandfather of modern yoga, held degrees in all six Indian *darśanas*, or philosophies, and was a great teacher and healer through yoga and Āyurveda. His legacy lives on through the teachings of his students, including Śrī K. Pattabhi Jois, B.K.S. Iyengar, his son T.K.V. Desikachar, Indra Devi, and A. G. Mohan.

### L. *Haṭhapradīpikā* 1.23

Note that the words in the second *pāda* should be read with निवेश्य in the third *pāda*.

पद्मासनं तु संस्थाप्य जानूर्वोरन्तरे करौ ।
निवेश्य भूमौ संस्थाप्य व्योमस्थं कुक्कुटासनम् ॥

Vocabulary
सं√स्था 1Ā, to dwell or live in, stand close together; caus. to establish, settle, raise up
जानूर्वोः of the knees and the thighs (m. gen. du.)
अन्तर mfn. interior, in the middle, between
नि√विश् 6Ā, to enter, be fixed on; caus. to put, place, keep
व्योमस्थ mfn. in the sky
कुक्कुटः m. rooster

## Review Exercises

### M. *Bhagavadgītā* 6.11–12

These verses describe how one should prepare to practice yoga. आत्मनः in the second *pāda* can be translated as "for oneself."

शुचौ देशे प्रतिष्ठाप्य स्थिरमासनमात्मनः ।
नात्युच्छ्रितं नातिनीचं चैलाजिनकुशोत्तरम् ॥

तत्रैकाग्रं मनः कृत्वा यतचित्तेन्द्रियक्रियः ।
उपविश्यासने युञ्ज्याद्योगमात्मविशुद्धये ॥

Vocabulary
अत्युच्छ्रित mfn. too high
अतिनीच mfn. too low
चैलाजिनकुशोत्तरम् with a covering of cloth, antelope skin, and *kuśa* grass (n. acc. sg.)
 चैलम् n. a piece of cloth
 अजिनम् n. the hairy skin of a black antelope
 कुशः m. a kind of grass considered holy and used in religious ceremonies
 उत्तरम् n. the upper surface or cover
एकाग्र mfn. one-pointed, concentrated on a single object
यतचित्तेन्द्रियक्रियः m. whose activity of mind and senses is controlled
उप√विश् 6P, to sit down
आत्मविशुद्धिः f. purification of the self, true knowledge of Soul
 विशुद्धिः f. purification, true knowledge

### N. *Bhagavadgītā* 2.22

वासांसि जीर्णानि यथा विहाय नवानि गृह्णाति नरोऽपराणि ।
तथा शरीराणि विहाय जीर्णान्यन्यानि संयाति नवानि देही ॥

Vocabulary
वासस् n. garment, clothes
जीर्ण mfn. old, worn-out
वि√हा 3P, to abandon, cast off
नव mfn. new
नरः m. man, person

संं√या 2P, to come to or into, attain
देही the Soul, Self, "possessing a body" (m. nom. sg. of देहिन्)

O. *Bṛhadāraṇyakopaniṣat* 1.3.28

In this verse, मा is translated as "me."

असतो मा सद्गमय ।
तमसो मा ज्योतिर्गमय ।
मृत्योर्मा अमृतं गमय ॥

Vocabulary
असत् n. nonexistence, the unreal, untruth
सत् n. existence, the real, truth

# 11
# Compounds: *Dvandva*; Passive Voice; Past Passive Participles

द्रष्टृदृश्ययोः संयोगो हेयहेतुः ॥ २.१७ ॥
**draṣṭṛ-dṛśyayoḥ saṃyogo heya-hetuḥ**
The cause of the future suffering which is to be avoided is the conjunction of the seer and the seen.
॥ *Yogasūtra* 2.17 ॥

## COMPOUNDS, समास

Compounds are one of the most fun, although initially intimidating, aspects of reading Sanskrit. Compounds are common in English, as well, for example:

bluebird: a bird that is blue
birdhouse: a house for birds
houseboat: a boat that is a house
lamplit: lit by a lamp
earthquake: a quake in the earth
facebook: a book of faces

Just as in English, in a Sanskrit compound, the meaning of the word is dependent upon the relationship between the two (or more) words of which the compound is made. However, compounds in Sanskrit are far more common and can combine an infinite number of words together.

There are four major types of compounds, distinguished by the ways in which the final member of the compound relates to the previous member, which is subordinated to it in various ways. Most compounds are made up of a series of undeclined nominals/nouns joined together. The compound is declined as a unit, so that only the last member of the compound is declined. When reading a compound, you work from right to left, first relating the last word to the word immediately preceding it, and then relating those two words to the word preceding them, and so forth, so that you are really only working with two nominal units at a time.

Compounds take time, patience, and common sense to decipher. They are one of the main reasons for the extensive commentaries that accompany most primary Sanskrit texts and attempt to help decipher and explain their intent. The analysis of a compound into its component parts is called its *vigraha*.

## *DVANDVAS*

In a *dvandva* compound, two or more members are joined together as a unit, each member standing as an equally important subject, like a god with multiple heads. There are two types of *dvandvas*; the most common is the *itaretara* (one with another) *dvandva*, in which the gender of the compound is determined by the final member, but the number is the cumulative number of all the members of the compound. All *itaretara dvandvas* are therefore either dual or plural, and can be declined in any case. All that is necessary for the *vigraha* (analysis) is the addition of the word च (and) after each member of the compound.

### Examples

Note the dual endings of the following examples:

सुखदुःखे n. nom. du. happiness and suffering; pleasure and pain ⇒ सुखम् n. happiness, pleasure + दुःखम् n. suffering, pain
*Vigraha*: सुखं च दुःखं च ⇒ सुखदुःखे

लाभालाभौ m. nom. du. gain and loss ⇒ लाभः m. gain + अलाभः m. loss
*Vigraha*: लाभश्चालाभश्च ⇒ लाभालाभौ

सिद्ध्यसिद्धी f. nom. du. success and failure ⇒ सिद्धिः f. success + असिद्धिः f. failure
*Vigraha*: सिद्धिश्चासिद्धिश्च ⇒ सिद्ध्यसिद्धी

### Example: *Yogasūtra* 1.7

Note that in this example, the entire compound is masculine because its final member, आगमः, is masculine.

प्रत्यक्षानुमानागमाः प्रमाणानि ।

*Vigraha*: प्रत्यक्षं चानुमानं चागमश्च ⇒ प्रत्यक्षानुमानागमाः

Vocabulary

प्रत्यक्षम् n. direct perception
अनुमानम् n. inference
आगमः m. verbal testimony
प्रमाणम् n. right knowledge

Right knowledge (प्रमाणानि) **consists of direct perception, inference, and verbal testimony** (प्रत्यक्षानुमानागमाः).

## Translate

### A. *Bhagavadgītā* 2.38

Note that the verb युज्यस्व goes with the dative युद्धाय, which can be translated as "to/in battle."

सुखदुःखे समे कृत्वा लाभालाभौ जयाजयौ ।
ततो युद्धाय युज्यस्व नैवं पापमवाप्स्यसि ॥

Vocabulary

सम mfn. same, equal
जयः m. victory
अजयः m. defeat
पापम् n. evil, misfortune
अव√आप् 5P, to attain, obtain

### B. *Bhagavadgītā* 12.18

समः शत्रौ च मित्रे च तथा मानापमानयोः ।
शीतोष्णसुखदुःखेषु समः सङ्गविवर्जितः ॥

Vocabulary

शत्रुः m. enemy
मित्रः m. friend

मान mn. respect, honor
अपमान mn. dishonor, disgrace
उष्ण mn. heat
सङ्गविवर्जितः m. freed from attachment

### C. *Dattātreyayogaśāstra* 145

Note that गत्वा in the third *pāda* goes with the words in the second *pāda* and यच्छतः is the present indicative, third-person dual form of √यम्.

प्राणापानौ नादबिन्दू मूलबन्धेन चैकताम्।
गत्वा योगस्य संसिद्धिं यच्छतो नात्र संशयः॥

Vocabulary
प्राणः m. upward breath
अपानः m. downward breath
नादः m. internal resonance, sound
बिन्दुः m. seed, semen
एकता f. oneness, unity
संसिद्धिः f. complete accomplishment or fulfillment, attainment, success
√यम् 1P, to bestow

### D. *Yogasūtra* 2.29

यमनियमासनप्राणायामप्रत्याहारधारणाध्यानसमाधयोऽष्टावङ्गानि।

Vocabulary
अष्टौ eight (n. nom. pl.)

## *Samāhāra Dvandva*

The second and less common type of *dvandva* is the *samāhāra* (aggregation) *dvandva*, which indicates a collective unity. It is always neuter singular, no matter how many members the compound has. This is in contrast to the *itaretara dvandva* we learned earlier, in which compounds are always either dual or plural, reflecting the number of members in the compound, and the gender is determined by the final member. This makes the *samāhāra dvandva*, with its अम् ending, easily recognizable.

### Examples

चराचरम् n. all created things, moving and unmoving, the world
अहर्निशम् n. day and night

### E. *Yogasūtra* 2.46

In the entire *Yogasūtra*, there are only three *sūtras* that speak about *āsana*, or postural practice, the third limb of *aṣṭāṅgayoga*, which is the predominant form of yoga known to most people today.

स्थिरसुखमासनम् ।

Vocabulary
स्थिर mfn. steady

### F. *Bhagavadgītā* 6.13

This verse occurs in a series of verses giving instruction on yoga practice, culminating in the attainment of *nirvāṇa*, "liberation."

समं कायशिरोग्रीवं धारयन्नचलं स्थिरः ।
संप्रेक्ष्य नासिकाग्रं स्वं दिशश्चानवलोकयन् ॥

Vocabulary
सम mfn. even, straight, on a level
शिरस् n. the head
ग्रीवः m. the neck
धारयन् holding (m. nom. sg. caus. present participle √धृ)
अचल mfn. not moving
सं√प्रेक्ष् 1Ā, to look at, concentrate the eyes, gaze
नासिकाग्रम् n. tip of the nose
    नासिका f. the nose
स्व mfn. one's own
अनवलोकयन् not looking (m. nom. sg. present participle अनव√लोक्)

### G. *Gheraṇḍasaṃhitā* 5.6

A verse about the yogī's practice place.

वापीकूपतडागं च प्राचीरमध्यवर्ति च ।
नात्युच्चं नातिनिम्नं च कुटीरं कीटवर्जितम् ॥

Vocabulary

वापी f. pond, large reservoir of water
कूपः m. well
तडागः m. tank, pool
प्राचीरमध्यवर्ति situated in the middle of the enclosure (n. acc. sg.)
    प्राचीर mn. an enclosure
अत्युच्च mfn. too high
    उच्च mfn. high, elevated
अतिनिम्न mfn. too low
    निम्न mfn. low, deep
कुटीरम् n. hut
कीटवर्जित mfn. free from insects
    कीटः m. a worm, insect

## PASSIVE CONSTRUCTION

So far, all of the verbs we have studied have been in the active voice. The passive voice forms a coextensive system of verbs, including the present indicative, imperfect, imperative, and optative, where the subject is no longer of primary importance and the emphasis is instead shifted to the object or the action. The passive is formed from the root + य, similarly to fourth class verbs, and is always conjugated with *ātmanepada* endings. Both *parasmaipada* and *ātmanepada* verbs can be made passive.

**√पत् 1P, to fall**

| | Present Tense | | | Past Imperfect | | |
|---|---|---|---|---|---|---|
| | Singular | Dual | Plural | Singular | Dual | Plural |
| 3 | पत्यते | पत्येते | पत्यन्ते | अपत्यत | अपत्येताम् | अपत्यन्त |
| 2 | पत्यसे | पत्येथे | पत्यध्वे | अपत्यथाः | अपत्येथाम् | अपत्यध्वम् |
| 1 | पत्ये | पत्यावहे | पत्यामहे | अपत्ये | अपत्यावहि | अपत्यामहि |

| | Imperative | | | Optative | | |
|---|---|---|---|---|---|---|
| | Singular | Dual | Plural | Singular | Dual | Plural |
| 3 | पत्यताम् | पत्येताम् | पत्यन्ताम् | पत्येत | पत्येयाताम् | पत्येरन् |
| 2 | पत्यस्व | पत्येथाम् | पत्यध्वम् | पत्येथाः | पत्येयाथाम् | पत्येध्वम् |
| 1 | पत्यै | पत्यावहै | पत्यामहै | पत्येय | पत्येवहि | पत्येमहि |

Sometimes the root undergoes changes before adding the infix य.

1. Final इ or उ is lengthened.
   √जि to win ⇒ जीयते is won
   √श्रु to hear ⇒ श्रूयते is heard

2. Final आ or ऐ becomes ई.
   √दा to give ⇒ दीयते is given
   √पा to drink ⇒ पीयते is drunk
   √गै to sing ⇒ गीयते is sung

   Exception:
   √ज्ञा to know ⇒ ज्ञायते is known

3. Final ऋ becomes रि.
   √कृ to do ⇒ क्रियते is done

4. Final ऋ after a conjunct consonant takes गुण.
   √स्मृ to remember ⇒ स्मर्यते is remembered

5. A nasal in the penultimate position (before a final stop) is dropped.
   √बन्ध् to bind ⇒ बध्यते is bound
   √रञ्ज् to redden ⇒ रज्यते is reddened

6. In many roots with the combination of a semivowel (य्, र्, ल्, व्) + अ, that combination is replaced by the simple vowel corresponding to the semivowel (इ, ऋ, ऌ, उ), a change called संप्रसारण, or "squeezing out."
   √वच् to say ⇒ उच्यते is said
   √वस् to live ⇒ उष्यते is lived
   √स्वप् to sleep ⇒ सुप्यते is slept
   √यज् to sacrifice ⇒ इज्यते is sacrificed
   √ग्रह् to grasp ⇒ गृह्यते is grasped

7. The root पश् is replaced by दृश्.
   √पश् to see ⇒ दृश्यते is seen

### Conjugate

√गम्, √बन्ध्

## PASSIVE OF A TRANSITIVE VERB

The passive can be formed from both transitive and intransitive verbs. A transitive verb is one that requires a direct object to form a complete sentence, whereas an intransitive verb only requires a subject, but stands on its own without an object. When the passive is formed from a transitive verb, the nominative subject in the active clause becomes the agent, and is written in the instrumental case, and the accusative object in the active clause becomes the nominative subject.

### Example

Active: सा बध्नाति मरीच्यासनं दी। She binds *marīcyāsana* D.
Passive: मरीच्यासनं दी तया बध्यते। *Marīcyāsana* D is bound by her.

### Translate

#### H. *Haṭhapradīpikā* 4.21

पवनो बध्यते येन मनस्तेनैव बध्यते।
मनश्च बध्यते येन पवनस्तेन बध्यते॥

Vocabulary
पवनः m. wind, breath, "purifier"

#### I. *Bhagavadgītā* 5.5

स्थानम्, that "state" or "place," here refers to मोक्षः or "liberation."

यत्सांख्यैः प्राप्यते स्थानं तद्योगैरपि गम्यते।
एकं सांख्यं च योगं च यः पश्यति स पश्यति॥

Vocabulary
सांख्यम् n. one of the six systems of Hindu philosophy, followers of Sāṃkhya

सांख्य (*Sāṃkhya*), which literally means "relating to number," is so titled because it "enumerates" the twenty-five *tattvas* or true principles, all of which evolve out of *prakṛti*, except *puruṣa*. As laid out by Kapila, the final aim is to move beyond the bounds of the first twenty-four categories and liberate *puruṣa* from *prakṛti*.

प्र√आप् 5P, to obtain, attain
योगैः by the yogīs (used in epic Sanskrit for योगिभिः, m. inst. pl.)
यः पश्यति स पश्यति Who sees this truly sees.

J. *Śivasaṃhitā* 1.79

चक्षुषा गृह्यते रूपं गन्धो घ्राणेन गृह्यते ।
रसो रसनया स्पर्शस्त्वचा संगृह्यते परम् ।
श्रोत्रेण गृह्यते शब्दो नियतं भाति नान्यथा ॥

Vocabulary
रूपम् n. form
गन्धः m. smell
घ्राणम् n. nose
रसः m. taste
रसना f. tongue
स्पर्शः m. touch
परम् ind. simply, nothing but, merely
नियतम् ind. always, surely
√भा 2P, to exist, manifest
न अन्यथा ind. not otherwise

## PASSIVE OF AN INTRANSITIVE VERB, भावे प्रयोग

Any intransitive verb or a transitive verb used without a direct object can use this construction. Here, the subject is neither the agent nor the object. The action itself is the focus and is always given in the third-person singular, while the agent, if there is one, is given in the instrumental case. There is no object.

K. *Yogarahasya* 1.21

इमं क्रमं परित्यज्य यथेच्छं यदि गम्यते ।
न तस्याष्टाङ्गयोगेन फलसिद्धिः प्रजायते ॥

Vocabulary
क्रमः m. order, sequence
यथेच्छम् n. according to desire

यदि ind. if
फलसिद्धिः f. attainment of fruits

## PARTICIPLES

In addition to the large variety of conjugatable verbal forms in Sanskrit, there is also a wealth of nominalized verbal forms (verbs turned into nouns) and, most important, participles. These participles have the form of an adjective and are used just as any adjective, to modify nouns; however, in their meaning, they perform a verbal function.

The *Yogarahasya*, "The Secret of Yoga," was composed by the ninth-century yogī and Vaisnavite saint Nāthamuni, but was lost soon after he died. In the early twentieth century, Krishnamacharya, a direct descendant of Nāthamuni, at the age of sixteen, went on a pilgrimage to Ālvār Tirunagarī, where Nāthamuni was thought to have received these teachings from the saint Nanmālvār. When Krishnamacharya was sitting in a mango grove, in a meditative trance, Nāthamuni came to him and taught him the *Yogarahasya*. It contains many teachings on *āsana* and *prāṇāyāma* and their various therapeutic applications, including instruction on yoga during pregnancy. This verse discusses the importance of practicing the eight limbs of *aṣṭāṅgayoga* in sequence.

## PAST PASSIVE PARTICIPLES (PPPs)

The past passive participle is used quite commonly to replace a passive verb. Like an adjective, it agrees with the noun it modifies in gender, case, and number. It is generally formed with one of the suffixes -त, -इत, or -न, although there are some exceptions. Below is a list of some of the most common past passive participles and the rules they derive from. It is not necessary to learn all of these forms, but it is important to learn to be able to recognize the past passive participle in its different incarnations.

1. Often, -त is added directly to the root.
   √कृ to do, make ⇒ कृत done, made
   √श्रु to hear ⇒ श्रुत heard

2. Other roots take the ending -इत.
   √पत् to fall ⇒ पतित fell
   √पूज् to worship ⇒ पूजित worshipped
   √जीव् to live ⇒ जीवित lived
   √चिन्त् to think ⇒ चिन्तित thought

3. Some roots ending in a nasal lose the final nasal before the ending -त.
   √गम् to go ⇒ गत gone
   √हन् to kill ⇒ हत killed

4. For other roots ending in a nasal, the vowel is lengthened and म् becomes न्.
   √शम् to pacify, calm, soothe ⇒ शान्त appeased, tranquil, calm

5. Roots starting with a semivowel followed by अ take संप्रसारण.
   √वच् to speak ⇒ उक्त spoke

6. Some roots take the ending -न or -ण.
   √भिद् to break ⇒ भिन्न broke
   √पॄ to fill ⇒ पूर्ण full

7. Roots ending in च् or ज् become क्; roots ending in श् become ष् and the final त becomes ट.
   √युज् to yoke ⇒ युक्त yoked, engaged in, proper, suitable, appropriate
   √दृश् to see ⇒ दृष्ट seen

8. If there is a weak form of the root, it is used to form the PPP.
   √बन्ध् to bind ⇒ बद्ध bound

9. In general, final -आ and complex vowels become -ई.
   √गै to sing ⇒ गीत sung

   Exceptions:
   √ज्ञा to know ⇒ ज्ञात known
   √स्था to stand, be situated ⇒ स्थित stood, situated
   √दा to give ⇒ दत्त given
   √धा to place ⇒ हित placed

10. Roots ending with a voiced aspirate lose their aspiration and the added -त becomes voiced and aspirated.
   √बुध् to awaken ⇒ बुद्ध awakened
   √लभ् to obtain ⇒ लब्ध obtained

11. The PPP of a causative verb is formed by replacing the -अय with -इत.
√कृ ⇒ कारयति causes to do ⇒ कारित caused to do
√दृश् ⇒ दर्शयति causes to see, shows ⇒ दर्शित caused to see, showed

Just like the passive verb, the past passive participle has two different functions depending on whether it is transitive or intransitive. Most commonly, it is formed from transitive roots and used as an adjective, agreeing with the noun (the direct object) it modifies in gender, case, and number. The agent (if there is one) appears in the instrumental case.

### Example

तया मरीच्यासनं दी बद्धम्। *Marīcyāsana* D was bound by her.

Past passive participles formed from intransitive verbs modify the subject (rather than the object) and can have an active meaning. The agent (if there is one) appears in the instrumental case.

### Example: *Yogasūtra* 2.16

हेयं दुःखमनागतम्।

#### Vocabulary

हेय mfn. to be avoided
अनागत mfn. not come, not arrived, future

Suffering (दुःखम्) **that has not yet come** (अनागतम्) is to be avoided (हेयम्).

There is also a rare भावे form in which there is no object. The action itself is the focus and is always given in the third-person singular, while the agent is given in the instrumental case. The past passive participle is also frequently found inside of compounds, as we will see in the following chapters.

### Translate

#### L. *Haṭhapradīpikā* 3.55

येन in the first *pāda* means "by this [practice]."

बद्धो येन सुषुम्नायां प्राणस्तूड्डीयते यतः।
तस्मादुड्डीयनाख्योऽयं योगिभिः समुदाहृतः॥

Vocabulary

सुषुम्ना f. the central *nāḍī* or channel of the nervous system
उड्√डी 4Ā, to fly up, soar
उड्डीयनाख्यः m. with the name *uḍḍīyana*
    उड्डीयनः m. abdominal energy lock
अयम् this [*bandha*] (m. nom. sg.)
योगिभिः by yogīs (m. inst. sg.)
समुदा√हृ 1U, to call, pronounce, declare, teach

### M. *Bhagavadgītā* 2.39

एषा तेऽभिहिता सांख्ये बुद्धिर्योगे त्विमां शृणु ।
बुद्ध्या युक्तो यया पार्थ कर्मबन्धं प्रहास्यसि ॥

Vocabulary

अभि√धा 3P, to set forth, explain, declare
इमाम् this (f. acc. sg.)
कर्मबन्धः m. the bondage of action
प्र√हा 3P, to give up, forsake, abandon, avoid

### N. *Bhagavadgītā* 2.58

This verse comes in a series of verses in which Kṛṣṇa describes someone who is steady-minded.

यदा संहरते चायं कूर्मोऽङ्गानीव सर्वशः ।
इन्द्रियाणीन्द्रियार्थेभ्यस्तस्य प्रज्ञा प्रतिष्ठिता ॥

Vocabulary

सं√हृ 1U, to draw together, unite
अयम् he, one (m. nom. sg.)
कूर्मः m. a tortoise
अङ्गम् n. limb
सर्वशस् ind. wholly, completely, entirely
इन्द्रियार्थः m. an object of sense
प्रति√स्था 1P, to stand firm, be established

## Review Exercises

### O. *Bhagavadgītā* 2.48

योगस्थः कुरु कर्माणि सङ्गं त्यक्त्वा धनंजय ।
सिद्ध्यसिद्ध्योः समो भूत्वा समत्वं योग उच्यते ॥

Vocabulary
योगस्थः m. situated/established in yoga
समत्वम् n. equanimity

### P. *Dhyānabindūpaniṣat* 7

This verse occurs in a series of verses discussing the nature of the soul. स in the fourth *pāda* refers to आत्मन्.

तिलानां तु यथा तैलं पुष्पे गन्ध इवाश्रितः ।
पुरुषस्य शरीरे तु स बाह्याभ्यन्तरे स्थितः ॥ ७ ॥

Vocabulary
तिलः m. sesame seed
तैलम् n. sesame oil
गन्धः m. scent, fragrance
आ√श्रि 1P, to inhabit, dwell in, reside, exist in

The *Dhyānabindūpaniṣat* is part of the group of *Yoga Upaniṣads* that emerged around the seventeenth century C.E. They are all largely compilations, drawing on the older tradition of Patañjali's *aṣṭāṅgayoga*, as well as on the more recent *haṭhayoga* texts, with influences from tantra and Vedanta too.

### Q. *Vivekamārtaṇḍa* 66

पीड्यते न स शोकेण लिप्यते न स कर्मणा ।
बाध्यते न स कालेन यो मुद्रां वेत्ति खेचरीम् ॥

Vocabulary
√पीड् 10U, to pain, torment
√लिप् 6U, to smear, stain
√बाध् 1Ā, to harass, oppress

*Khecarī mudrā* in its full expression involves cutting the frenulum of the tongue so that it can be drawn back above the soft palate and into the nasal cavity, in order to capture the *aṃrta* and become immortal.

# 12
# COMPOUNDS: *TATPURUṢA*, *KARMADHĀRAYA*

वितर्कबाधने प्रतिपक्षभावनम् ॥ २.३३ ॥
**vitarka-bādhane pratipakṣa-bhāvanam**
When there is obstruction by negative impulses, one should contemplate the opposite.
॥ *Yogasūtra* 2.33 ॥

## *TATPURUṢA* COMPOUNDS

In this type of compound, the final member is predominant. The gender and number of the entire compound is determined by the last member. *Tatpuruṣa* compounds can be subdivided and analyzed according to the relationship between the two words. These relationships are the same as those represented by the case endings for individual nouns. However, the relationship is no longer explicit and must be inferred according to context. That relationship can be shown by a *vigraha*. The most common relationship in compounds is through the genitive case. The past passive participle makes a frequent appearance in *tatpuruṣa* compounds, particularly those in the instrumental case.

### Examples (with Reference to Compound XY)

#### Accusative: Y to X

धातुप्रपोषणम् nourishing the constituent elements of the body ⇒ धातुः constituent element of the body + प्रपोषण nourishing
*Vigraha*: धातून् प्रपोषणम् ⇒ धातुप्रपोषणम्

पुष्टिवर्धनम् increasing prosperity/welfare ⇒ पुष्टिः prosperity, welfare + वर्धन increasing
*Vigraha*: पुष्टिं वर्धनम् ⇒ पुष्टिवर्धनम्

#### Instrumental: Y by Means of X

परम्पराप्राप्तम् received by succession ⇒ परम्परा succession + प्राप्त obtained, received
*Vigraha*: परम्परया प्राप्तम् ⇒ परम्पराप्राप्तम्

अहंकारविमूढः bewildered by egotism ⇒ अहंकारः egotism + विमूढ bewildered
*Vigraha*: अहंकारेण विमूढः ⇒ अहंकारविमूढः

### Dative: Y for/to X

गुर्वष्टकम् an octet for the teacher ⇒ गुरुः teacher + अष्टक consisting of eight parts
*Vigraha*: गुरवेऽष्टकम् ⇒ गुर्वष्टकम्

शान्तिमन्त्रः prayer for peace ⇒ शान्तिः peace + मन्त्रः prayer
*Vigraha*: शान्तये मन्त्रः ⇒ शान्तिमन्त्रः

### Ablative: Y from/because of X

द्वैतविवर्जितः free from duality ⇒ द्वैतम् duality + विवर्जित free from
*Vigraha*: द्वैताद्विवर्जितः ⇒ द्वैतविवर्जितः

श्रमजातः born from fatigue ⇒ श्रमः fatigue + जात born
*Vigraha*: श्रमाद् जातः ⇒ श्रमजातः

### Genitive: Y of X

भगवद्गीता song of the Lord ⇒ भगवद् Lord + गीता song
*Vigraha*: भगवस्य गीता ⇒ भगवद्गीता

योगसूत्रम् thread of yoga ⇒ योगः yoga + सूत्रम् thread
*Vigraha*: योगस्य सूत्रम् ⇒ योगसूत्रम्

हठयोगः yoga of force ⇒ हठः force + योगः yoga
*Vigraha*: हठस्य योगः ⇒ हठयोगः

### Locative: Y in/on/about X

साधनपादः chapter on practice ⇒ साधनम् practice + पादः chapter
*Vigraha*: साधनौ पादः ⇒ साधनपादः

क्रियायुक्तः yoked/absorbed in action ⇒ क्रिया action + युक्त yoked/absorbed
*Vigraha*: क्रियायां युक्तः ⇒ क्रियायुक्तः

हठप्रदीपिका a small lamp on *haṭhayoga* ⇒ हठः *haṭhayoga* + प्रदीपिका small lamp
*Vigraha*: हठो प्रदीपिका ⇒ हठप्रदीपिका

## Pronomial Stems in Compounds

A pronomial stem can be used as the first member of a *tatpuruṣa* compound, as exemplified in the name *tatpuruṣa*, itself. Because it must appear in stem form, there are multiple possibilities as to what the pronomial stem may stand for and what relationship may be expressed, which must be inferred from context or understood with the help of a commentary.

तत्पुरुषः his man ⇒ तत् his + पुरुषः man
*Vigraha*: तस्य पुरुषः ⇒ तत्पुरुषः

मत्कर्म my work/action ⇒ मत् my + कर्म work, action
*Vigraha*: मम कर्म ⇒ मत्कर्म

### Example: *Dhyānabindūpaniṣat* 5–6

पुष्पमध्ये यथा गन्धः पयोमध्ये यथा घृतम् ।
तिलमध्ये यथा तैलं पाषाणाष्विव काञ्चनम् ॥

एवं सर्वाणि भूतानि मणौ सूत्र इवात्मनि ।
स्थिरबुद्धिरसंमूढो ब्रह्मविद् ब्रह्मणि स्थितः ॥

Vocabulary
पयस् n. milk
पाषाणः m. stone
काञ्चनम् n. gold
मणिः m. jewel, gem, pearl
स्थिरबुद्धिः f. one whose understanding is steady, steady-minded
असंमूढ mfn. not confused

As (यथा) **in the midst of a flower** (पुष्पमध्ये) there is fragrance (गन्धः),
As (यथा) **in the midst of milk** (पयोमध्ये) there is ghee (घृतम्),
As (यथा) **in the midst of sesame seeds** (तिलमध्ये) there is oil (तैलम्),
As (इव) in a stone (पाषाणाषु) there is gold (काञ्चनम्).

Thus (एवम्) all (सर्वाणि) beings (भूतानि) [exist] in the Soul (आत्मनि),
As (इव) a thread (सूत्र) through a jewel (मणौ).
Steady-minded (स्थिरबुद्धिः), unconfused (असंमूढः),
Knowing *Brahman* (ब्रह्मविद्), situated (स्थितः) in *Brahman* (ब्रह्मणि).

## Translate

### A. *Yogasūtra* 1.1

अथ योगानुशासनम्।

Vocabulary
अनुशासनम् n. instruction

### B. *Aparokṣānubhūti* 112

Note the relative and correlative clauses, indicated by यस्मिन्, "in which," and तद्, "that," in the first and third *pādas*, respectively.

सुखेनैव भवेद्यस्मिन्नजस्रं ब्रह्मचिन्तनम्।
आसनं तद्विजानीयान्नेतरत्सुखनाशनम्॥

Sandhi Rule: A final न्, ण्, or ङ् is doubled after a short vowel, before any initial vowel.

Ex. यस्मिन् अजस्रम् ⇒ यस्मिन्नजस्रम्

Vocabulary
सुखेन ind. easily, comfortably, joyfully
अजस्रम् ind. perpetually, constantly, forever, always
चिन्तनम् n. meditation, reflection on
इतरद् n. other, i.e., another posture
नाशन mfn. destroying

### C. *Gheraṇḍasaṃhitā* 5.7

Another verse about the yogī's hut.

सम्यग्गोमयलिप्तं च कुटीरं रन्ध्रवर्जितम्।
एवं स्थाने हि गुप्ते च प्राणायामं समभ्यसेत्॥

Vocabulary

सम्यक् ind. completely
गोमयम् n. cow dung
लिप्त mfn. smeared
रन्ध्रम् n. hole

## *UPAPADA TATPURUṢA* COMPOUNDS

In these compounds, which are usually in the accusative case, the second member is not a freestanding, seperable word, but a bound or reduced form of a verbal root. An example in English is "ghostbusters." You would not use the word "busters" on its own and yet, in a compound, it is clear that a "buster" is "one who busts." Similarly, we use the word "dustbuster" for "something that busts dust." Thus, in the *vigraha*, it is not possible to simply separate the components. The second member always represents the agent of action and is analyzed in terms of a finite verb, which is quoted with the particle इति.

### Examples

योगदः one who bestows yoga, name for Patañjali ⇒ योगम् yoga + √दा to give ⇒ द
*Vigraha*: योगं ददातीति योगदः

वेदवित् one who knows the Vedas ⇒ वेदम् Vedas + √विद् to know ⇒ विद्
*Vigraha*: वेदान् वेत्तीति वेदविद्

पङ्कजम् born from mud, lotus ⇒ पङ्क mud + √जन् to be born ⇒ ज
*Vigraha*: पङ्काज्जायत इति पङ्कजम्

गृहस्थः one who lives in the house, a householder ⇒ गृहम् house + √स्था to stay ⇒ स्थ
*Vigraha*: गृहे तिष्ठतीति गृहस्थः

खगः one who goes/moves in the sky, a bird ⇒ खम् sky + √गम् to go ⇒ ग
*Vigraha*: खं गच्छतीति खगः

तमोघ्नः one who destroys darkness ⇒ तमस् darkness + √हन् to destroy ⇒ घ्न
*Vigraha*: तमो हन्तीति तमोघ्नः

### D. *Śivapañcākṣarīstotram* 1

ॐकारं बिन्दुसंयुक्तं नित्यं ध्यायन्ति योगिनः ।
कामदं मोक्षदं चैव ॐकाराय नमो नमः ॥

The sacred syllable ॐ, sometimes called *praṇava*, is considered the primordial sound, made up of a-u-ṃ and *turiya* (silent part). It is thought to encompass everything in the universe—creation, sustenance, destruction, and liberation (the part beyond).

Vocabulary

कारः m. a letter, sound, syllable
बिन्दुः m. dot, drop
संयुक्त mfn. endowed with, full of
√ध्यै 1P, to meditate on, contemplate
योगिनः the yogīs (m. nom. pl.)

### E. *Haṭhapradīpikā* 3.82

वलितं पलितं चैव षण्मासोर्ध्वं न दृष्यते ।
याममात्रं तु यो नित्यमभ्यसेत्स तु कालजित् ॥

The ability to hold an *āsana* or *mudrā* for three hours is considered a sign of perfection. This *sūtra* is referring to *viparītakaraṇī mudrā*, which was probably an inverted posture, such as a shoulderstand.

Vocabulary

वलित mfn. wrinkles
पलितम् n. gray hair
षण्मासोर्ध्व mfn. after six months
मासः m. a month
यामः m. a period of three hours, an eighth of the day
मात्र mfn. having the measure of

### F. *Haṭhapradīpikā* 4.2

अथेदानीं प्रवक्ष्यामि समाधिक्रममुत्तमम् ।
मृत्युघ्नं च सुखोपायं ब्रह्मानन्दकरं परम् ॥

Vocabulary

इदानीम् ind. now, at this moment
प्र√वच् 2P, to teach, explain
क्रमः m. method

## *KARMADHĀRAYA* (NOMINAL) COMPOUNDS

These compounds are a subtype of *tatpuruṣa* compound, in which both members are in the nominative case. In all cases, the first component modifies the second component.

1. In the most common type of *karmadhāraya*, the first word is an adjective describing the second word, which is a noun. These are the most frequently used compounds in English, for example, bluebird.

### Examples

नीलकमलम् blue lotus ⇒ नील blue + कमलम् lotus
*Vigraha*: नीलं च तद् कमलं च ⇒ नीलकमलम्
It is both blue and a lotus ⇒ blue lotus

सर्वभूतानि all beings ⇒ सर्व all + भूतानि beings
*Vigraha*: सर्वाणि च तानि भूतानि च ⇒ सर्वभूतानि

समस्थितिः equal standing ⇒ सम equal + स्थितिः standing
*Vigraha*: समा च ता स्थितिश्च ⇒ समस्थितिः

2. The second type of *karmadhāraya* contains two nouns and is often used for names or titles.

राजर्षिः royal seer ⇒ राजन् king + ऋषिः seer
*Vigraha*: राजा स च ऋषिश्च ⇒ राजर्षिः

शङ्कराचार्यः Teacher Śaṅkara ⇒ शङ्करः Śaṅkara + आचार्यः teacher
*Vigraha*: शङ्करः स चाचार्यश्च ⇒ शङ्कराचार्यः

लक्ष्मीपुरम् the town of Lakṣmī ⇒ लक्ष्मी Lakṣmī + पुरम् town
*Vigraha*: लक्ष्म्येव पुरम् or लक्ष्मी नाम्ना पुरम् ⇒ लक्ष्मीपुरम्

3. Other types of noun–noun *karmadhārayas* involve a comparison or simile and are glossed with the word इव or एव.

चरणारविन्दम् lotus-like foot ⇒ चरण foot + अरविन्दम् lotus
*Vigraha*: चरणमरविन्दमिव ⇒ चरणारविन्दम्

नरसिंहः lionlike man ⇒ नरः man + सिंहः lion
*Vigraha*: नरः सिंह इव ⇒ नरसिंहः

4. Many *karmadhārayas* have a particle or prefix as the first component.

अधर्मः injustice, unrighteousness ⇒ अ non-, without + धर्मः justice, righteousness
*Vigraha*: धर्मादन्यः ⇒ अधर्मः

अनुत्तमः unsurpassed ⇒ अन् non- + उत्तमः highest, most excellent
*Vigraha*: उत्तमादन्यत् ⇒ अनुत्तमः

सुमधुरः very sweet ⇒ सु good, well, very + मधुरः sweet
*Vigraha*: सुष्ठु मधुरः ⇒ सुमधुरः

### *Dvi-gu Samāsas*

These "two-cow" compounds are a type of *karmadhāraya* compound in which the first component is a number. They are used mainly to indicate sets of things in which the relationship of the number to the given set is well known. See Chapter 15 for the declension of numerals.

त्रिगुणम् a group of three qualities
*Vigraha*: त्रायाणां गुणानां समाहारः ⇒ त्रिगुणम्

त्रिभुवनम् a group of three worlds
*Vigraha*: त्रायाणां भुवनानां समाहारः ⇒ त्रिभुवनम्

सप्ताहः a group of seven days
*Vigraha*: सप्तानामाह्नां समाहारः ⇒ सप्ताहः

### *Madhyama-pada-lopin Samāsas*

These are compounds whose "middle word has been dropped." Thus, another word is needed in the *vigraha* in order to properly gloss the compound.

शाकपार्थिवः a king [who loves] vegetables ⇒ शाकम् vegetable + पार्थिवः king
*Vigraha*: शाकप्रियः पार्थिवः ⇒ शाकपार्थिवः

**Example:** ***Bhagavadgītā* 6.29**

Note that ईक्षते, "[one] sees," in the third *pāda*, applies to both the first and second lines.

सर्वभूतस्थमात्मानं सर्वभूतानि चात्मनि ।
ईक्षते योगयुक्तात्मा सर्वत्र समदर्शनः ॥

Vocabulary
योगयुक्तात्मा one whose Soul/Self is absorbed in yoga (m. nom. sg.)
समदर्शनः m. one who sees the same aspect/essence [everywhere]
दर्शनम् n. aspect, appearance, vision

[One] who sees (ईक्षते) Soul (आत्मानम्) **present in all beings** (सर्वभूतस्थम्),
And (च) all beings (सर्वभूतानि) in Soul (आत्मनि).
[That one], whose Soul is absorbed in yoga (योगयुक्तात्मा),
Sees everywhere (सर्वत्र) the same essence (समदर्शनः).

**G.** ***Aparokṣānubhūti* 116**

This verse expresses an *advaitavedantin* viewpoint on knowledge and yoga practice.

दृष्टिं ज्ञानमयीं कृत्वा पश्येद् ब्रह्ममयं जगत् ।
सा दृष्टिः परमोदारा न नासाग्रावलोकिनी ॥

Vocabulary
मय / मयी mfn. made up of, consisting of (at the end of a compound)
उदार mfn. great, noble
अवलोकिनी f. looking

**H.** ***Dhyānabindūpaniṣat* 1**

यदि शैलसमं पापं विस्तीर्णं बहुयोजनम् ।
भिद्यते ध्यानयोगेन नान्यो भेदो कदाचन ॥

Vocabulary
यदि ind. if (note that here it has the meaning of यद्यपि, "even if")
पापम् n. evil, sin, misfortune

शैलः m. mountain
विस्तीर्ण mfn. spread out, extending
योजनम् n. mile
√भिद् 7P, to break, pierce, destroy
भेदः m. breaking open, piercing

### I. *Yogayājñavalkya* 2.15cd–16

उच्चैर्जपादुपांशुश्च सहस्रगुण उच्यते ॥
मानसस्तु तथोपांशोः सहस्रगुण उच्यते ।
मानसाच्च तथा ध्यानं सहस्रगुणमुच्यते ॥

Vocabulary
उच्चैस् ind. loud
जपः m. repetition of a mantra
उपांशुः m. a prayer/mantra uttered in a low voice
सहस्रगुण mfn. a thousand times [more powerful than . . .]
मानस mfn. pertaining to the mind, mental, spiritual, expressed only in the mind, performed in thought, silent

### J. *Yogasūtra* 2.42

सन्तोषादनुत्तमः सुखलाभः ।

Vocabulary
लाभः m. attainment

## *Aluk Samāsas*: Compounds That Do Not Lose Their Case Endings

The first member of these compounds retains its case ending, even when compounded.

युधिष्ठिरः firm/steady in battle, the eldest Pāṇḍava brother ⇒ युधि in battle (locative) + स्थिर firm, steady

*Vigraha*: युधि स्थिरः ⇒ युधिष्ठिरः

धनंजयः conqueror of wealth, Arjuṇa ⇒ धनम् wealth (accusative) + जय conquering
*Vigraha*: धनं जयः ⇒ धनंजयः

परंतपः scorcher of enemies, Arjuṇa ⇒ परम् enemy (accusative) + तप consuming by heat
*Vigraha*: परं तपः ⇒ परंतपः

परस्मैपदम् word for another ⇒ परस्मै another (dative) + पदम् word
*Vigraha*: परस्मै पदम् ⇒ परस्मैपदम्

आत्मनेपदम् word for oneself ⇒ आत्मने oneself (dative) + पदम् word
*Vigraha*: आत्मने पदम् ⇒ आत्मनेपदम्

### K. *Bhagavadgītā* 4.2

एवं परम्पराप्राप्तमिमं राजर्षयो विदुः ।
स कालेनेह महता योगो नष्टः परंतप ॥

> परम्परा (*Paramparā*) is the method of passing on knowledge from teacher to student through direct transmission. In this way, a tradition is kept vibrant and alive from generation to generation.

Vocabulary

परम्परा f. succession, tradition
प्राप्त mfn. obtained, received
इमम् this [yoga] (m. acc. sg.)
विदुः they knew (3rd p. sg. perfect √विद्)
महत् mfn. great, large, long
नष्ट mfn. lost, destroyed

### L. *Bhagavadgītā* 7.7

मत्तः परतरं नान्यत् किंचिदस्ति धनंजय ।
मयि सर्वमिदं प्रोतं सूत्रे मणिगणा इव ॥

Vocabulary

परतरम् n. higher than, superior
सर्वमिदम् this whole universe (n. nom. sg.)
प्रोत mfn. sewed, strung
मणिगणः m. (group of) pearls

## COMPLEX COMPOUNDS

An infinite number of words can potentially be joined together in compound. In the *vigraha*, two units are analyzed at a time.

सर्वदेवनमस्करः salutations to all the gods ⇒ सर्व all + देवः god + नमस्करः salutations
*Vigraha*: सर्वाश्च ताः देवाश्च ⇒ सर्वदेवाः, सर्वदेवेभ्यः नमस्करः ⇒ सर्वदेवनमस्करः

कंसचाणूरमर्दनः destroyer of Kaṃsa and Cāṇūra (i.e., Kṛṣṇa) ⇒ कंसः Kaṃsa + चाणूरः Cāṇūra + मर्दन destroyer
*Vigraha*: कंसश्च चाणूरश्च ⇒ कंसचाणूर, कंसचाणूरं मर्दनः ⇒ कंसचाणूरमर्दनः

### *Tatpuruṣa* Compounds Ending in अर्थम्

The word अर्थम् at the end of a *tatpuruṣa* compound turns it into an indeclinable adverb, which expresses the purpose of something.

भोगापवर्गार्थम् for the purpose of enjoyment and liberation ⇒ भोगः enjoyment + अपवर्गः liberation + अर्थम् purpose
*Vigraha*: भोगस्य चापवर्गस्य चार्थम् ⇒ भोगापवर्गार्थम्

धर्मसंस्थापनार्थम् for the purpose of establishing justice ⇒ धर्मः justice + संस्थापन establishing + अर्थम् purpose
*Vigraha*: धर्मं संस्थापनम् ⇒ धर्मसंस्थापनम्, धर्मसंस्थापनस्य अर्थम् ⇒ धर्मसंस्थापनार्थम्

### Example: *Yogasūtra* 1.2

योगश्चित्तवृत्तिनिरोधः ⇒ योगः is चित्त mind + वृत्ति fluctuation + निरोधः restraint, control, stilling
*Vigraha*: चित्तस्य वृत्तयः ⇒ चित्तवृत्तयः, चित्तवृत्तीनां निरोधः ⇒ चित्तवृत्तिनिरोधः

Yoga is **the stilling of the fluctuations of the mind**.

#### M. *Haṭhapradīpikā* 2.16

प्राणायामेन युक्तेन सर्वरोगक्षयो भवेत्।
अयुक्ताभ्यासयोगेन सर्वरोगसमुद्भवः॥

Vocabulary

युक्त mfn. fit, suitable, appropriate, proper
क्षयः m. loss, wane, diminution
अयुक्त mfn. unsuitable, inappropriate, improper
समुद्भवः m. origin, arising

N. *Bhagavadgītā* 4.27

This verse comes in a series of verses describing different sacrifices performed by yogīs. The अपरे here is referring to followers of Sāṃkhya. The main verb is in the fourth *pāda*.

सर्वाणीन्द्रियकर्माणि प्राणकर्माणि चापरे ।
आत्मसंयमयोगाग्नौ जुह्वति ज्ञानदीपिते ॥

Vocabulary

संयमः m. *dhāraṇā* + *dhyāna* + *samādhi*, profound meditation, control, restraint
दीपित mfn. set on fire, illuminated, kindled

## Review Exercises

### O. *Śivasaṃhitā* 1.39–40

रज्जुज्ञानाद्यथा सर्पो मिथ्याभूतो निवार्तते ।
आत्मज्ञानात्तथा याति मिथ्याभूतमिदं जगत् ॥

रौप्यभ्रान्तिरियं याति शुक्तिज्ञानाद्यथा खलु ।
जगद्भ्रान्तिरियं याति चात्मज्ञानात्सदा तथा ॥

Vocabulary
सर्पः m. snake, serpent
मिथ्याभूत mfn. false, illusory
इदम् this (n. nom. sg.)
रौप्य mfn. silver
भ्रान्तिः f. mistaken perception
इयम् this (f. nom. sg.)
√या 2P, to disappear
शुक्तिः f. pearl oyster
खलु ind. indeed, certainly, as you know

### P. *Yogabīja* 148–49

प्रतीतिर्वायुयोगाच्च जायते पश्चिमे पथि ।
हकारेण तु सुर्योऽसौ ठकारेणेन्दुरुच्यते ॥

सूर्याचन्द्रमसोर्योगाद् हठयोगोऽभिधीयते ।
हठेन ग्रस्यते जाड्यं सर्वदोषसमुद्भवम् ॥

The *Yogabīja*, attributed to Gorakṣanātha in the thirteenth to fourteenth century C.E., is in the form of a dialogue between Śiva and Devī, mostly consisting of Devī's questions about yoga and Śiva's answers. It is most famous for the definition of the word *haṭha*, given in this verse, which was frequently repeated in later texts. Note that the sun and moon probably refer to the *piṅgalā* and *iḍā nāḍīs*, respectively.

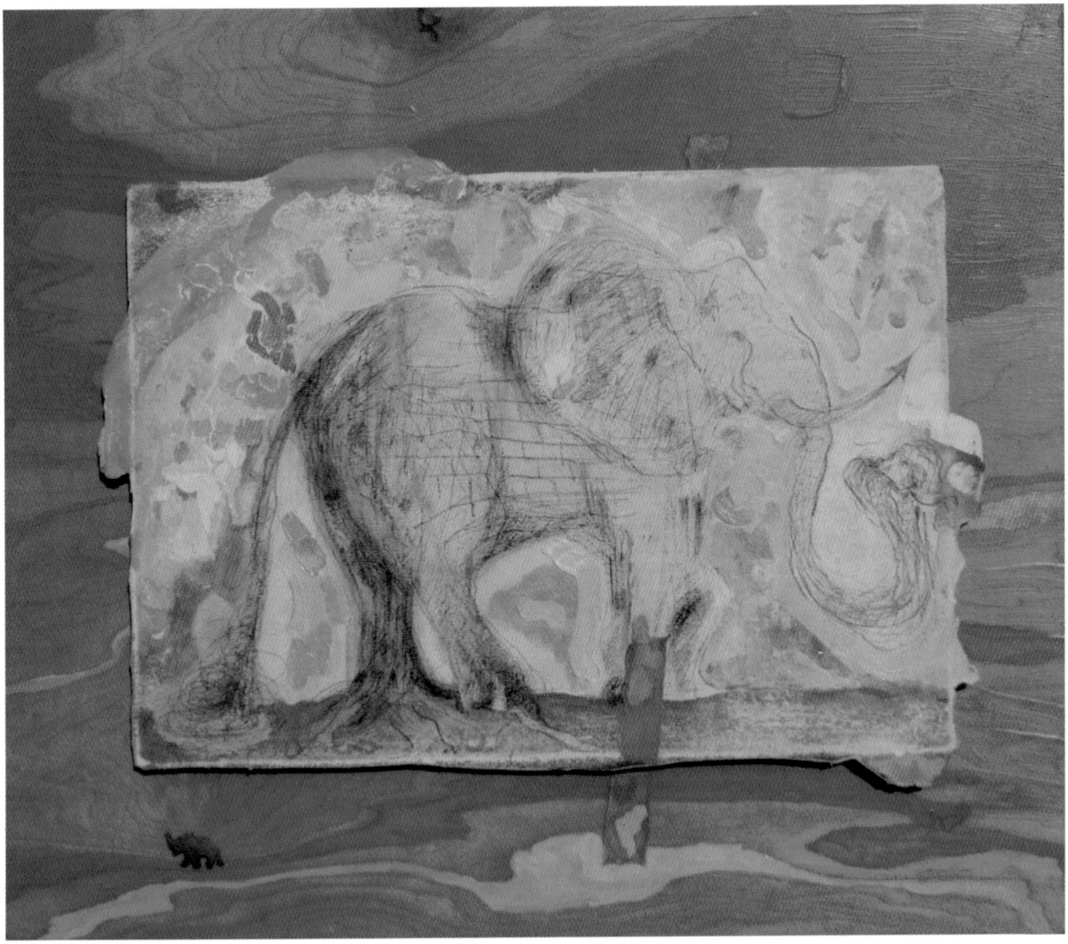

There is a well-known Indian parable of six blind men and an elephant. Each perceives the elephant differently depending on which part they touch: the man on the side feels it is like a wall; the one touching the tail imagines a rope; the trunk—a snake; the tusk—a spear; the leg—a tree; the ear—a fan. The moral is that our perception can be misguided if we only look at what is narrowly in front of us and that there are many ways to perceive the same truth.

Vocabulary

प्रतीतिः f. clear apprehension, complete understanding
पश्चिमे पथि on the western/back path, probably meaning in the *suṣumṇā nāḍī* (m. loc. sg.)
असौ that (m. nom. sg.)
सूर्याचन्द्रमसौ m. sun and moon (note the long आ in सूर्या, a relic of strict rules in Vedic Sanskrit for *dvandvas)*
अभि√धा pass. to be named or called
√ग्रस् 1P, to swallow, devour
जाड्यम् n. apathy, sluggishness, inactivity, dullness, stupidity
दोषः m. fault, defect, disease, the 3 humors when in a disordered state

Q. *Yogatattvopaniṣat* 14–16

The previous two verses list many of the possible disturbances to reaching मोक्ष.

तस्माद्दोषविनाशार्थमुपायं कथयामि ते ।
योगहीनं कथं ज्ञानं मोक्षदं भवति ध्रुवम् ॥

योगो हि ज्ञानहीनस्तु न क्षमो मोक्षकर्मणि ।
तस्माज्ज्ञानं च योगं च मुमुक्षुर्दृढमभ्यसेत् ॥

अज्ञानादेव संसारो ज्ञानादेव विमुच्यते ।
ज्ञानस्वरूपमेवादौ ज्ञानं ज्ञेयैकसाधनम् ॥

The *Yogatattvopaniṣat* is a member of the syncretic seventeenth-century *Yoga Upaniṣads* mentioned earlier. In this text, Brahmā approaches Viṣṇu, asking him to tell him about *yogatattva*, the true nature of yoga, and Viṣṇu replies with the teachings contained in this text.

Vocabulary

हीन mfn. without, deprived of
ध्रुवम् ind. certainly, surely
क्षम mfn. adequate, enough, appropriate (takes the locative)
मुमुक्षु mfn. desiring freedom/liberation
दृढम् ind. steadily
वि√मुच् pass. to be freed, liberated
स्वरूपम् n. one's own form, natural state
आदौ ind. in the beginning, at first
ज्ञेय mfn. to be known

# 13

# COMPOUNDS: *BAHUVRĪHI*; POSSESSIVE NOUNS ENDING IN मत् OR वत्; PRESENT PARTICIPLES

विवेकख्यातिरविप्लवा हानोपायः ॥ २.२६ ॥
**viveka-khyātir aviplavā hānopāyaḥ**
The means to liberation is uninterrupted discriminative discernment.
॥ *Yogasūtra* 2.26 ॥

## BAHUVRĪHI COMPOUNDS

These are possessive exocentric compounds where neither the first nor second member of the compound is predominant and the entire compound is used as an adjective to describe an outside entity. For example, Śiva is often called नीलकण्ठः, which, when used as a *bahuvrīhi*, means "he who has a blue throat." These compounds are always written in the same case, gender, and number as the word they are describing.

The word बहुव्रीहिः literally means "much rice," and is a perfect example of this kind of compound. Although by itself it is a *karmadhāraya* compound, if used to describe a person or a pot, it comes to mean "one who possesses much rice." *Bahuvrīhi* compounds often end with the suffix -क (m.) or -इका (f.), or are seen with a gender other than their natural one. These are sure signs that they are possessive compounds.

1. The most common type of *bahuvrīhi* is a *karmadhāraya* compound in the form "adjective-noun," used to describe an outside entity.

बहुव्रीहिः possessing much rice ⇒ बहु much + व्रीहिः rice
*Vigraha*: बहुव्रीहिर्यस्य स बहुव्रीहिः

नीलकण्ठः possessing a blue throat ⇒ नीलम् blue + कण्ठः throat
*Vigraha*: नीलं कण्ठं यस्य स नीलकण्ठः

Recall the Gaṇeśa mantra we learned in Chapter 3:

वक्रतुण्ड महाकाय सूर्यकोटिसमप्रभ ।
निर्विघ्नं कुरु मे देव सर्वकार्येषु सर्वदा ॥

The epithets given in the first line are all *bahuvrīhi* compounds describing the word देव in the third *pāda*. Since देव is in the vocative case, these descriptive compounds are as well.

वक्रतुण्डः one who has a curved trunk ⇒ वक्र curved + तुण्डम् trunk
*Vigraha*: वक्रं तुण्डं यस्य स वक्रतुण्डः

महाकायः one who has a great body ⇒ महत् great + कायः body
*Vigraha*: महा कायं यस्य स महाकायः

सूर्यकोटिसमप्रभः one whose brilliance is equal to 10 million suns ⇒ सूर्यः sun + कोटिः 10 million + सम equal + प्रभा brilliance
*Vigraha*: सूर्यकोट्याः समप्रभा यस्य स सूर्यकोटिसमप्रभः

2. Another type of *bahuvrīhi* compound has a prefix or preposition as its first component (like its *karmadhāraya* cousin).

निरामयः someone who is free from disease ⇒ निर्गत without + आमयः disease
*Vigraha*: निर्गतामय यस्मात्स निरामयः

सस्मितः someone with a smile ⇒ सहित with + स्मितम् smile
*Vigraha*: सहितः स्मितो यस्य स सस्मितः

3. Other *bahuvrīhi* compounds consist of a past passive participle as the first component and a noun or adjective that is the object of the participle's action as the second component.

स्थितप्रज्ञः one whose wisdom is steady ⇒ स्थित steady + प्रज्ञा wisdom
*Vigraha*: स्थिता प्रज्ञा येन स स्थितप्रज्ञः

Example: पतञ्जलिः स्थितप्रज्ञः ।

*Note that even though प्रज्ञा is feminine, if the compound is referring to a masculine noun, as it is in this case, the compound takes on a masculine ending.

जितेन्द्रियः one by whom the senses have been conquered ⇒ जित conquered + इन्द्रियम् sense
*Vigraha*: जितेन्द्रिया येन स जितेन्द्रियः

4. There is also a *bahuvrīhi* application of the *dvigu samāsa*, used for names or epithets.

अष्टाङ्गः having eight limbs ⇒ अष्टौ eight + अङ्गः limb
*Vigraha*: अष्टावङ्गानि यस्य सोऽष्टाङ्गः

त्र्यम्बकः having three eyes, Śiva ⇒ त्रीणि three + अम्बकः eye
*Vigraha*: त्रीण्यम्बकानि यस्य स त्र्यम्बकः

दशरथः having ten chariots ⇒ दश ten + रथः chariot
*Vigraha*: दश रथा यस्य स दशरथः

### Example: *Mahābhārata* 12.289.53

योगमार्गं तथासाद्य यः कश्चिद्भजते द्विजः ।
क्षेमेणोपरमेन्मार्गाद्बहुदोषो हि स स्मृतः ॥

Vocabulary
आसाद्य mfn. attainable, to be attained
√भज् 1Ā, to pursue, practice
कश्चिद् ind. someone, anyone
द्विजः m. twice born, a man of the first three classes, esp. a Brahmin (born for the second time after the sacred thread ceremony, the *upanayana*)
क्षेमेण ind. easily, with ease
उप√रम् 1U, to give up, renounce (takes the ablative)

If some (यः कश्चिद्) Brahmin (द्विजः) pursues (भजते) the path of yoga (योगमार्गम्),
And (तथा) it is attained (आसाद्य) with ease (क्षेमेण),

He should give up (उपरमेत्) that path (मार्गात्),
For (हि) it is thought (स्मृतः) that he (स) must **have many faults** (बहुदोषः).

### A. *Viṣṇu Mantra* II

This chant is also often used to address Gaṇeśa as well. The main verb is in the third *pāda*.

शुक्लाम्बरधरं विष्णुं शशिवर्णं चतुर्भुजम् ।
प्रसन्नवदनं ध्यायेत्सर्वविघ्नोपशान्तये ॥

Vocabulary
शुक्ल mfn. white
अम्बरम् n. clothes, garment
धर mfn. holding, bearing, wearing (from √धृ, in an *upapada tatpuruṣa* compound)
विष्णुः m. all-pervading
शशिन् m. "containing a hare, rabbit," the moon
वर्णः m. appearance, form
चतुर् mfn. four
भुजः m. arm
वदनम् n. the face, mouth
उपशान्तम् n. pacifying, quelling

### B. *Viṣṇu Mantra* III

This verse is in the *Mandākrāntā* meter, which has seventeen syllables in each *pāda*. The main sentence and verb are in the fourth *pāda*.

शान्ताकारं भुजगशयनं पद्मनाभं सुरेशं
विश्वाधारं गगनसदृशं मेघवर्णं शुभाङ्गम् ।
लक्ष्मीकान्तं कमलनयनं योगिभिर्ध्यानगम्यं
वन्दे विष्णुं भवभयहरं सर्वलोकैकनाथम् ॥

Vocabulary
शान्त mfn. tranquil
भुजगः m. snake, serpent
शयनम् n. bed, sleeping place

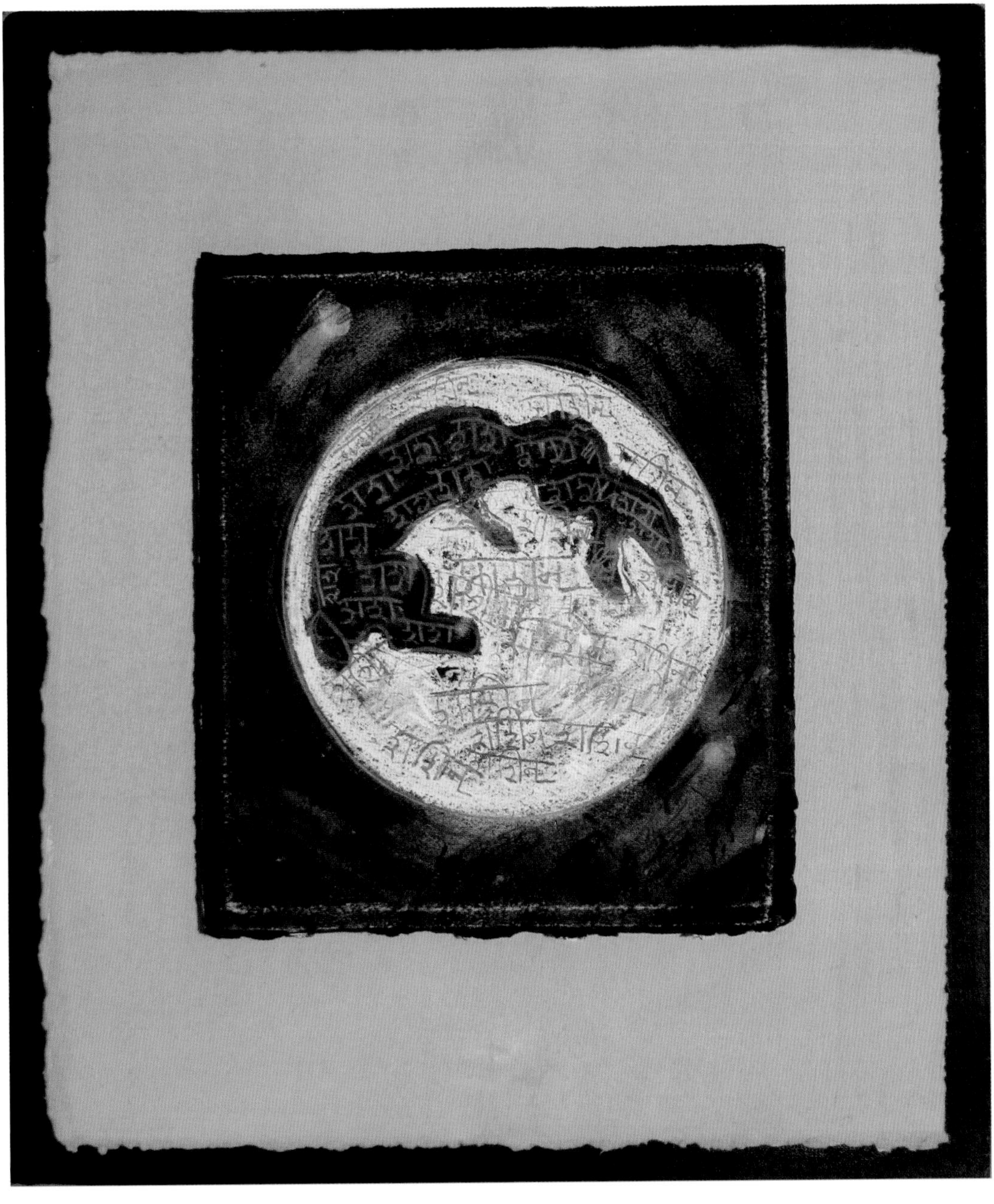

In India, people have traditionally seen a hare or rabbit, as opposed to a man, in the moon.

नाभ mfn. navel
सुरः m. god
ईशः m. lord
विश्वम् n. the whole world, universe
आधारः m. support
गगनम् n. sky
सदृश् mfn. like, resembling
मेघः m. cloud
शुभ mfn. beautiful
कान्तः m. beloved, lover, husband
कमल mn. lotus
नयनम् n. eye
योगिभिः by the yogīs (m. inst. pl.)
गम्य mfn. approachable, attainable
भवः m. existence
नाथः m. lord

### C. *Śivasaṃhitā* 1.75–76

These verses are a good example of the way in which *bahuvrīhi* compounds change depending on the gender of the noun they modify.

खं शब्दलक्षणं वायुश्चञ्चलः स्पर्शलक्षणः।
स्याद्रूपलक्षणं तेजः सलिलं रसलक्षणम्॥

गन्धलक्षणिका पृथ्वी नान्यथा भवति ध्रुवम्।
विशेषगुणाः स्फुरन्ति यतः शास्त्राद्विनिर्णयः॥

> The five elements, or *pañca-mahābhūtas*, play a prominent role in the Indian conception of the Universe. Space gives birth to air, which produces fire, which leads to water, which gives rise to earth. The five elements correspond to the five senses as illustrated in this verse.

Vocabulary

खम् n. ether, space
लक्षणम् n. mark, sign, characteristic, attribute
चञ्चल mfn. moving to and fro, unsteady, shaky
तेजस् n. fire
सलिलम् n. water
पृथ्वी f. the earth
विशेषः m. distinction, difference

गुणः m. characteristic, quality
√स्फुर् 6P, to shine, be evident, or manifest
विनिर्णयः m. certainty, a settled rule

### D. *Yogayājñavalkya* 1.43

ज्ञानं योगात्मकं विद्धि योगश्चाष्टाङ्गसंयुतः ।
संयोगो योग इत्युक्तो जीवात्मपरमात्मनोः ॥

Vocabulary
संयुत mfn. endowed with, contains, consists of
संयोगः m. conjunction, union, combination (to be read with जीवात्मपरमात्मनोः)
जीवात्मन् m. individual Soul
परमात्मन् m. universal Soul, Supreme Spirit

### E. *Bhagavadgītā* 15.1

ऊर्ध्वमूलमधःशाखमश्वत्थं प्राहुरव्ययम् ।
छन्दांसि यस्य पर्णानि यस्तं वेद स वेदवित् ॥

Vocabulary
ऊर्ध्व mfn. rising upward, elevated, above
अधस् ind. below, under
शाखा f. branch
अश्वत्थः m. the holy fig tree
प्राहुर् they say (3 p. pl. perfect)
अव्यय mfn. imperishable, undecaying, eternal
छन्दस् n. sacred hymn, Vedic hymn
पर्णम् n. leaf

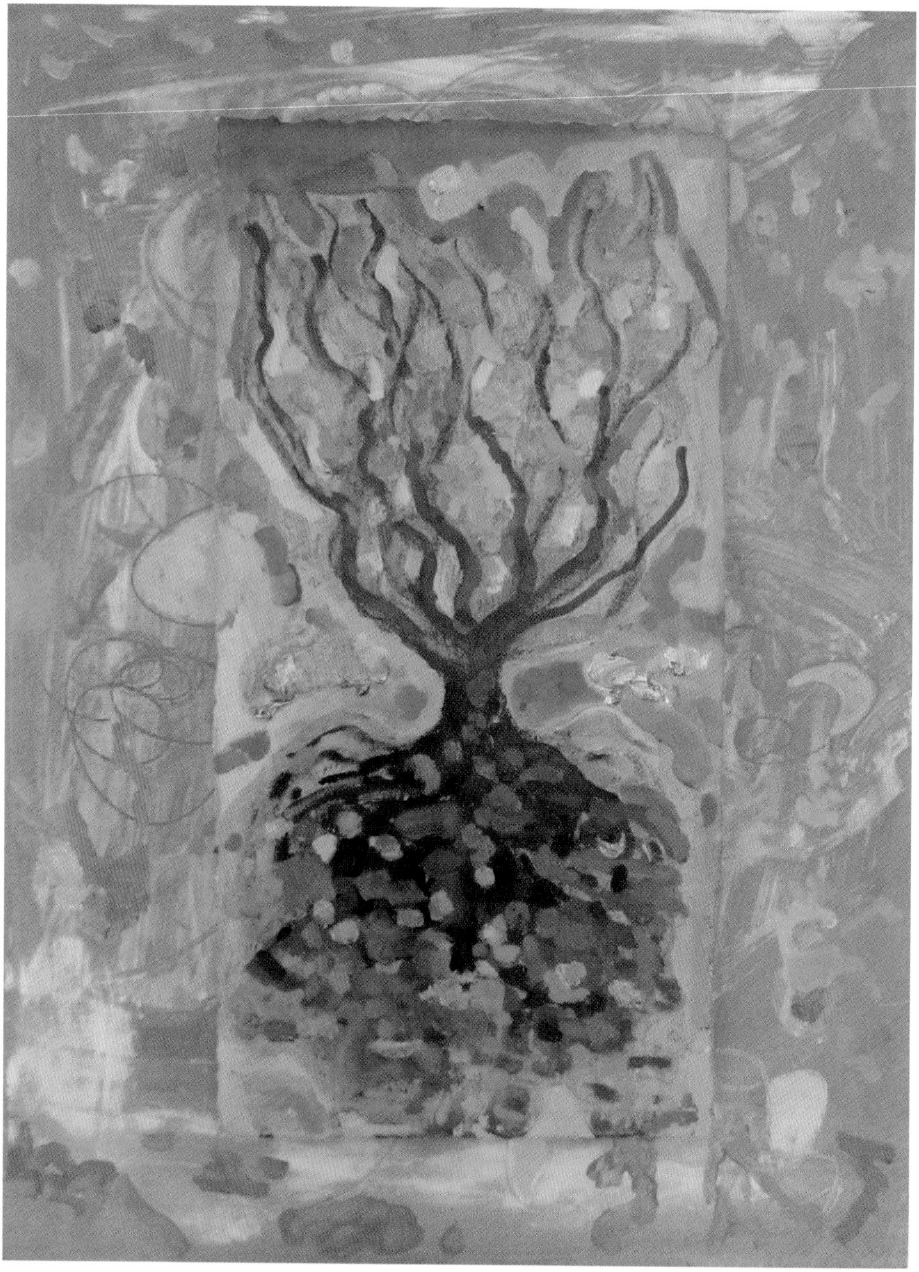

The *aśvattha* is the sacred fig tree, imagined to grow downward, with its roots in the heavens. This illustrates the idea of an immortal soul, an invisible essence in everyone, reborn into the world according to *karma*.

## POSSESSIVE NOUNS ENDING IN -मत् OR -वत्

Nouns ending in -मत् or -वत् indicate possession. The strong stems end in -अन्त् (the final त् drops off and the अ is lengthened in the masculine nominative singular). The weak stems end in -अत्. The feminine is formed by dropping the न् and adding ई and is declined like नदी.

**भगवत् m. fortunate, possessing fortune (भगः)**

| | Singular | Dual | Plural |
|---|---|---|---|
| **Nominative** | भगवान् | भगवन्तौ | भगवन्तः |
| **Accusative** | भगवन्तम् | भगवन्तौ | भगवतः |
| **Instrumental** | भगवता | भगवद्भ्याम् | भगवद्भिः |
| **Dative** | भगवते | भगवद्भ्याम् | भगवद्भ्यः |
| **Ablative** | भगवतः | भगवद्भ्याम् | भगवद्भ्यः |
| **Genitive** | भगवतः | भगवतोः | भगवताम् |
| **Locative** | भगवति | भगवतोः | भगवत्सु |
| **Vocative** | भगवन् | भगवन्तौ | भगवन्तः |

**भगवत् n. fortunate, possessing fortune (भगः)**

| | Singular | Dual | Plural |
|---|---|---|---|
| **Nom./Acc./Voc.** | भगवत् | भगवती | भगवन्ति |

**भगवती f. fortunate, possessing fortune (भगः)**

| | Singular | Dual | Plural |
|---|---|---|---|
| **Nominative** | भगवती | भगवत्यौ | भगवत्यः |
| **Accusative** | भगवतीम् | भगवत्यौ | भगवतीः |
| **Instrumental** | भगवत्या | भगवतीभ्याम् | भगवतीभिः |
| **Dative** | भगवत्यै | भगवतीभ्याम् | भगवतीभ्यः |
| **Ablative** | भगवत्याः | भगवतीभ्याम् | भगवतीभ्यः |
| **Genitive** | भगवत्याः | भगवत्योः | भगवतीनाम् |
| **Locative** | भगवत्याम् | भगवत्योः | भगवतीषु |
| **Vocative** | भगवति | भगवत्यौ | भगवत्यः |

Vocabulary

ज्योतिष्मत् mfn. luminous, possessing light (ज्योतिस्)
धनवत् mfn. wealthy, possessing wealth (धनम्)
धीमत् mfn. intelligent, possessing intelligence (धी)
बलवत् mfn. strong, possessing strength (बलम्)
बुद्धिमत् mfn. endowed with understanding, wise, possessing wisdom (बुद्धिः)
विद्यावत् mfn. learned, possessing knowledge (विद्या)
श्रद्धावत् mfn. full of faith (श्रद्धा)
हनुमत् m. Hanumān, possessing a jaw (हनुः)
हिमवत् mfn. snowy, possessing snow (हिमः), m. Himālaya

## Conjugate

बुद्धिमत्, श्रद्धावत्

## Translate

### F. *Bhagavadgītā* 18.71

The object of the verb शृणुयाद् is given in the previous verse—इमं धर्म्यं संवादम्—"this virtuous dialogue."

श्रद्धावाननसूयश्च शृणुयादपि यो नरः।
सोऽपि मुक्तः शुभाँल्लोकान्प्राप्नुयात्पुण्यकर्मणाम्॥

Vocabulary

अनसूय mfn. not spiteful, not envious

Sandhi Rule: A final न् before an initial ल् changes to ल् and *candrabindu* (ँ), the special mark of nasalization, is added.

Example. शुभान् लोकान् ⇒ शुभाँल्लोकान्

### G. *Aparokṣānubhūti* 33

अहम् refers to "the Soul" and is in contrast to देहः / देहकः, "the body."

अहं विकारहीनस्तु देहो नित्यं विकारवान्।
इति प्रतीयते साक्षात्कथं स्याद्देहकः पुमान्॥

Vocabulary

विकारः m. change, transformation, disease
प्रति√इ 2P, to recognize; pass. to be recognized
पुमान् Soul (m. nom. sg. पुंस्)

### H. *Kaṭhopaniṣat* 3.5–6

यस्त्वविज्ञानवान्भवत्ययुक्तेन मनसा सदा ।
तस्येन्द्रियाण्यवश्यानि दुष्टाश्वा इव सारथेः ॥

यस्तु विज्ञानवान्भवति युक्तेन मनसा सदा ।
तस्येन्द्रियाणि वश्यानि सदश्वा इव सारथेः ॥

Vocabulary
अविज्ञानम् n. lack of discernment, without understanding
अवश्य mfn. disobedient
दुष्ट mfn. bad
अश्वः m. horse
सारथिः m. charioteer
विज्ञानम् n. discernment, understanding

### I. *Yogasūtra* 1.36

This *sūtra* comes in a series of *sūtras* providing different methods for preventing and eliminating the disturbances of the mind. Infer "Or [there is clarity of mind, when . . .]"

विशोका वा ज्योतिष्मती ।

Vocabulary
विशोक mfn. free from sorrow

## PRESENT PARTICIPLES (*PARASMAIPADA*)

Present participles denote an action that is occurring continuously in the present moment, in relation to the main verb. They are conjugated just like nouns ending in अन्त्, with the exception of the nominative singular, where the final vowel is shortened.

### पतत् m. (He who is) falling

| | Singular | Dual | Plural |
|---|---|---|---|
| **Nominative** | पतन् | पतन्तौ | पतन्तः |
| **Accusative** | पतन्तम् | पतन्तौ | पततः |
| **Instrumental** | पतता | पतद्भ्याम् | पतद्भिः |
| **Dative** | पतते | पतद्भ्याम् | पतद्भ्यः |
| **Ablative** | पततः | पतद्भ्याम् | पतद्भ्यः |
| **Genitive** | पततः | पततोः | पतताम् |
| **Locative** | पतति | पततोः | पतत्सु |
| **Vocative** | पतन् | पतन्तौ | पतन्तः |

### पतत् n. (That which is) falling

| | Singular | Dual | Plural |
|---|---|---|---|
| **Nom./Acc./Voc.** | पतत् | पतन्ती | पतन्ति |

### पतन्ती f. (She who is) falling

| | Singular | Dual | Plural |
|---|---|---|---|
| **Nominative** | पतन्ती | पतन्त्यौ | पतन्त्यः |
| **Accusative** | पतन्तीम् | पतन्त्यौ | पतन्तीः |
| **Instrumental** | पतन्त्या | पतन्तीभ्याम् | पतन्तीभिः |
| **Dative** | पतन्त्यै | पतन्तीभ्याम् | पतन्तीभ्यः |
| **Ablative** | पतन्त्याः | पतन्तीभ्याम् | पतन्तीभ्यः |
| **Genitive** | पतन्त्याः | पतन्त्योः | पतन्तीनाम् |
| **Locative** | पतन्त्याम् | पतन्त्योः | पतन्तीषु |
| **Vocative** | पतन्ति | पतन्त्यौ | पतन्त्यः |

## Translate

### J. *Bhagavadgītā* 5.8–9

युक्तः in this verse refers to one who is योगयुक्तः, "yoked/absorbed/engaged in yoga." Infer "while" at the beginning of the second line, referring to all of the following activities.

नैव किञ्चित्करोमीति युक्तो मन्यते तत्त्ववित् ।
पश्यञ्शृण्वन्स्पृशञ्जिघ्रन्नश्नन्गच्छन्स्वपञ्श्वसन् ॥

प्रलपन्विसृजन्गृह्णन्नुन्मिषन्निमिषन्नपि ।
इन्द्रियाणीन्द्रियार्थेषु वर्तन्त इति धारयन् ॥

Vocabulary

न किञ्चित् ind. nothing, not anything
तत्त्वम् n. true nature
√घ्रा 3P, to smell
प्र√लप् 1P, to talk idly
वि√सृज् 6P, to eliminate
उन्√मिष् 6P, to open the eyes
नि√मिष् 6P, to close the eyes
धारयन् holding fast [to the thought], bearing in mind, remembering (caus. pres. part. m. nom. sg.√धृ)

K. *Bhagavadgītā* 6.16

नात्यश्नतस्तु योगोऽस्ति न चैकान्तमनश्नतः ।
न चातिस्वप्नशीलस्य जाग्रतो नैव चार्जुन ॥

Vocabulary

अत्य्√अश् 1Ā, to eat too much
एकान्तम् ind. absolutely, solely, at all
अति ind. beyond, too much, excessive
शीलम् n. habit

The present participle of the irregular verb √अस्, "to be," is सत्, and is declined as on the previous page. सत् is often translated as "the real" or "existent" and असत् as "the unreal" or "nonexistent."

L. *Bhagavadgītā* 2.16

नासतो विद्यते भावो नाभावो विद्यते सतः ।
उभयोरपि दृष्टोऽन्तस्त्वनयोस्तत्त्वदर्शिभिः ॥

Vocabulary

भावः m. being, existence
अभावः m. nonexistence
अन्तः m. end, limit, boundary, certainty
तत्त्वदर्शिभिः by seers of true nature/truth (inst. pl.)

## PRESENT PARTICIPLES (*ĀTMANEPADA*)

Present participles of *Ātmanepada* verbs are formed by taking the third person singular form, taking away the suffix -ते and adding the suffix -मान. They are conjugated as masculine or neuter nouns ending in -अ or as feminine nouns ending in -आ.

### Translate

#### M. *Dattātreyayogaśāstra* 39

Translate the second and third *pādas* together.

सांकृते शृणु सत्त्वस्थो योगाभ्यासक्रमं मया ।
वक्ष्यमाणं प्रयत्नेन योगिनां सर्वलक्षणैः ॥

Vocabulary
सत्त्वस्थ mfn. resolutely, energetically
प्रयत्नेन ind. with special effort, diligently, carefully
योगिनाम् of/for yogīs (m. gen. pl.)

#### N. *Gheraṇḍasaṃhitā* 1.8

In the first verse of the *Gheraṇḍasaṃhitā*, Caṇḍa asks Gheraṇḍa to teach him घटस्थयोग, "the yoga of the body." In this text, घटः, usually translated as "pot," means "body."

आमकुम्भ इवाम्भःस्थो जीर्यमाणः सदा घटः ।
योगानलेन संदह्य घटशुद्धिं समाचरेत् ॥

Vocabulary
आम mfn. unbaked
कुम्भः m. jar, pot
अम्भःस्थ mfn. situtated in water
अम्भस् n. water
√जॄ 1,4 U, to grow old, decay
सं√दह् 1U, to burn up, bake

## Review Exercises

One of the two great epics, the *Rāmāyaṇa*, literally "The Path of Rāma," was composed by the sage Vālmīki around the fifth to fourth century B.C.E. It tells the story of Rāma, who was an incarnation of Viṣṇu, his exile from Ayodhya, the abduction of his wife, Sītā, by Rāvaṇa, and how he rescued her with the help of Hanumān and returned to rule Ayodhya.

### O. *Rāmāyaṇa* 1.8–9

इक्ष्वाकुवंशप्रभवो रामो नाम जनैः श्रुतः ।
नियतात्मा महावीर्यो द्युतिमान्धृतिमान्वशी ॥

बुद्धिमान्नीतिमान्वाग्मी श्रीमाञ्शत्रुनिबर्हणः ।
विपुलांशो महाबाहुः कम्बुग्रीवो महाहनुः ॥

#### Vocabulary

इक्ष्वाकुः m. first king of the solar dynasty, son of Manu Vaivasvata
वंशः m. lineage
श्रुत mfn. known, famous, celebrated
नियत mfn. restrained, controlled
द्युतिः f. splendor, brightness, luster
धृतिः f. constancy, resolution
वशी having will or power, mastery (m. nom. sg. वशिन्)
नीतिः f. conduct, propriety, prudence
वाग्मी speaking well, eloquent (m. nom. sg. वाग्मिन्)
श्री f. radiance, beauty, grace
निबर्हण mfn. crushing, destroying, removing
विपुल mfn. large, extensive, wide
अंशः m. shoulder
कम्बु mn. conch shell

### P. *Bhāgavatapurāṇa* 3.28.10

मनोऽचिरात्स्याद्विरजं जितश्वासस्य योगिनः ।
वाय्वग्निभ्यां यथा लोहं ध्मातं त्यजति वै मलम् ॥

#### Vocabulary

अचिरात् ind. not long, soon
विरज mfn. free from dust
जित mfn. controlled
श्वासः m. breath

योगिनः of the yogī (m. nom. sg.)
लोहः m. gold
ध्मात mfn. blown, fanned

Q. *Bhagavadgītā* 6.19

यथा दीपो निवातस्थो नेङ्गते सोपमा स्मृता ।
योगिनो यतचित्तस्य युञ्जतो योगमात्मनः ॥

Vocabulary
दीपः m. a light, lamp, lantern
निवातम् n. a place sheltered from the wind, calm, stillness
√इङ्ग् 1U, to move, agitate, flicker
उपमा f. comparison, simile (to be read with योगिनः, of/to the yogī)

R. *Bhagavadgītā* 3.27

प्रकृतेः क्रियमाणानि गुणैः कर्माणि सर्वशः ।
अहंकारविमूढात्मा कर्ताहमिति मन्यते ॥

Vocabulary
सर्वशस् ind. always, universally
अहंकारः m. "I-maker," egotism
विमूढात्मन् mfn. bewildered, perplexed in mind

# 14
# Compounds: *Avyayībhāva*; the Suffix इन्; Gerundives; Locative and Genitive Absolute

**शान्तोदिताव्यपदेश्यधर्मानुपाती धर्मी ॥ ३.१४ ॥**
**śāntoditāvyapadeśya-dharmānupātī dharmī**
Any object contains within it the characteristics of past, present, and future.
‖ *Yogasūtra* 3.14 ‖

## *AVYAYĪBHĀVA* COMPOUNDS

*Avyayībhāva* compounds are indeclinable adverbial compounds, in which the first member is predominant. The word *avyayībhāva* literally means "the state of being unchangeable." The first word is usually an indeclinable particle or preposition, modified by the second word. The first component can be (a) a preposition, (b) स = सहः, or (c) a relative adverb. The final member is a nominal stem, always with a neuter accusative singular ending. Sometimes, other words are needed in order to gloss the compound.

### Examples

(a) a preposition as the first component

अनुरूपम् in accordance with form, fittingly
*Vigraha*: रूपयोग्यम् ⇒ अनुरूपम्

आमुक्ति until liberation
*Vigraha*: आ मुक्तेः ⇒ आमुक्ति

प्रतिदिनम् every day
*Vigraha*: दिने दिने ⇒ प्रतिदिनम्

(b) स = सहः as the first component

सकामम् with desire
*Vigraha*: सह कामेन ⇒ सकामम्

सस्मितम् with a smile
*Vigraha*: सह स्मितेन ⇒ सस्मितम्

सादरम् with respect
*Vigraha*: सहादरेण ⇒ सादरम्

(c) a relative adverb as the first component

यथाशक्ति in accordance with one's ability
*Vigraha*: शक्तिमनतिक्रम्य ⇒ यथाशक्ति

यथाकामम् in accordance with one's desire
*Vigraha*: काममनतिक्रम्य ⇒ यथाकामम्

यथागतम् in accordance with the way one arrived
*Vigraha*: गतमनतिक्रम्य ⇒ यथागतम्

यथायोग्यम् in accordance with what is suitable
*Vigraha*: योग्यमनतिक्रम्य ⇒ यथायोग्यम्

यावत्संवत्सरम् for as long as a year
*Vigraha*: यावत्संवत्सरो वर्तते तावत् ⇒ यावत्संवत्सरम्

यावज्जीवम् for as long as one lives
*Vigraha*: यावज्जीवो वर्तते तावत् ⇒ यावज्जीवम्

**A. *Ādityahṛdayam* 27**

Here, महाबाहो refers to Rāma.

अस्मिन्क्षणे महाबाहो रावणं त्वं वधिष्यसि ।
एवमुक्त्वा तदागस्त्यो जगाम च यथागतम् ॥

Vocabulary

क्षण mn. an instant, moment
√वध् 1P, to slay, kill
जगाम he/she went, left (3rd p. sg. perfect √गम्)

B. *Dattātreyayogaśāstra* 37

The object of समाकृष्य is पवनम्, the breath, in the fourth *pāda*.

यथाशक्ति समाकृष्य पूरयेदुदरं शनैः ।
यथाशक्त्येव पश्चात्तु रेचयेत्पवनं शनैः ॥

Vocabulary

समा√कृष् 1P, to draw together, draw in
√पॄ 3P, to fill; caus. to fill with wind, inhale
पश्चात् ind. afterward
√रिच् 7U, 1, 10P, to empty; caus. to make empty (of breath), exhale

C. *Dattātreyayogaśāstra* 93

Note that कर्तुः in the fourth *pāda* is the genitive singular form of the agent noun कर्तृ, "the doer, practitioner."

एकबारं प्रतिदिनं कुर्यात्केवलकुम्भकम् ।
प्रत्याहारो हि एवं स्यादेवं कर्तुर्हि योगिनः ॥

Vocabulary

बारः (वारः) m. time
केवलकुम्भकः m. pure/absolute breath retention
    केवल mfn. pure, absolute
    कुम्भकः m. a pot, stopping the breath
योगिनः of/for the yogī (m. gen. sg.)

## NOUNS ENDING IN -इन्

The suffix -इन् is primarily used to form possessive nouns. This suffix is added to the original noun, with its final vowel removed. For nouns ending in स्, the suffix becomes -विन् or -मिन्. The feminine forms are conjugated like नदी.

**योगिन् m. practitioner of yoga, one who possesses union**

| | Singular | Dual | Plural |
|---|---|---|---|
| **Nominative** | योगी | योगिनौ | योगिनः |
| **Accusative** | योगिनम् | योगिनौ | योगिनः |
| **Instrumental** | योगिना | योगिभ्याम् | योगिभिः |
| **Dative** | योगिने | योगिभ्याम् | योगिभ्यः |
| **Ablative** | योगिनः | योगिभ्याम् | योगिभ्यः |
| **Genitive** | योगिनः | योगिनोः | योगिनाम् |
| **Locative** | योगिनि | योगिनोः | योगिषु |
| **Vocative** | योगिन् | योगिनौ | योगिनः |

**तेजस्विन् n. brilliant, one who possesses light (तेजस्)**

| | Singular | Dual | Plural |
|---|---|---|---|
| **Nom./Acc./Voc.** | तेजस्वि | तेजस्विनी | तेजस्वीनि |

**योगिनी f. female practitioner of yoga, one who possesses union**

| | Singular | Dual | Plural |
|---|---|---|---|
| **Nominative** | योगिनी | योगिन्यौ | योगिन्यः |
| **Accusative** | योगिनीम् | योगिन्यौ | योगिनीः |
| **Instrumental** | योगिन्या | योगिनीभ्याम् | योगिनीभिः |
| **Dative** | योगिन्यै | योगिनीभ्याम् | योगिनीभ्यः |
| **Ablative** | योगिन्याः | योगिनीभ्याम् | योगिनीभ्यः |
| **Genitive** | योगिन्याः | योगिन्योः | योगिनीनाम् |
| **Locative** | योगिन्याम् | योगिन्योः | योगिनीषु |
| **Vocative** | योगिनि | योगिन्यौ | योगिन्यः |

Vocabulary

गुणिन् mfn. virtuous, one who possesses virtue (गुणः)
तपस्विन् mfn. one who practices austerities (तपस्), m. ascetic
तेजस्विन् mfn. brilliant, one who possesses light (तेजस्)
धनिन् mfn. wealthy, one who possesses wealth (धनम्)
बलिन् mfn. strong, one who possesses strength (बलम्)
शशिन् m. the moon, one who possesses a rabbit (शशः)
सुखिन् mfn. happy, one who possesses happiness (सुखम्)
हस्तिन् mfn. elephant, one who possesses a hand (हस्तः)

## Conjugate

सुखिन्

The suffix -इन् can also be added to verbal roots to form nouns that serve as the final component of an *upapada* compound, indicating the agent of an action.

√गम् ⇒ गामिन् one who goes, going
√वद् ⇒ वादिन् one who speaks, speaking

## Example: *Kaṭhopaniṣat* 3.3–4

Note that although in 3a, आत्मन् means Soul, in 4c, in the compound आत्मेन्द्रियमनः, आत्मन् means body.

आत्मानँ रथिनं विद्धि शरीरँ रथमेव तु ।
बुद्धिं तु सारथिं विद्धि मनः प्रग्रहमेव च ॥

इन्द्रियाणि हयानाहुर्विषयाँस्तेषु गोचरान् ।
आत्मेन्द्रियमनोयुक्तं भोक्तेत्याहुर्मनीषिणः ॥

### Vocabulary

रथः m. chariot
प्रग्रहः m. rein, bridle
आहुः they say (3 p. pl. perfect)
गोचरः m. range, field for action
मनीषिन् m. teacher, one who is wise

Know (विद्धि) the Soul (आत्मानम्) as **the chariot owner** (रथिनम्),
And (तु) the body (शरीरम्) as merely (एव) the chariot (रथम्).
Know (विद्धि) understanding (बुद्धिम्) as **the charioteer** (सारथिम्),
And (च) the mind (मनः) as merely (एव) the reins (प्रग्रहम्).

The senses (इन्द्रियाणि) are the horses (हयान्), they say (आहुः),
The sense objects (विषयान्) are the fields for action (गोचरान्).
One who is yoked to body, senses, and mind (आत्मेन्द्रियमनोयुक्तम्),
**The wise** (मनीषिणः) pronounce as (इति आहुः) one who enjoys (भोक्ता).

## Translate

### D. *Śivasaṃhitā* 3.30

All of the compounds in the third line are descriptions of the yogī.

चिह्नानि योगिनो देहे दृश्यन्ते नाडिशुद्धितः ।
कथ्यन्ते तु समन्तात्तान्यंगे संक्षेपतो मया ।
समकायः सुगन्धिश्च सुकान्तिः सुररसाधारः ॥

Vocabulary

चिह्नम् n. mark, sign, characteristic
नाडिशुद्धितः ind. from, as a result of the purification of the subtle channels
समन्तात् ind. on all sides, wholly, completely
अंगम् n. the body
संक्षेपतः ind. briefly, concisely, shortly
सुगन्धि mfn. sweet-smelling, fragrant
सुकान्ति mfn. very beautiful
सुरः m. a god
रसः m. essence, nectar
आधारः m. vessel, receptacle

### E. *Śivasaṃhitā* 3.33

प्रौढवह्निः सुभोजी च सुखी सर्वाङ्गसुन्दरः ।
संपूर्णहृदयो योगी सर्वोत्साहबलान्वितः ।
जायन्ते योगिनोऽवश्यमेते सर्वे कलेवरे ॥

Vocabulary

प्रौढ mfn. mighty, strong
वह्निः m. fire, digestive fire
सुभोजिन् mfn. one who eats well
सुन्दर mfn. beautiful, lovely
संपूर्ण mfn. completely filled or full
अन्वित mfn. endowed with, possessed of
अवश्यम् ind. inevitably, certainly, by all means
कलेवर mn. the body

### F. *Yogarahasya* 1.39

The first word and the last word should be read together as the subject of the verse.

रोगिणो धनिनो वा स्युः राजानः सुधियोऽपि वा ।
न कदापि मनः शान्तिं लभन्ते भूतले नराः ॥

Vocabulary
सुधियः very wise (m. gen. sg.)
न कदापि ind. not at any time
भूतलम् n. the earth

### G. *Bhagavadgītā* 6.46

तपस्विभ्योऽधिको योगी ज्ञानिभ्योऽपि मतोऽधिकः ।
कर्मिभ्यश्चाधिको योगी तस्माद्योगी भवार्जुन ॥

Vocabulary
अधिक mfn. surpassing, superior (takes the ablative)

## GERUNDIVES OR FUTURE PASSIVE PARTICIPLES

The gerundive is a passive participle, used in nominal form, which has a similar meaning to the optative, for example, something "is to be, should be, or ought to be done." It is formed by adding the suffix -तव्य, -य, or -अनीय to the root, which takes गुण, or sometimes वृद्धि.

### Examples

√गुप् 1P, to guard, protect, hide, conceal ⇒ गोपनीय to be guarded, protected, hidden
√छिद् 7P, to cut, pierce, divide ⇒ छेद्य to be cut off, divided, pierced
√युज् 7P, to yoke, join, unite ⇒ योक्तव्य to be yoked/concentrated/absorbed, to be practiced

### Translate

### H. *Bhagavadgītā* 2.24–25

Note in these verses that the addition of the letter अ at the beginning of the gerundive is not an augment but indicates negation.

अच्छेद्योऽयमदाह्योऽयमक्लेद्योऽशोष्य एव च ।
नित्यः सर्वगतः स्थाणुरचलोऽयं सनातनः ॥

अव्यक्तोऽयमचिन्त्योऽयमविकार्योऽयमुच्यते ।
तस्मादेवं विदित्वैनं नानुशोचितुमर्हसि ॥

Vocabulary
अयम् this [Soul] (m. nom. sg.)
√दह् 1P, to burn
स्थाणुः m. fixed, stationary, immovable
सनातन mfn. eternal, everlasting
अव्यक्त mfn. unmanifest
वि√कृ 8P, to change, transform
एनम् this [Soul] (m. nom. sg.)

### I. *Bhagavadgītā* 6.23

Note that विद्यात् in the first *pāda* is the optative of √विद्.

तं विद्याद्दुःखसंयोगवियोगं योगसंज्ञितम् ।
स निश्चयेन योक्तव्यो योगोऽनिर्विण्णचेतसा ॥

Vocabulary
वियोगः m. disjunction, separation, absence of
संज्ञित mfn. known as, called, named
अनिर्विण्ण mfn. not downcast, depressed, despondent

### J. *Śivasaṃhitā* 5.41

Note that the subject is in the fourth *pāda*.

गोपनीयः प्रयत्नेन सद्यःप्रत्ययकारकः ।
निर्वाणदायको लोके योगोऽयं मम वल्लभः ॥

Vocabulary
प्रयत्नः m. great care, effort
सद्यस् ind. on the same day, in the very moment, at once, immediately

प्रत्ययः m. trust, faith, proof, confidence
कारक mfn. who or what produces or creates
निर्वाणम् n. liberation
दायक mfn. giving, granting, bestowing
अयम् this (m. nom. sg.)
वल्लभ mfn. beloved above all, dear to

## LOCATIVE ABSOLUTE (सति सप्तमि)

An absolute clause is used to express two time-related actions (e.g., when X happens, Y happens). The locative absolute requires a noun and a participle in the locative case. The noun in the locative absolute is always different from the subject of the main verb, and that is why a locative absolute is used instead of a gerund. Often, the word सति (locative of the present participle सत् from the verb √अस्, "to be") is either used or implied.

### Example: *Yogasūtra* 2.49

तस्मिन्सति श्वासप्रश्वासयोर्गतिविच्छेदः प्राणायामः ।

तस्मिन्सति is a locative absolute, referring back to the previous three *sūtras* concerning *āsana* practice. "When that [*āsana*] is established, then . . ."

Vocabulary
श्वासः m. exhalation
प्रश्वासः m. inhalation
गतिः f. movement
विच्छेदः m. cutting off

**When that [*āsana*] is established** (तस्मिन्सति), then there is the cutting off (विच्छेदः) of the movement (गतिः) of the inhalation and exhalation (श्वासप्रश्वासयो), [called] *prāṇāyāma* (प्राणायामः).

## Translate

### K. *Haṭhapradīpikā* 1.42

तथैकस्मिन्नेव दृढे सिद्धे सिद्धासने सति ।
बन्धत्रयमनायासात्स्वयमेवोपजायते ॥

#### Vocabulary

सिद्ध mfn. perfected
बन्धत्रयम् n. the triad of *bandhas*, locks (i.e., *mūlabandha*, *uḍḍīyānabandha*, *jālandhara-bandha*)
अनायास mfn. ease, absence of exertion
स्वयम् ind. spontaneously, of one's own accord

### L. *Haṭhapradīpikā* 2.2

Note that in the first *pāda*, the present participle सति has to be inferred. In the second *pāda*, वाते सति and चित्तम् must be inferred.

चले वाते चलं चित्तं निश्चले निश्चलं भवेत् ।
योगी स्थाणुत्वमाप्नोति ततो वायुं निरोधयेत् ॥

#### Vocabulary

चल mfn. moving, unsteady, fluctuating
वातः m. wind, breath
स्थाणुत्वम् n. motionlessness, stableness
नि√रुध् 7P, to control, hold back, stop, restrain

### M. *Bhajagovindam* (Refrain)

This verse is the refrain to a hymn composed by Ādi Śaṅkarācārya. In addition to the refrain, the hymn is composed of a cluster of twelve blossoms (verses), *dvādaśa-mañjarīka-stotra*, written by Śaṅkara, plus fourteen blossoms (verses), *caturdaśa-mañjarīka-stotra*, written, one each, by his disciples.

भज गोविन्दं भज गोविन्दं भज गोविन्दं मूढमते ।
सम्प्राप्ते संनिहिते काले न हि न हि रक्षति डुकृङ्करणे ॥

Vocabulary

गोविन्दः m. Kṛṣṇa, cow herder
मूढमतिः m. foolish person
सम्प्राप्त mfn. attained, reached, arrived
संनिहित mfn. near, at hand
कालः m. time, death
न हि ind. surely not, by no means, not at all
√रक्ष् 1P, to protect, save
डुकृङ्करणे rules of grammar

## Genitive Absolute

The genitive absolute is used much more rarely. Like the locative absolute, it is used to indicate actions occurring simultaneously, except that it uses the genitive case instead of the locative. It is used to express that the main action is occurring "in spite of" some other background action.

One day Śaṅkara was walking through the streets of Varanasi and saw an old man teaching the grammatical rules of Pāṇini to some students. Śaṅkara felt pity for this man who had spent his life obsessed with intellectual accomplishment, but never really understood the essence of what he was studying. Śaṅkara then wrote these verses, advising him not to continue to waste his time and to turn his mind to divine contemplation. *Bhajagovindam* is also known as *Mohamudgaraḥ*, the hammer [that shatters] delusion.

## Review Exercises

### N. *Haṭhapradīpikā* 1.11

हठविद्या परं गोप्या योगिना सिद्धिमिच्छता।
भवेद्वीर्यवती गुप्ता निर्वीर्या तु प्रकाशिता॥

Vocabulary
परम् ind. in a high degree, absolutely, completely
√इष् 6P, to desire, wish for (pres. part. इच्छत्)
निर्वीर्य mfn. powerless, impotent
प्रकाशित mfn. displayed, revealed

### O. *Haṭhapradīpikā* 2.1

The present participle सति should be assumed in the first *pāda*.

अथासने दृढे योगी वशी हितमिताशनः।
गुरूपदिष्टमार्गेण प्राणायामान्समभ्यसेत्॥

Vocabulary
वशिन् m. possessing self-control
हित mfn. beneficial, wholesome
मित mfn. measured, moderate
अशनम् n. eating
उपदिष्ट mfn. taught
समभ्यु√अस् 4P, to practice

### P. *Haṭhapradīpikā* 2.7

बद्धपद्मासनो योगी प्राणं चन्द्रेण पूरयेत्।
धारयित्वा यथाशक्ति भूयः सूर्येण रेचयेत्॥

Vocabulary
चन्द्रः m. the moon, i.e., the lunar channel, *iḍā nāḍī*
भूयस् ind. again, besides, then
सूर्यः m. the sun, i.e., the solar channel, *piṅgalā nāḍī*

Q. *Yogarahasya* 1.32–33

In the second *pāda*, infer that the कारणानि [are explained].

यथायोग्यं विचार्याथ कारणानि मनीषिणा ।
प्रयोज्यानीति ऋषिभिः प्रोक्तानि प्रविभागतः ॥

अभ्याससमये नित्यं रेचपूरककुम्भकान् ।
यथाशक्ति प्रकुर्वीत रीत्योज्जाय्या विलम्बितः ॥

Vocabulary
वि√चर् 1P, to examine, investigate, ascertain
कारणम् n. means
प्रयोज्य mfn. [the postures] to be practiced
प्रविभागतः ind. proportionately, according to [people's] differences
समयः m. proper time, time
रीतिः f. custom, practice, method
उज्जायी f. victorious breath
विलम्बित mfn. slowly

# Part II Review: *Bhagavadgītā*, Chapter 12

अर्जुण उवाच ।

एवं सततयुक्तो ये भक्तास्त्वां पर्युपासते ।
ये चाप्यक्षरमव्यक्तं तेषां के योगवित्तमाः ॥ १ ॥

श्रीभगवानुवाच ।

मय्यावेश्य मनो ये मां नित्ययुक्ता उपासते ।
श्रद्धया परयोपेतास्ते मे युक्ततमा मताः ॥ २ ॥

ये त्वक्षरमनिर्देश्यमव्यक्तं पर्युपासते ।
सर्वत्रगमचिन्त्यं च कूटस्थमचलं ध्रुवम् ॥ ३ ॥

संनियम्येन्द्रियग्रामं सर्वत्र समबुद्धयः ।
ते प्राप्नुवन्ति मामेव सर्वभूतहिते रताः ॥ ४ ॥

क्लेशोऽधिकतरस्तेषामव्यक्तासक्तचेतसाम् ।
अव्यक्ता हि गतिर्दुःखं देहवद्भिरवाप्यते ॥ ५ ॥

ये तु सर्वाणि कर्माणि मयि संन्यस्य मत्पराः ।
अनन्येनैव योगेन मां ध्यायन्त उपासते ॥ ६ ॥

तेषामहं समुद्धर्ता मृत्युसंसारसागरात् ।
भवामि नचिरात्पार्थ मय्यावेशितचेतसाम् ॥ ७ ॥

मय्येव मन आधत्स्व मयि बुद्धिं निवेशय ।
निवसिष्यसि मय्येवात ऊर्ध्वं न संशयः ॥ ८ ॥

अथ चित्तं समाधातुं न शक्नोषि मयि स्थिरम् ।
अभ्यासयोगेन ततो मामिच्छाप्तुं धनंजय ॥ ९ ॥

अभ्यासेऽप्यसमर्थोऽसि मत्कर्मपरमो भव ।
मदर्थमपि कर्माणि कुर्वन्सिद्धिमवाप्स्यसि ॥ १० ॥

अथैतदप्यशक्तोऽसि कर्तुं मद्योगमाश्रितः ।
सर्वकर्मफलत्यागं ततः कुरु यतात्मवान् ॥ ११ ॥

श्रेयो हि ज्ञानमभ्यासाज् ज्ञानाद्ध्यानं विशिष्यते ।
ध्यानात्कर्मफलत्यागस्त्यागाच्छान्तिरनन्तरम् ॥ १२ ॥

अद्वेष्टा सर्वभूतानां मैत्रः करुण एव च ।
निर्ममो निरहंकारः समदुःखसुखः क्षमी ॥ १३ ॥

संतुष्टः सततं योगी यतात्मा दृढनिश्चयः ।
मय्यर्पितमनोबुद्धिर्यो मद्भक्तः स मे प्रियः ॥ १४ ॥

यस्मान्नोद्विजते लोको लोकान्नोद्विजते च यः ।
हर्षामर्षभयोद्वेगैर्मुक्तो यः स च मे प्रियः ॥ १५ ॥

अनपेक्षः शुचिर्दक्ष उदासीनो गतव्यथः ।
सर्वारम्भपरित्यागी यो मद्भक्तः स मे प्रियः ॥ १६ ॥

यो न हृष्यति न द्वेष्टि न शोचति न काङ्क्षति ।
शुभाशुभपरित्यागी भक्तिमान्यः स मे प्रियः ॥ १७ ॥

समः शत्रौ च मित्रे च तथा मानापमानयोः ।
शीतोष्णसुखदुःखेषु समः सङ्गविवर्जितः ॥ १८ ॥

तुल्यनिन्दास्तुतिर्मौनी संतुष्टो येन केनचित् ।
अनिकेतः स्थिरमतिर्भक्तिमान्मे प्रियो नरः ॥ १९ ॥

ये तु धर्म्यामृतमिदं यथोक्तं पर्युपासते ।
श्रद्दधाना मत्परमा भक्तास्तेऽतीव मे प्रियाः ॥ २० ॥

Vocabulary

अक्षर mfn. imperishable, unchangeable
अत ऊर्ध्वम् ind. from then forward
अतीव ind. exceedingly
अद्वेष्टृ mfn. one who has no hatred

अधिकतर mfn. greater
अनन्तर mfn. uninterrupted, continuous, immediately following
अनन्य mfn. no other [object]
अनपेक्ष mfn. indifferent, impartial
अनिकेत mfn. houseless, having no fixed abode
अनिर्देश्य mfn. undefinable
अमर्षः m. impatience, indignation
अमृतम् n. nectar, ambrosia
अशक्त mfn. unable, incapable
अशुभ mfn. unpleasant, disagreeable
असमर्थ mfn. unable, incapable
आ√धा 1Ā, to place
आ√विश् 6P, to enter, approach; caus. to cause to enter or approach
आवेशित mfn. entered into
आश्रित mfn. resorting to
आसक्त mfn. attached to
इच्छा f. desire, wish, endeavor
इदम् this (n. acc. sg.)
उदासीन mfn. sitting apart, indifferent, neutral, open-minded
उद्√विज् 1Ā, to tremble, fear, shrink from
उद्वेगः m. agitation, anxiety
उप√आस् 1Ā, to honor, worship, meditate upon
उपेत mfn. accompanied by, endowed with, possessing
उवाच he/she spoke (3rd p. sg. perfect √वच्)
करुण mfn. compassionate
√काङ्क्ष् 1P, to desire, lust
कूटस्थ mfn. immovable, unchangeable
क्लेशः m. affliction
क्षमिन् mfn. patient, possessing patience
गतिः m. path
ग्रामः m. a multitude, class, collection
त्यागः m. giving up, abandoning
दक्ष mfn. able, adroit, dexterous
दृढ mfn. firm, strong
देहवत् m. living creature, man, embodied being, one who identifies with the body
धर्म्य mfn. just, righteous, fair
धान mfn. holding

√ध्यै 1P, think of, contemplate
ध्रुव mfn. fixed, immovable, unchangeable, eternal
नचिरात् ind. shortly, soon
निन्दा f. blame, reproach
निरहंकार mfn. free from egotism, unselfish
निर्मम mfn. unselfish, free from worldly attachment
परित्यागिन् mfn. renouncing, unattached
पर्युप√आस् 1Ā, to approach respectfully, attend upon, worship, meditate on
प्रिय mfn. dear, beloved
भक्तः m. a worshipper, adorer, devotee
भक्तिमत् mfn. filled with devotion
भगवत् mfn. possessing fortune, glorious, divine
मैत्र mfn. friendly
मौनिन् mfn. observing silence, silent, taciturn
युक्ततम mfn. most intent upon, most devoted
रत mfn. delighting in, intent upon
वित्तम mfn. most knowing, having the best knowledge
वि√शिष् 7P, to be better than, distinguish, excel
व्यथा f. agitation, anguish, fear
शुभ mfn. pleasant
श्री mfn. sacred, holy, revered
श्रेयस् mfn. better
सततम् ind. constantly, always, ever
संतुष्ट mfn. quite satisfied or contented
समा√धा 3P, to place, direct, keep
समुद्धर्तृ mfn. one who lifts up or raises or extricates from
संनि√यम् 1P, to hold together, restrain, control
सं√न्यस् 2P, to place together
सर्वत्रग mfn. all-pervading, omnipresent
स्तुतिः f. praise
हर्षः m. lustfulness
हितम् n. welfare
√हृष् 4P, to rejoice, exult, gloat

# Part III

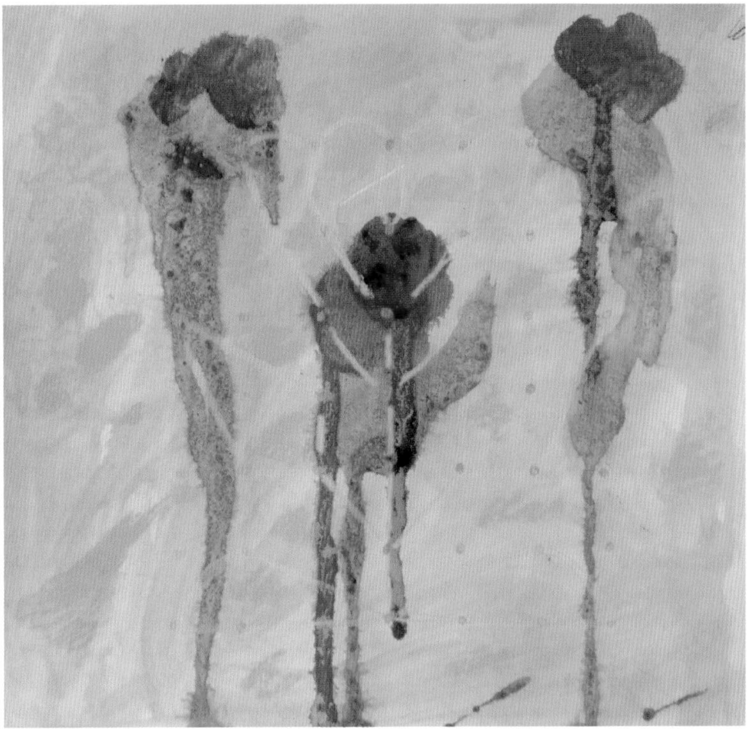

# 15
# Sanskrit Numerals; Degrees of Comparison; आदि, अद्य, and प्रभृति

त्रयमेकत्र संयमः ॥ ३.४ ॥
These three (*dhāraṇā*, *dhyāna*, and *samādhi*), when practiced all together, are called *saṃyama*.
॥ *Yogasūtra* 3.4 ॥

## SANSKRIT NUMERALS (*SAṂKHYĀ*)

We have encountered some numerals already, including the pronomial declension of the number one, एक, and numbers within compounds, *dvigu samāsas*. We will now look at numbers in a more comprehensive manner. Sanskrit numerals can appear as either cardinals ("one," "two," "three") or as ordinals ("first," "second," "third"). The *devanāgarī* numerals are the source of our "Arabic" numbers and combine in a similar manner (see below).

## CARDINAL NUMBERS

Cardinal numbers are adjectives, such as "one," "two," and "three," which are singular, dual, and plural, respectively. The first four numerals agree in gender, number, and case with the noun they are accompanying. There are no vocative forms.

**एक one**

| | Masculine | Neuter | Feminine |
|---|---|---|---|
| **Nominative** | एकः | एकम् | एका |
| **Accusative** | एकम् | एकम् | एकाम् |
| **Instrumental** | एकेन | एकेन | एकया |
| **Dative** | एकस्मै | एकस्मै | एकस्यै |
| **Ablative** | एकस्मात् | एकस्मात् | एकस्यात् |
| **Genitive** | एकस्य | एकस्य | एकस्याः |
| **Locative** | एकस्मिन् | एकस्मिन् | एकस्याम् |

**द्वि two**

| | Masculine | Neuter | Feminine |
|---|---|---|---|
| **Nom., Acc.** | द्वौ | द्वे | द्वे |
| **Inst., Dat., Abl.** | द्वाभ्याम् | द्वाभ्याम् | द्वाभ्याम् |
| **Gen., Loc.** | द्वयोः | द्वयोः | द्वयोः |

**त्रि three**

| | Masculine | Neuter | Feminine |
|---|---|---|---|
| **Nominative** | त्रयः | त्रीणि | तिस्रः |
| **Accusative** | त्रीन् | त्रीणि | तिस्रः |
| **Instrumental** | त्रिभिः | त्रिभिः | तिसृभिः |
| **Dat., Abl.** | त्रिभ्यः | त्रिभ्यः | तिसृभ्यः |
| **Genitive** | त्रयाणाम् | त्रयाणाम् | तिसृणाम् |
| **Locative** | त्रिषु | त्रिषु | तिसृषु |

**चतुर् four**

| | Masculine | Neuter | Feminine |
|---|---|---|---|
| **Nominative** | चत्वारः | चत्वारि | चतस्रः |
| **Accusative** | चतुरः | चत्वारि | चतस्रः |
| **Instrumental** | चतुर्भिः | चतुर्भिः | चतसृभिः |
| **Dat., Abl.** | चतुर्भ्यः | चतुर्भ्यः | चतसृभ्यः |
| **Genitive** | चतुर्णाम् | चतुर्णाम् | चतसृणाम् |
| **Locative** | चतुर्षु | चतुर्षु | चतसृषु |

The remaining numbers are not differentiated by gender, although they still must agree in case with the accompanying noun and are all plural through the number nineteen. The numbers from five to nineteen are all declined just like **पञ्चन्** (five), with the exception of **षष्** (six) and **अष्टन्** (eight). The numbers from twenty onward are declined as singular nouns.

| | पञ्चन् five | षष् six | अष्टन् eight |
|---|---|---|---|
| **Nom., Acc.** | पञ्च | षट् | अष्ट / अष्टौ |
| **Instrumental** | पञ्चभिः | षड्भिः | अष्टभिः / अष्टाभिः |
| **Dat., Abl.** | पञ्चभ्यः | षड्भ्यः | अष्टभ्यः / अष्टाभ्यः |
| **Genitive** | पञ्चानाम् | षण्णाम् | अष्टानाम् |
| **Locative** | पञ्चसु | षट्सु | अष्टसु / अष्टासु |

## ORDINAL NUMBERS

Ordinal numbers in masculine and neuter forms end in -अ and in the feminine form end in -आ or -ई. The first three ordinals—प्रथम (first), द्वितीय (second), and तृतीय (third)—can be optionally declined as pronouns. For numbers higher than twenty, there are two ordinal forms: a longer form ending with the suffix -तम and a shorter form that reduces the cardinal back to its final -अ or, if its final vowel is -इ, replaces it with -अ (see below). Note that for cardinal and ordinal numbers above ten ending in nine (i.e., nineteen, twenty-nine, thirty-nine, etc.), the word एकोन, meaning "one less than," is usually used before the following number (i.e., एकोनविंशति, "one less than twenty," nineteen).

| | | Cardinals | Ordinals (m/n) | Ordinals (f) |
|---|---|---|---|---|
| 1 | १ | एक | प्रथम | प्रथमा |
| 2 | २ | द्वि | द्वितीय | द्वितीया |
| 3 | ३ | त्रि | तृतीय | तृतीया |
| 4 | ४ | चतुर् | चतुर्थ / तुरीय / तुर्य | चतुर्थी / तुरीया / तुर्या |
| 5 | ५ | पञ्चन् | पञ्चम | पञ्चमी |
| 6 | ६ | षष् | षष्ठ | षष्ठी |
| 7 | ७ | सप्तन् | सप्तम | सप्तमी |
| 8 | ८ | अष्टन् | अष्टम | अष्टमी |
| 9 | ९ | नवन् | नवम | नवमी |
| 10 | १० | दशन् | दशम | दशमी |
| 11 | ११ | एकादशन् | एकादश | एकादशी |
| 12 | १२ | द्वादशन् | द्वादश | द्वादशी |
| 13 | १३ | त्रयोदशन् | त्रयोदश | त्रयोदशी |
| 14 | १४ | चतुर्दशन् | चतुर्दश | चतुर्दशी |
| 15 | १५ | पञ्चदशन् | पञ्चदश | पञ्चदशी |
| 16 | १६ | षोदशन् | षोदश | षोदशी |
| 17 | १७ | सप्तदशन् | सप्तदश | सप्तदशी |
| 18 | १८ | अष्टादशन् | अष्टादश | अष्टादशी |
| 19 | १९ | नवदशन् / एकोनविंशति / ऊनविंशति | नवदश / एकोनविंश / ऊनविंश | नवदशी / एकोनविंशी / ऊनविंशी |
| 20 | २० | विंशति | विंश / विंशतितम | विंशी / विंशतितमी |
| 21 | २१ | एकविंशति | एकविंश / एकविंशतितम | एकविंशी / एकविंशतितमी |
| 30 | ३० | त्रिंशत् | त्रिंश / त्रिंशत्तम | त्रिंशी / त्रिंशत्तमी |
| 40 | ४० | चत्वारिंशत् | चत्वारिंश / चत्वारिंशत्तम | चत्वारिंशी / चत्वारिंशत्तमी |
| 50 | ५० | पञ्चाशत् | पञ्चाश / पञ्चाशत्तम | पञ्चाशी / पञ्चाशत्तमी |

| | | | | |
|---|---|---|---|---|
| 60 | ६० | षष्टि | षष्टितम | षष्टितमी |
| 61 | ६१ | एकषष्टि | एकषष्ट / एकषष्टितम | एकषष्टी / एकषष्टितमी |
| 70 | ७० | सप्तति | सप्ततितम | सप्ततितमी |
| 71 | ७१ | एकसप्तति | एकसप्तत / एकसप्ततितम | एकसप्तती / एकसप्ततितमी |
| 80 | ८० | अशीति | अशीतितम | अशीतितमी |
| 81 | ८१ | एकाशीति | एकाशीत / एकाशीतितम | एकाशीती / एकाशीतितमी |
| 90 | ९० | नवति | नवतितम | नवतितमी |
| 91 | ९१ | एकनवति | एकनवत / एकनवतितम | एकनवती / एकनवतितमी |
| 100 | १०० | शत | शततम | शततमी |
| 1,000 | १००० | सहस्र | सहस्रतम | सहस्रतमी |
| 100,000 | १००००० | लक्ष | लक्षतम | लक्षतमी |
| 10,000,000 | १०००००००० | कोटि | कोटितम | कोटितमी |

## Translate

### A. *Yogatattvopaniṣat* 134cd–136ab

The three letters here, referred to as the त्र्याक्षर, are the three letters अ, उ, म् (a, u, m) that make up ॐ and are thought to contain the entire universe within them.

त्रयो लोकास्त्रयो वेदास्तिस्रः सन्ध्यास्त्रयः स्वराः ॥
त्रयोऽग्नयश्च त्रिगुणाः स्थिताः सर्वे त्र्याक्षरे ।
त्रयाणामक्षराणां च योऽधीतेऽप्यर्धमक्षरम् ॥
तेन सर्वमिदं प्रोतं तत्सत्यं तत्परं पदम् ।

Vocabulary

सन्ध्या f. juncture of the three divisions of the day (morning, noon, and night)
स्वरः m. sound, tone, accent
अक्षरम् n. letter, syllable
अधि√इ 1Ā, to learn, understand
अर्ध mfn. half
सर्वम् इदम् this whole [universe] (n. nom. sg.)
प्रोत mfn. strung, contained in, pervaded by

### B. *Gheraṇḍasaṃhitā* 5.22

In this verse, instructions regarding the four quarters of the उदरम्, "stomach," in the third *pāda* are being described. अर्ध, "half," represents two quarters.

अन्नेन पूरयेदर्धं तोयेन तु तृतीयकम् ।
उदरस्य तुरीयांशं संरक्षेद्वायुचारणे ॥

Vocabulary
अन्नम् n. food
सं√रक्ष् 1P, to protect, preserve, keep
वायुचारणे (the locative is being used in place of the dative, probably for metrical reasons)

### C. *Śivasaṃhitā* 3.19–20

This verse comes in a sequence of verses explaining how to attain सिद्धि, "fulfillment, success, or perfection," in yoga. The preceding verses speak of the importance of honoring one's guru for attaining सिद्धि in yoga. The subject of फलिष्यति is "one's practice."

फलिष्यतीति विश्वासः सिद्धेः प्रथमलक्षणम् ।
द्वितीयं श्रद्धया युक्तं तृतीयं गुरुपूजनम् ॥

चतुर्थं समताभावः पंचमेन्द्रियनिग्रहः ।
षष्ठं च प्रमिताहारः सप्तमं नैव विद्यते ॥

Vocabulary
विश्वासः m. confidence, trust, belief in
पूजनम् n. honoring
समता f. equanimity
भावः m. state
निग्रहः m. restraining, holding fast
प्रमिताहारः m. a measured diet

### D. *Bṛhadāraṇyakopaniṣat* 3.9.1

Janaka, king of Videha, decided to perform a sacrifice, which Brahmins from all over the region came to attend. Janaka wanted to find out who among the Brahmins was most learned in the Vedas, so he corralled one thousand cows, with ten pieces of gold tied to the horns of each cow. He then asked that the most learned man among the Brahmins drive the cows away, but no one dared. Then Yājñavalkya told his student to drive away the cows. The Brahmins were angry, thinking him arrogant, and proceeded to question him in turn. In this section, Vidagdha Śākalya is questioning him.

अथ हैनं विदग्धः शाकल्यः पप्रच्छ । कति देवा याज्ञवल्क्येति ।
स हैतयैव निविदा प्रतिपेदे यावन्तो वैश्वदेवस्य निविद्युच्यन्ते ।

त्रयश्च त्री च शता त्रयश्च त्री च सहस्रेति ।
ओमिति होवाच । कत्येव देवा याज्ञवल्क्येति । त्रयस्त्रिँशदिति ।
ओमिति होवाच । कत्येव देवा याज्ञवल्क्येति । षडिति ।
ओमिति होवाच । कत्येव देवा याज्ञवल्क्येति । त्रय इति ।
ओमिति होवाच । कत्येव देवा याज्ञवल्क्येति । द्वाविति ।
ओमिति होवाच । कत्येव देवा याज्ञवल्क्येति । अध्यर्ध इति ।
ओमिति होवाच । कत्येव देवा याज्ञवल्क्येति । एक इति ।

Vocabulary

ह ind. indeed, assuredly, verily, of course
एनम् m. him (Yājñavalkya)
विदग्धः शाकल्यः m. "the clever grammarian"
पप्रच्छ questioned (3rd p. sg. perfect √प्रछ्)
कति ind. how many
स हैतयैव निविदा प्रतिपेदे यावन्तो वैश्वदेवस्य निविद्युच्यन्ते ।
Translate the second half of this line first:
"It is said there are as many as are in the ritual invocation to all of the gods."
He answered in accordance with this very ritual injunction:

निविद् f. ritual invocation
प्रतिपेदे answered (3rd p. sg. perfect प्रति√पद्)
वैश्वदेव mfn. relating or sacred to all the gods

ओम् ind. yes, verily, so be it
उवाच he/she said (3rd p. sg. perfect √वच्)
अध्यर्ध mfn. having an additional half, one, and a half

After this passage, Vidagdha Śākalya continues to question Yājñavalkya about the gods and about *Brahman*. Finally, Yājñavalkya turns the exchange on its head and asks Vidagdha Śākalya a question. He asks about the person who provides the hidden connection, the *upaniṣad*, saying that if Vidagdha Śākalya cannot answer his question, his head would shatter apart. Vidagdha Śākalya had no idea of the answer and indeed his head shattered apart. Robbers then came and stole his bones, mistaking them for something else. After that no one else dared to question Yājñavalkya.

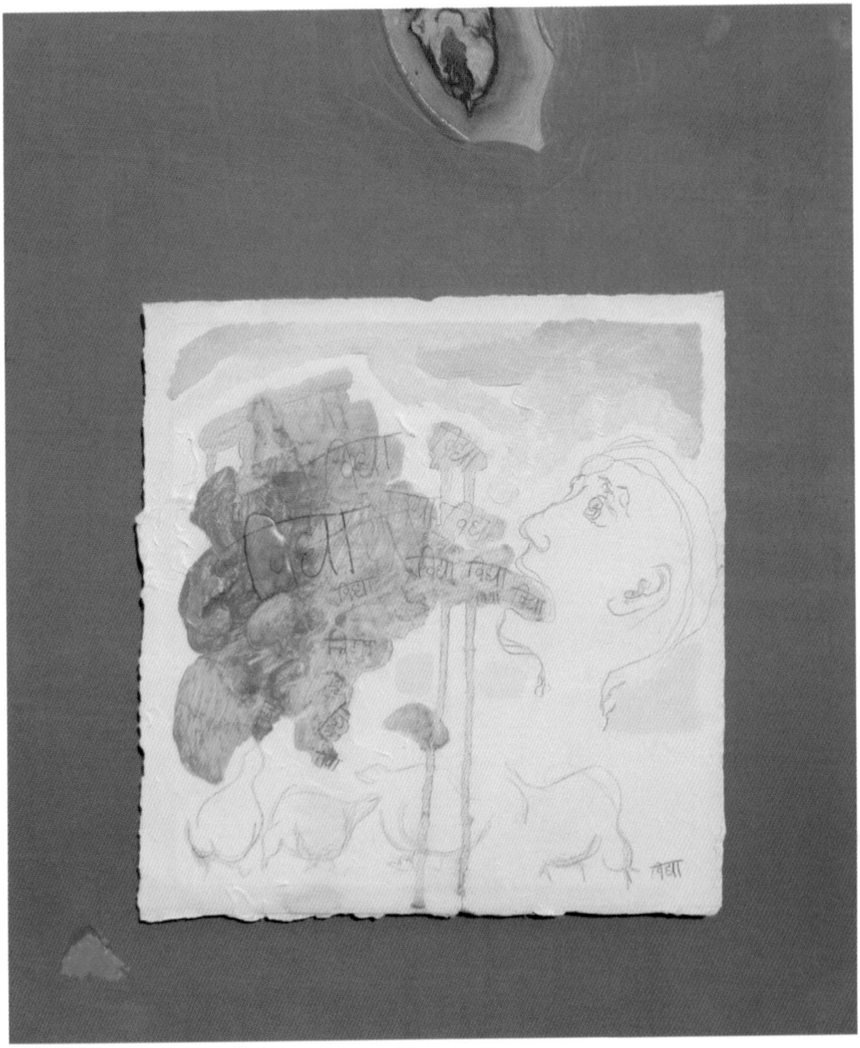

Yājñavalkya was a famous seer, known for his great wisdom. He was a pupil of Vaiśampayana, who, one day, in a fit of anger, asked Yājñavalkya to return the knowledge he'd imparted to him. Yājñavalkya vomited the knowledge he'd received from his teacher in the form of digested food (simplified knowledge), which was immediately eaten by the other disciples who'd taken the form of *tittiri* (partridge) birds. This became the *Taittirīya Yajurveda*, also known as the *Kṛṣṇayajurveda* or *Black Yajurveda*. Yājñavalkya then determined not to have a human guru and worshipped Sūrya, the Sun God, who was pleased and, assuming the form of a horse, taught him unknown portions of knowledge that became the *Śuklayajurveda* or *White Yajurveda*.

## DEGREES OF COMPARISON

The comparative is the form of an adjective or adverb used to indicate a "greater" degree of some quality, expressed in English by the suffix -er. The superlative is the form used to express a degree that is the "greatest" degree possible, expressed in English with the suffix -est. In Sanskrit, the comparative and superlative can be formed in two ways. The simplest way is by adding the suffix -**तर** for the comparative or -**तम** for the superlative to the end of an adjective or noun and then declining as any noun ending in अ (m/n) or in आ (f).

### Examples

| Adjective | Comparative | Superlative |
|---|---|---|
| गुरु heavy | गुरुतर heavier | गुरुतम heaviest |
| प्रिय dear | प्रियतर dearer | प्रियतम dearest |

### Translate

E. *Dattātreyayogaśāstra* 76–77

The practice of *kevala kumbhaka*, pure breath retention, is being spoken of. In the first stage of practice (as explained in the previous verse), sweat is produced, which the yogī should rub into the body. "Then slowly, by degrees, increasing the retention of the breath . . ." In the stage after the one described in these verses, the yogī starts to levitate.

कम्पो भवति देहस्य आसनस्थस्य योगिनः ।
ततोऽधिकतराभ्यासाद् दर्दुरी जायते ध्रुवम् ॥

यथा तु दर्दुरो गच्छेदुत्पत्योत्पत्य भूतले ।
पद्मासनस्थितो योगी तथा गच्छति भूतले ॥

Vocabulary

दर्दुरी f. frog-like
दर्दुरः m. frog
उत्√पत् 1P, to jump
भूतलम् n. the ground

### F. *Śivasaṃhitā* 3.101

This verse is speaking of *siddhāsana.*

नातः परतरं गुह्यमासनं विद्यते भुवि ।
येनानुध्यानमात्रेण योगी पापाद्विमुच्यते ॥

Vocabulary

अतस् ind. than this
भूः f. the earth
अनुध्यानम् n. meditation

### G. *Yogayājñavalkya* 4.49

The तेषु in this verse is referring to the ten *prāṇas* named in verse 47, of which (as verse 48 explains) five are most important. नरोत्तमे is a vocative referring to Gārgī.

तेषु मुख्यतमावेतौ प्राणापानौ नरोत्तमे ।
प्राण एवेतयोर्मुख्यः सर्वप्राणभृतां सदा ॥

Vocabulary

प्राणभृत् mfn. filled with *prāṇa* (i.e., a living being)

## THE COMPARATIVE SUFFIX ENDING IN -(ई)यांस्

The more complex comparative forms are made by adding the suffix -(ई)यांस् for the comparative or -इष्ठ for the superlative. The stem usually takes *guṇa* strengthening or is changed slightly (or sometimes completely) before the addition of these endings.

### Examples

| Adjective | Comparative | Superlative |
|---|---|---|
| गुरु heavy | गरीयांस् heavier | गरिष्ठ heaviest |
| प्रिय dear | प्रेयांस् dearer | प्रेष्ठ dearest |
| बहु many | भूयांस् more | भूयिष्ठ most |
| लघु small | लघीयांस् smaller | लघिष्ठ smallest |

| | | |
|---|---|---|
| वृद्ध old | ज्ययांस् older | ज्येष्ठ oldest |
| श्री splendor | श्रेयांस् better | श्रेष्ठ best, most splendid |

The strong form is -(ई)यांस् and the weak form is -(ई)यस्. The feminine is formed from the weak form + -ई and is declined like नदी.

**श्रेयान् m. better**

| | Singular | Dual | Plural |
|---|---|---|---|
| **Nominative** | श्रेयान् | श्रेयांसौ | श्रेयांसः |
| **Accusative** | श्रेयांसम् | श्रेयांसौ | श्रेयसः |
| **Instrumental** | श्रेयसा | श्रेयोभ्याम् | श्रेयोभिः |
| **Dative** | श्रेयसे | श्रेयोभ्याम् | श्रेयोभ्यः |
| **Ablative** | श्रेयसः | श्रेयोभ्याम् | श्रेयोभ्यः |
| **Genitive** | श्रेयसः | श्रेयसोः | श्रेयसाम् |
| **Locative** | श्रेयसि | श्रेयसोः | श्रेयःसु |
| **Vocative** | श्रेयन् | श्रेयांसौ | श्रेयांसः |

**श्रेयस् n. better**

| | Singular | Dual | Plural |
|---|---|---|---|
| **Nom./Acc./Voc.** | श्रेयः | श्रेयसी | श्रेयांसि |

**श्रेयसी f. better**

| | Singular | Dual | Plural |
|---|---|---|---|
| **Nominative** | श्रेयसी | श्रेयस्यौ | श्रेयस्याः |
| **Accusative** | श्रेयसीम् | श्रेयस्यौ | श्रेयसीः |
| **Instrumental** | श्रेयस्या | श्रेयसीभ्याम् | श्रेयसीभिः |
| **Dative** | श्रेयस्यै | श्रेयसीभ्याम् | श्रेयसीभ्यः |
| **Ablative** | श्रेयस्याः | श्रेयसीभ्याम् | श्रेयसीभ्यः |
| **Genitive** | श्रेयस्याः | श्रेयस्योः | श्रेयसीनाम् |
| **Locative** | श्रेयस्याम् | श्रेयस्योः | श्रेयसीषु |
| **Vocative** | श्रेयसि | श्रेयस्यौ | श्रेयस्याः |

The comparative forms are generally accompanied by a word in the ablative case, to indicate the thing that the subject is being compared to.

## Translate

### H. *Bhagavadgītā* 3.35

श्रेयान्स्वधर्मो विगुणः परधर्मात्स्वनुष्ठितात् ।
स्वधर्मे निधनं श्रेयः परधर्मो भयावहः ॥

Vocabulary
विगुण mfn. deficient, imperfect
स्वनुष्ठित mfn. performed well
निधनम् n. settling down, residence, death
आवह mfn. brings, produces

### I. *Bhagavadgītā* 11.37

Arjuna is speaking to Kṛṣṇa, who has just revealed his true form. Note that ब्रह्मणः in the second *pāda* refers to Brahmā, the God of Creation.

कस्माच्च ते न नमेरन्महात्मन्गरीयसे ब्रह्मणोऽप्यादिकर्त्रे ।
अनन्त देवेश जगन्निवास त्वमक्षरं सदसत्तत्परं यत् ॥

Vocabulary
आदिकर्तृ m. the original creator
निवासः m. dwelling place, abode

### J. *Bhagavadgītā* 3.21

यद्यदाचरति श्रेष्ठस्तत्तदेवेतरो जनः ।
स यत्प्रमाणं कुरुते लोकस्तदनुवर्तते ॥

Vocabulary
आ√चर् 1P, to act, undertake, practice, perform
प्रमाणम् n. measure, standard
अनु√वृत् 1Ā, to follow

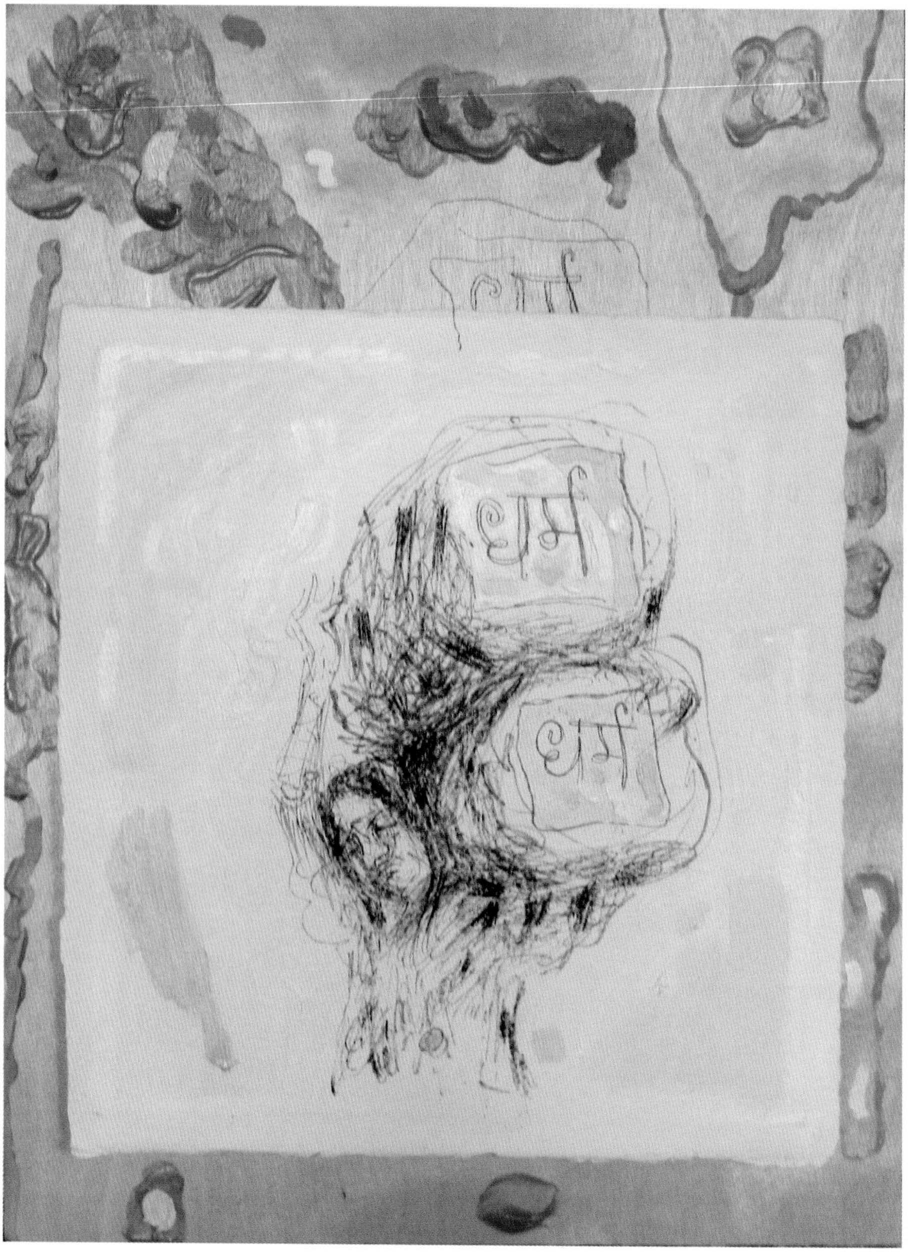


The word धर्म (*dharma*) comes from the root √धृ (*dhṛ*), "to hold, bear, carry." This is cognate with the Greek root *dher*, of the same meaning, which is the root of the word "therapy." So *dharma*, commonly translated as "duty" (one's calling in the world), and therapy both provide paradigms of support.

## आदि, अद्य, AND प्रभृति

These words can be used at the end of a *bahuvrīhi* compound to mean "et cetera" or "and so forth." They all literally mean "beginning with" and denote a list of things of which only the first member is given. आदि is the most common.

### Example: *Gheraṇḍasaṃhitā* 1.5

अभ्यासात्कादिवर्णानां यथा शास्त्राणि बोधयेत् ।
तथा योगं समासाद्य तत्त्वज्ञानं च लभ्यते ॥

Vocabulary

अभ्यासः m. repeated practice, study
कादिवर्णाः m. nom. pl. letters, beginning with "ka" (i.e., the alphabet)
  वर्णः m. letter
समासाद्य ind. by means of, on account of

Just as (यथा) from the repeated study (अभ्यासात्) of **the alphabet** (कादिवर्णानाम्),
One may come to understand (बोधयेत्) sacred texts (शास्त्राणि).
So (तथा), too (च), by means of (समासाद्य) yoga (योगम्),
One may attain (लभ्यते) knowledge of the real truth (तत्त्वज्ञानम्).

### Translate

#### K. *Yogasūtra* 3.23–24

In this sequence of *sūtras*, [by *saṃyama*] on X, [one attains] Y.

मैत्र्यादिषु बलानि ।
बलेषु हस्तिबलादीनि ।

Vocabulary

बलम् n. strength, power

#### L. *Bhagavadgītā* 4.26

This verse comes in a sequence of different sacrifices performed by yogīs.

श्रोत्रादीनीन्द्रियाण्यन्ये संयमाग्निषु जुह्वति ।
शब्दादीन्विषयानन्य इन्द्रियाग्निषु जुह्वति ॥

M. *Dattātreyayogaśāstra* 130cd–131

कविमार्गोऽयमुक्तस्ते सांकृतेऽष्टाङ्गयोगतः ॥
सिद्धानां कपिलादीनां मतं वक्ष्ये ततः परम् ।
अभ्यासभेदतो भेदः फलं तु सममेव हि ॥

Vocabulary

कविः m. poet, seer
अयम् this (m. nom. sg.)
अष्टाङ्गयोगतः ind. as the yoga with eight limbs, in accordance with the eight limbs
सिद्धः m. an inspired sage or seer, a semidivine being of great purity and perfection, perfected one
मतम् n. doctrine, thought, beliefs, ideology
ततः परम् ind. besides that, thereupon, afterward

## Review Exercises

### N. Dawn Prayer

सप्तार्णवाः सप्तकुलाचलाश्च सप्तर्षयो द्वीपवनानि सप्त ।
भूरादि कृत्वा भुवनानि सप्त कुर्वन्तु सर्वे मम सुप्रभातम् ॥

Vocabulary
अर्णवः m. sea, ocean
कुलाचलः m. chief mountain range
द्वीप mn. island
वनम् n. forest
भूर् ind. the earth
प्रभातम् n. daybreak, dawn

### O. *Bhagavadgītā* 9.1

इदं तु ते गुह्यतमं प्रवक्ष्याम्यनसूयवे ।
ज्ञानं विज्ञानसहितं यज्ज्ञात्वा मोक्ष्यसेऽशुभात् ॥

Vocabulary
इदम् this (n. nom. sg.)
अनसूयु mfn. not spiteful or envious
विज्ञानम् n. understanding, discernment, experience
अशुभम् n. inauspiciousness, misfortune

### P. *Śivasaṃhitā* 3.8

नागादिवायवः पंच कुर्वन्ति ते च विग्रहे ।
उद्गारोन्मीलनं क्षुत्तृड्जृम्भां हिक्कां च पंचमीम् ॥

Vocabulary
नागः m. one of the five winds of the body
विग्रहः m. individual form, figure, the body
उद्गारः m. belching
उन्मीलनम् n. opening the eyes, raising the eyelids
क्षुत्तृड् hunger and thirst

जृम्भः m. yawning
हिक्का f. hiccup

## Q. *Yogayājñavalkya* 12.33

Yājñavalkya is addressing Gārgī. Note the feminine form विहीनशोका in the last *pāda*.

अणोरणीयान्महतो महीयान्
आत्मा गुहायां निहितोऽस्य जन्तोः ।
तमक्रतुं पश्य विशुद्धबुद्ध्या
प्रयाणकाले च विहीनशोका ॥

Vocabulary
अणु mfn. minute, small, subtle
गुहा f. hiding place, cave, heart
निहित mfn. placed, situated, entrusted
अक्रतु mfn. free from desire, beyond understanding
प्रयाणम् n. departure, death

# 16
# Perfect Tense; Periphrastic Perfect; Periphrastic Future; Perfect Active Participle

अतीतानागतं स्वरूपतोऽस्त्यध्वभेदाद्धर्माणाम् ॥ ४.१२ ॥

**atītānāgataṃ svarūpato 'sty adhva-bhedād dharmāṇām**

The past and future exist, according to their own form, because of the difference in the time of manifestation of their characteristics.

॥ *Yogasūtra* 4.12 ॥

## PERFECT TENSE

The perfect tense is the second type of past tense. Although in common usage it is undistinguished from the other past tenses, it originally referred to the distant past, unobserved by the speaker. Because of this, it is usually only found in the third person. The perfect is a nonconjugational tense, which means verbs of all *gaṇas* are treated the same. It is divided into two categories: reduplicative and periphrastic.

## REDUPLICATIVE PERFECT

The reduplicative perfect is used for all monosyllabic roots beginning with a consonant or with the vowels अ, आ, इ, उ, and ऋ. It is formed by a reduplicated root + (frequently) the augment इ + final terminations. In the *parasmaipada* singular forms, the stem is strong; in all other forms it is weak. Refer to pages 162–63 for the general rules of reduplication. The rules for the formation of the reduplicative perfect presented in the following pages are to help you learn to recognize the perfect when you see it. It is not necessary to memorize these rules.

| | Parasmaipada Endings | | | Ātmanepada Endings | | |
|---|---|---|---|---|---|---|
| | Singular | Dual | Plural | Singular | Dual | Plural |
| 3rd | -अ | -अतुः | -उः | -ए | -आते | -इरे |
| 2nd | -थ | -अथुः | -अ | -से | -आथे | -ध्वे |
| 1st | -अ | -व | -म | -ए | -वहे | -महे |

1. The most common syllable for reduplication is अ.

**√दृश् to see**

| | Parasmaipada | | | Ātmanepada | | |
|---|---|---|---|---|---|---|
| | Singular | Dual | Plural | Singular | Dual | Plural |
| 3rd | ददर्श | ददृशतुः | ददृशुः | ददृशे | ददृशाते | ददृशिरे |
| 2nd | ददर्शिथ | ददृशथुः | ददृश | ददृशिषे | ददृशाथे | ददृशिध्वे |
| 1st | ददर्श | ददृशिव | ददृशिम | ददृशे | ददृशिवहे | ददृशिमहे |

2. In roots ending with आ, the first- and third-person singular *parasmaipada* forms end in औ. In weak forms, the आ is dropped.

**√दा to give**

| | Parasmaipada | | | Ātmanepada | | |
|---|---|---|---|---|---|---|
| | Singular | Dual | Plural | Singular | Dual | Plural |
| 3rd | ददौ | ददतुः | ददुः | ददे | ददाते | ददिरे |
| 2nd | ददाथ/ददिथ | ददथुः | दद | ददिषे | ददाथे | ददिध्वे |
| 1st | ददौ | ददिव | ददिम | ददे | ददिवहे | ददिमहे |

3. In roots with the vowel ऋ, the vowel अ is used in the reduplicative syllable.

**√कृ to do**

| | Parasmaipada | | | Ātmanepada | | |
|---|---|---|---|---|---|---|
| | Singular | Dual | Plural | Singular | Dual | Plural |
| 3rd | चकार | चक्रतुः | चक्रुः | चक्रे | चक्राते | चक्रिरे |
| 2nd | चकर्थ | चक्रथुः | चक्र | चकृषे | चक्राथे | चकृध्वे |
| 1st | चकर/चकार | चकृव | चकृम | चक्रे | चकृवहे | चकृमहे |

4. In some roots beginning with a semivowel followed by अ, there is *samprasāraṇa*.

**√वच् to speak**

| | Parasmaipada | | | Ātmanepada | | |
|---|---|---|---|---|---|---|
| | Singular | Dual | Plural | Singular | Dual | Plural |
| 3rd | उवाच | ऊचतुः | ऊचुः | ऊचे | ऊचाते | ऊचिरे |
| 2nd | उवचिथ / उवक्थ | ऊचथुः | ऊच | ऊचिषे | ऊचाथे | ऊचिध्वे |
| 1st | उवच / उवाच | ऊचिव | ऊचिम | ऊचे | ऊचिवहे | ऊचिमहे |

5. In roots containing the vowel इ / उ this vowel is repeated in the reduplicating syllable.

√मुच् to liberate ⇒ मुमोच liberated (3rd p. sg.)

6. In roots containing the vowel ई / ऊ this vowel is shortened in the reduplicating syllable.

√दीप् to shine ⇒ दिदीपे shone (3rd p. sg.)

7. In roots that contain the vowel अ between two single consonants (with an initial consonant that would be unchanged by reduplication), in the weak form, instead of reduplication, अ becomes ए.

√तप् to heat ⇒ तताप (3rd p. sg.); तेपुः (3rd p. pl.)
√पत् to fall ⇒ पपात (3rd p. sg.); पेतुः (3rd p. pl.)

8. The common verb √अह्, "to say, speak," is defective, and only has a few forms, and is used with present meaning.

| | Singular | Dual | Plural |
|---|---|---|---|
| 3rd | आह | आहतुः | आहुः |
| 2nd | आत्थ | आहथुः | |

9. The perfect forms of the verb √विद्, "to know," are also used with present meaning, but without reduplication.

| | Singular | Plural |
|---|---|---|
| 3rd | वेद | विदुः |

## Conjugate in the Perfect Tense

√अस् (आस 3rd p. sg.), √भू (बभूव 3rd p. sg.), √गम् (जगाम 3rd p. sg.)

## Example: *Bṛhadāraṇyakopaniṣat* 4.5.1–3

अथ ह याज्ञवल्क्यस्य द्वे भार्ये बभूवतुर्मैत्रेयी च कात्यायनी च ।
Now, **there were** two wives of Yājñavalkya: Maitreyī and Kātyayanī.

तयोर्ह मैत्रेयी ब्रह्मवादिनी बभूव । स्त्रीप्रज्ञैव तर्हि कात्यायनी ।

Of the two, Maitreyī **was** a woman who discoursed on sacred texts.
Kātyayanī only had knowledge of womanly matters.

अथ ह याज्ञवल्क्योऽन्यद्वृत्तमुपाकरिष्यन् ॥ १ ॥
One day, Yājñavalkya was preparing to embark on another mode of life.

मैत्रेयीति होवाच याज्ञवल्क्यः । प्रव्रजिष्यन्वा अरेऽहमस्मात्स्थानादस्मि ।

Yājñavalkya **said**, "Maitreyī, my dear, I am going forth from this place.

हन्त तेऽनया कात्यायन्यान्तं करवाणीति ॥ २ ॥
Look, I will make a settlement between you and Kātyayanī."

सा होवाच मैत्रेयी यन्नु म इयं भगोः सर्वा पृथिवी वित्तेन पूर्णा स्यात्स्यां न्वहं तेनामृताहो३ नेति ।
Then Maitreyī **asked**, "Sir, if I were to have this whole world, filled with wealth, Would I become immortal through that or not?"

नेति होवाच याज्ञवल्क्यः । यथैवोपकरणवतां जीवितं तथैव ते जीवितँ स्यात् ।

"No," **said** Yājñavalkya.
"Just as one living with means, in that way would you live.

अमृतत्वस्य तु नाशास्ति वित्तेनेति ॥ ३ ॥
There is no hope of immortality through wealth."

> The number ३ after a word is called प्लुत and indicates that a vowel should be prolated or lengthened to three *mātrās* (metrical units, length of time required to pronounce a short vowel; note that a long vowel is two *mātrās*).

### Vocabulary

ब्रह्मवादिन् mfn. one who discourses on sacred texts/theology
स्त्रीप्रज्ञा f. woman with knowledge of womanly matters
  स्त्री f. woman
तर्हि ind. then, in that case

वृत्तम् n. mode of life
उपाकरिष्यन् undertaking, preparing to embark (m. nom. sg. future participle उप√कृ)
प्रव्रजिष्यन् going forth (m. nom. sg. future participle प्र√व्रज्)
अरे ind. interjection of affection, "my dear"
हन्त ind. interjection of exhortation to do something, "Look," "Listen"
अनया with her/this (f. inst. sg.)
आन्त mfn. end, settlement
नु ind. so now, indeed (indicates a question)
भगोः sir, holy one (m. voc. pl. भगवत्)
इयम् this (f. nom. sg.)
वित्तम् n. wealth, acquisition, money, power
स्यां न्वहं . . . नेति would I become . . . or not?
उपकरणवत् mfn. furnished with means
अमृतत्वम् n. immortality
आशा f. hope, expectation, wish

## Translate

### A. *Yogatattvopaniṣat* 3–4

Brahmā is speaking to Viṣṇu.

तमाराध्य जगन्नाथं प्रणिपत्य पितामहः।
पप्रच्छ योगतत्त्वं मे ब्रूहि चाष्टाङ्गसंयुतम्॥

तमुवाच हृषीकेषो वक्ष्यामि शृणु तत्त्वतः।
सर्वे जीवाः सुखैर्दुःखैर्मायाजालेन वेष्टिताः॥

Vocabulary
आ√राध् 5P, to honor, worship, propitiate
जगन्नाथः m. Lord of the universe, Viṣṇu
प्रणि√पत् 1P, to bow respectfully to, to throw oneself down before
पितामहः m. grandfather (here referring to Brahmā)
हृषीकेषः m. Lord of the senses, Viṣṇu
तत्त्वतः ind. truly, really, accurately
वेष्टित mfn. enveloped, covered with, veiled in

### B. *Rāmāyaṇa* 1.41–2

At the beginning of the *Rāmāyaṇa*, the whole story is told in brief by the sage Nārada to the ascetic Vālmīki. This excerpt alludes to the pivotal moment when the ten-headed demon Rāvaṇa kidnaps Rāma's wife, Sītā, with the help of the *rākṣasa* (demon), Mārīca, who turns into a golden deer in order to lure Rāma and his brother Lakṣmaṇa away from protecting Sītā. The तु in the first *pāda* refers back to the previous verse, in which Mārīca tries to dissuade Rāvaṇa from fighting with the mighty Rāma. In the first verse, तद् refers to Mārīca and तस्य refers to Rāma.

अनादृत्य तु तद्वाक्यं रावणः कालचोदितः ।
जगाम सह मारीचस्तस्याश्रमपदं तदा ॥

तेन मायाविना दूरमपवाह्य नृपात्मजौ ।
जहार भार्यां रामस्य गृध्रं हत्वा जटायुषम् ॥

Vocabulary
आ√दृ 1Ā, to regard with attention, attend to, be careful about
कालः m. time, death, fate
चोदित mfn. urged, impelled
आश्रमपदम् n. a hermitage
मायाविन् mfn. possessing illusion or magical powers, master of illusion
दूर mfn. far, a long way
अप√वह् 1P, lead away
आत्मज mf. born from oneself, son, daughter
गृध्रः m. vulture (named Jaṭāyu)

### C. *Bhagavadgītā* 1.14

Note that पाण्डवः in the third *pāda* refers to Arjuna.

ततः श्वेतैर्हयैर्युक्ते महति स्यन्दने स्थितौ ।
माधवः पाण्डवश्चैव दिव्यौ शङ्खौ प्रदध्मतुः ॥

Vocabulary
श्वेत mfn. white
हयः m. horse
स्यन्दन mfn. chariot, "moving swiftly"
माधवः m. descendant of Madhu, Kṛṣṇa
प्र√ध्मा 1P, to blow into

### D. *Kaṭhopaniṣat* 1.1–3

उशन्ह वै वाजश्रवसः सर्ववेदसं ददौ । तस्य ह नचिकेता नाम पुत्र आस ॥ १ ॥
तँ ह कुमारँ सन्तं दक्षिणासु नीयमानासु श्रद्धाविवेश । सोऽमन्यत ॥ २ ॥

पीतोदका जग्धतृणा दुग्धदोहा निरिन्द्रियाः ।
अनन्दा नाम ते लोकास्तान्स गच्छति ता ददत् ॥ ३ ॥
स होवाच पितरं तत कस्मै मां दास्यसीति । द्वितीयं तृतीयम् ।
तँ होवाच मृत्यवे त्वा ददामीति ॥ ४ ॥

Vocabulary

उशन् m. father of Naciketas, "desirous"
वाजश्रवसः m. son of Vājaśravas
वेदस् n. property, wealth
कुमारः m. a child, boy, youth
दक्षिणा f. cows presented as donation to the priest
पीत mfn. drunk, sipped
उदकम् n. water
√जक्ष् 2P, to eat, consume
तृणम् n. grass
√दुह् 4P, to give milk
दोहः m. milk
निरिन्द्रिय mfn. barren
अनन्द mfn. joyless, cheerless
ताः these [*dakṣināḥ*] (f. acc. pl.)
ततः m. father
द्वितीयं तृतीयम् [He asked a] second [time and a] third [time]

## PERIPHRASTIC PERFECT

"Periphrastic" means constructed through circumlocution or in a roundabout way. In Sanskrit, it entails the use of an auxiliary word, rather than an inflected form. The periphrastic perfect is formed by adding the ending -आम् to the root and adding to this base the reduplicated perfect forms of the verbs अस्, भू, or कृ.

The periphrastic perfect is mainly formed from:

1. polysyllabic verbs with stems ending in अय (i.e., tenth class roots, causatives, and denominatives [Chapter 17]).
2. monosyllabic roots beginning with long vowels except आ.
3. monosyllabic roots beginning with short vowels except अ, followed by more than one consonant.

## Examples

**√दृश् to see**

| | Parasmaipada | | |
|---|---|---|---|
| | Singular | Dual | Plural |
| 3rd | दर्शयामास | दर्शयामासतुः | दर्शयामासुः |
| 2nd | दर्शयामासिथ | दर्शयामासथुः | दर्शयामास |
| 1st | दर्शयामास | दर्शयामासिव | दर्शयामासिम |

**√कीर्त् 10U, to utter, recite, praise**

| | Parasmaipada | | | Ātmanepada | | |
|---|---|---|---|---|---|---|
| | Singular | Dual | Plural | Singular | Dual | Plural |
| 3rd | कीर्तयांबभूव | कीर्तयांबभूवतुः | कीर्तयांबभूवुः | कीर्तयाञ्चक्रे | कीर्तयाञ्चक्राते | कीर्तयाञ्चक्रिरे |
| 2nd | कीर्तयांबभूविथ | कीर्तयांबभूवथुः | कीर्तयांबभूव | कीर्तयाञ्चकृषे | कीर्तयाञ्चक्राथे | कीर्तयाञ्चकृढ्वे |
| 1st | कीर्तयांबभूव | कीर्तयांबभूविव | कीर्तयांबभूविम | कीर्तयाञ्चक्रे | कीर्तयाञ्चकृवहे | कीर्तयाञ्चकृमहे |

## Translate

### E. *Dattātreyayogaśāstra* 25

Dattātreya has just explained to Sāṃkṛti some of the secret practices of *layayoga* (the yoga of absorption into the cosmos), taught by Śaṅkara (Śiva). In the first line, infer "if [one practices]."

शिथिलो निर्जने देशे कुर्याच्चेत्सिद्धिमाप्नुयात् ।
एवं च बहुसंकेतान्<u>कथयामास</u> शङ्करः ॥

Vocabulary
शिथिल mfn. relaxed
संकेतः m. secret practice of *layayoga*, the yoga of cosmic absorption

### F. *Bhagavadgītā* 11.50

In this chapter, Kṛṣṇa reveals his powerful, divine form to Arjuna.

इत्यर्जुनं वासुदेवस्तथोक्त्वा स्वकं रूपं <u>दर्शयामास</u> भूयः ।
<u>आश्वासयामास</u> च भीतमेनं भूत्वा पुनः सौम्यवपुर्महात्मा ॥

Vocabulary
आ√श्वस् 2P, to breathe again, calm, console
भीत mfn. frightened
एनम् him (i.e., Arjuna) (m. acc. sg.)
सौम्य mfn. gentle, soft, "moonlike"
वपुस् n. form, figure

G. *Rāmāyaṇa* 1.64–65

With the help of the monkey king, Sugrīva, Rāma crossed the ocean to Laṅkā and killed Rāvaṇa. The subject of the first verse and the last two *pādas* of the second verse is Rāma.

ततः सुग्रीवसहितो गत्वा तीरं महोदधेः ।
समुद्रं क्षोभयामास शरैरादित्यसंनिभैः ॥

दर्शयामास चात्मानं समुद्रः सरितां पतिः ।
समुद्रवचनाच्चैव नलं सेतुमकारयत् ॥

Vocabulary
तीरम् n. shore, bank
उदधिः m. the ocean
समुद्रः m. the sea, ocean
√क्षुभ् 1Ā, to shake, tremble
संनिभ mfn. like, similar, resembling
सेतुः m. bridge

## PERIPHRASTIC FUTURE

The periphrastic future is traditionally used for the अनद्यतन, or "nontoday" future, although, like the perfect, there is no distinction in common usage. It is formed through the addition of the nominal forms of agent nouns in तृ (ending in ता) + the corresponding present tense form of the verb √अस्. In the third person, the finite form of √अस् is usually omitted. The *ātmanepada* forms are quite rare.

**√भू to be**

| | Parasmaipada | | | Ātmanepada | | |
|---|---|---|---|---|---|---|
| | Singular | Dual | Plural | Singular | Dual | Plural |
| 3rd | भविता | भवितारौ | भवितारः | भविता | भवितारौ | भवितारः |
| 2nd | भवितासि | भवितास्थः | भवितास्थ | भवितासे | भवितासाथे | भविताध्वे |
| 1st | भवितास्मि | भवितास्वः | भवितास्मः | भविताहे | भवितास्वहे | भवितास्महे |

## Translate

### H. *Bhagavadgītā* 2.52

यदा ते मोहकलिलं बुद्धिर्व्यतितरिष्यति ।
तदा गन्तासि निर्वेदं श्रोतव्यस्य श्रुतस्य च ॥

Vocabulary
कलिलम् n. a large heap, thicket, confusion
व्यति√तॄ 1P, to completely cross over
निर्वेदः m. disgust, loathing, complete indifference to worldly objects

### I. *Bhagavadgītā* 11.34

द्रोणं च भीष्मं च जयद्रथं च कर्णं तथान्यानपि योधवीरान् ।
मया हतांस्त्वं जहि मा व्यथिष्ठा युध्यस्व जेतासि रणे सपत्नान् ॥

Vocabulary
योधवीरः m. hero, warrior
मा व्यथिष्ठाः do not waver, hesitate (3rd p. sg. injunctive aorist √व्यथ्)
सपत्नः m. rival, adversary, enemy

### J. *Bhagavadgītā* 18.69

Kṛṣṇa is speaking. The तस्मात् refers to one who teaches this secret knowledge, as described in the previous verse.

न च तस्मान्मनुष्येषु कश्चिन्मे प्रियकृत्तमः ।
भविता न च मे तस्मादन्यः प्रियतरो भुवि ॥

Vocabulary
प्रियकृत्तम mfn. doing that which gives most pleasure

## PERFECT ACTIVE PARTICIPLE

The perfect active participle has a past active meaning. It is quite rare in occurrence, as it is only formed from a minimal number of roots. The most commonly used example is विद्वांस् (learned person), formed from the root √विद् (to know), which loses its past meaning as well as its reduplication.

The third-person plural *parasmaipada* perfect form is used in the weak form of the stem before endings beginning with a vowel, with its final consonant changed to ष्. For the weak stem before consonants the final उष् is changed to वद्, for the strong stem it becomes वांस्, and for the feminine stem it becomes उषी.

**चक्रवांस् m. had done**

| | Singular | Dual | Plural |
|---|---|---|---|
| **Nominative** | चकृवान् | चकृवांसौ | चकृवांसः |
| **Accusative** | चकृवांसम् | चकृवांसौ | चक्रुषः |
| **Instrumental** | चक्रुषा | चकृवद्भ्याम् | चकृवद्भिः |
| **Dative** | चक्रुषे | चकृवद्भ्याम् | चकृवद्भ्यः |
| **Ablative** | चक्रुषः | चकृवद्भ्याम् | चकृवद्भ्यः |
| **Genitive** | चक्रुषः | चक्रुषोः | चक्रुषाम् |
| **Locative** | चक्रुषि | चक्रुषोः | चकृवत्सु |
| **Vocative** | चकृवन् | चकृवांसौ | चकृवांसः |

**चक्रवांस् n. had done**

| | Singular | Dual | Plural |
|---|---|---|---|
| **Nom./Acc./Voc.** | चकृवत् | चक्रुषी | चकृवांसि |

चक्रुषी f. had done (same as नदी)

**विद्वांस् m. wise, learned, a seer**

| | Singular | Dual | Plural |
|---|---|---|---|
| **Nominative** | विद्वान् | विद्वांसौ | विद्वांसः |
| **Accusative** | विद्वांसम् | विद्वांसौ | विदुषः |
| **Instrumental** | विदुषा | विद्वद्भ्याम् | विद्वद्भिः |

| | | | |
|---|---|---|---|
| **Dative** | विदुषे | विद्वद्भ्याम् | विद्वद्भ्यः |
| **Ablative** | विदुषः | विद्वद्भ्याम् | विद्वद्भ्यः |
| **Genitive** | विदुषः | विदुषोः | विदुषाम् |
| **Locative** | विदुषि | विदुषोः | विद्वत्सु |
| **Vocative** | विद्वन् | विद्वांसौ | विद्वांसः |

**विद्वांस् n. wise, learned**

| | Singular | Dual | Plural |
|---|---|---|---|
| **Nom./Acc./Voc.** | विद्वत् | विदुषी | विद्वांसि |

विदुषी f. wise, learned (same as नदी)

## Translate

### K. *Bhagavadgītā* 3.25

सक्ताः कर्मण्यविद्वांसो यथा कुर्वन्ति भारत ।
कुर्याद्विद्वांस्तथासक्तश्चिकीर्षुर्लोकसंग्रहम् ॥

Vocabulary
अविद्वांस् m. unwise
असक्त mfn. unattached
चिकीर्षु mfn. intending to do, desiring to make
संग्रहः m. holding together

### L. *Bhāgavatapurāṇa* 10.24.6

ज्ञात्वाज्ञात्वा च कर्माणि जनोऽयमनुतिष्ठति ।
विदुषः कर्मसिद्धिः स्याद्यथा नाविदुषो भवेत् ॥

Vocabulary
अयं जनः these people, people, we (m. nom. sg.)
अनु√स्था 1P, to carry out, perform, practice
कर्मसिद्धिः m. attainment of a goal, accomplishment of an action

## Review Exercises

### M. *Rāmāyaṇa* 1.56–59

Taking Hanumān's advice, Rāma approached the monkey Sugrīva. After Rāma helped Sugrīva regain his rightful throne as king, Sugrīva, with Hanumān's assistance, helped him find Sītā.

स च सर्वान्समानीय वानरान्वानरर्षभः ।
दिशः प्रस्थापयामास दिदृक्षुर्जनकात्मजाम् ॥

ततो गृध्रस्य वचनात्सम्पातेर्हनुमान्बली ।
शतयोजनविस्तीर्णं पुप्लुवे लवणार्णवम् ॥

तत्र लङ्कां समासद्य पुरीं रावणपालिताम् ।
ददर्श सीतां ध्यायन्तीमशोकवनिकां गताम् ॥

निवेदयित्वाभिज्ञानं प्रवृत्तिं च निवेद्य च ।
समाश्वास्य च वैदेहीं मर्दयामास तोरणम् ॥

Sītā, Rāma's wife, whose name means "furrow," is so named because she was found by her adopted father, Janaka, while he was plowing the land. She is sometimes called *ayonijā*, which means "not born from a womb."

Vocabulary

समा√नी 1U, to collect, assemble
वानरः m. monkey
ऋषभः m. a bull, the best or most excellent of any kind or race
दिशः (for दिशो दिशः) in all directions
प्र√स्था 1U, to set out; caus. to send out
दिदृक्षु mfn. desirous of finding
जनकात्मजा f. daughter of Janaka, i.e., Sītā
वचनम् n. advice, instruction, direction
सम्पातिः m. name of a vulture, elder brother of Jaṭāyu
योजनम् n. measure of distance equal to eight to nine miles, league
विस्तीर्ण mfn. spread out, expanded, broad
√प्लु 1Ā, to leap, jump, spring
लवण mfn. salt
समा√सद् 1,6P to approach, arrive
पुरी f. city
पालित mfn. guarded, protected
वनिका f. little wood, grove
नि√विद् 2P, to tell, communicate; caus. to offer, present, give, deliver

अभिज्ञानम् n. token of remembrance/recognition
प्रवृत्तिः f. news, tidings
वैदेही f. name for Sītā, daughter of the king of Videha
√मृद् 9P, to crush, smash
तोरणम् n. arch, arched doorway

### N. *Kaṭhopaniṣat* 1.11

This verse is spoken to Naciketas by Death, who is agreeing to grant him the first of three wishes—that his father Auddālaki Āruṇi's anger be subdued. Auddālaki Āruṇi is the subject.

यथा पुरस्ताद्भविता प्रतीत
  औद्दालकिरारुणिर्मत्प्रसृष्टः ।
सुखँ रात्री शयिता वीतमन्युस्
  त्वां ददृशिवान्मृत्युमुखात्प्रमुक्तम् ॥

Vocabulary
पुरस्तात् ind. before
प्रतीत mfn. glad, pleased
प्रसृष्ट mfn. let loose, dismissed, set free
वीत mfn. gone away, departed
मन्युः mfn. rage, fury, anger

### O. *Kaṭhopaniṣat* 6.5

यथादर्शे तथात्मनि
  यथा स्वप्ने तथा पितृलोके ।
यथाप्सु परीव ददृशे
  तथा गन्धर्वलोके छायातपयोरिव ब्रह्मलोके ॥

Vocabulary
आदर्शः m. a looking glass, mirror
पितृलोकः m. world of the ancestors
अप्सु in water (f. loc. pl.)
गन्धर्वः m. a celestial musician
छाया f. shadow
आतपः m. sunshine, light

# 17
# Desideratives; Intensive/Frequentative Verbs; Denominatives

**तासामनादित्वं चाशिषो नित्यत्वात् ॥ ४.१० ॥**
**tāsām anāditvaṃ cāśiṣo nityatvāt**
These *samskāras* are beginningless, since desire is eternal.
॥ *Yogasūtra* 4.10 ॥

## SECONDARY VERBAL ROOTS

Secondary verbal roots are derived from primary verbal roots or nouns by adding a suffix. Secondary verbal roots can be conjugated in any mood or tense, although they are found most frequently in the present tense. We have already encountered causative verbs, the most common verbs in this category.

## DESIDERATIVES

Desiderative verbs are used to express one's own desire to do something. They are formed through reduplicating the verb and suffixing -स, -ष, or -इष. Additionally, two nominal forms can be derived from desiderative verbs: action nouns ending in -आ and agent adjectives ending in -उ.

| Verbal Root | Desiderative Stem | Action Noun | Agentive Adjective |
|---|---|---|---|
| √ज्ञा<br>to know | √जिज्ञास्<br>to want to know | जिज्ञासा<br>desire to know | जिज्ञासुः<br>inquisitive, curious |
| √पा<br>to drink | √पिपास्<br>to want to drink | पिपासा<br>thirst | पिपासुः<br>thirsty |
| √भुज्<br>to eat | √बुभुक्ष्<br>to want to eat | बुभुक्षा<br>hunger | बुभुक्षुः<br>hungry |

| | | | |
|---|---|---|---|
| √मुच् | √मुमुक्ष् | मुमुक्षा | मुमुक्षुः |
| to set free | to want to be set free | desire for liberation | wanting liberation |

## Translate

### A. *Bhagavadgītā* 2.6

Arjuna is speaking to Kṛṣṇa.

न चैतद्विद्मः कतरन्नो गरीयो यद्वा जयेम यदि वा नो जयेयुः ।
यानेव हत्वा न जिजीविषामस्तेऽवस्थिताः प्रमुखे धार्तराष्ट्राः ॥

Vocabulary

कतर mfn. which of the two
गरीयस् mfn. heavier, greater, preferable
अवस्थित mfn. standing near
प्रमुखम् n. before the face of, in front of, before
धार्तराष्ट्रः m. son of Dhṛtarāṣṭra

### B. *Bhagavadgītā* 2.14

The previous verse speaks of the transient nature of the body.

मात्रास्पर्शास्तु कौन्तेय शीतोष्णसुखदुःखदाः ।
आगमापायिनोऽनित्यास्तांस्तितिक्षस्व भारत ॥

Vocabulary

मात्रा f. material, measure
आगम mfn. coming, approaching
अपायिन् mfn. going
अनित्य mfn. not everlasting, transient
√तिज् 1U, to be or become sharp
√तितिक्ष् desire to become sharp, to bear with firmness, suffer with courage, endure

### C. *Bhagavadgītā* 6.3

Note that the desiderative agent adjectives can take an object.

आरुरुक्षोर्मुनेर्योगं कर्म कारणमुच्यते ।
योगारूढस्य तस्यैव शमः कारणमुच्यते ॥

Vocabulary

आ√रुह् 1P, to ascend, mount, climb, attain
मुनिः m. sage, seer, one who is moved by inward impulse, an inspired person
आरूढ mfn. ascended
शमः m. tranquillity, calmness

D. *Bhagavadgītā* 6.44

The previous verses speak of how the yogī's karma is carried on through many births.

पूर्वाभ्यासेन तेनैव ह्रियते ह्यवशोऽपि सः ।
जिज्ञासुरपि योगस्य शब्दब्रह्मातिवर्तते ॥

Vocabulary

पूर्वाभ्यासः m. previous practice (i.e., practice done in a previous life)
√हृ 1U, to carry
अवश mfn. not having one's free will, doing something against one's desire, unwillingly
शब्दब्रह्मन् n. *Brahman* in the form of sound (e.g., recitation of Vedic texts)
अति√वृत् 1Ā, to pass beyond

E. *Yogasūtra* 3.30

[By *saṃyama* . . .]

कण्ठकूपे क्षुत्पिपासानिवृत्तिः ।

Vocabulary

कण्ठः m. throat
कूपः m. hollow, cave
क्षुध् f. hunger (क्षुत् in compound)

## INTENSIVES/FREQUENTATIVES

Intensive or frequentative verbs are used (rarely) to express repeated or frequently performed actions. They can be formed from any verbal root of the first nine *gaṇas* through reduplication. When used in *parasmaipada* conjugations, there is no suffix before the endings; in *ātmanepada* conjugations, there is the addition of य between the reduplicated root and the endings.

### Examples

√कृ to go ⇒ चेक्रिय to do repeatedly
√गम् to go ⇒ जङ्गम्य to go zigzag
√दीप् to shine ⇒ देदीप्य to shine extremely brightly
√पा to drink ⇒ पेपीय to drink endlessly
√भू to do ⇒ बोभूय to become repeatedly
√लिह् to lick ⇒ लेलिह्य to lick vigorously

### Example: *Muṇḍakopaniṣat* 3.1.1

This well-known verse is speaking of *Ātman* and *Brahman*.

द्वा सुपर्णा सयुजा सखाया
समानं वृक्षं परिषस्वजाते ।
तयोरन्यः पिप्पलं स्वादु अत्ति
अनश्नन्यो अभिचाकशीति ॥

#### Vocabulary

सुपर्ण mfn. having beautiful wings, i.e., a bird
सयुज् mfn. a companion
सखः m. friend
समान mfn. same
परि√ष्वज् 1Ā, to embrace, clasp, nestle
पिप्पलः m. sacred fig tree, fig
स्वादु mfn. sweet, pleasant to taste
अनश्नत् mfn. not eating
अभि√चक्ष् 2Ā, to look at, view, perceive

Two (द्वा) birds (सुपर्णा), companions (सयुजा) and friends (सखाया),
Nestle (परिषस्वजाते) on the same (समानम्) tree (वृक्षम्).
Of the two (तयोर्), one (अन्यः) eats (अत्ति) a sweet (स्वादु) fig (पिप्पलम्),
The other (अन्यः), not eating (अनश्नन्), **watches intensely** (अभिचाकशीति).

## Translate

### F. *Bhagavadgītā* 11.30

लेलिह्यसे ग्रसमानः समन्ताल्लोकान्समग्रान्वदनैर्ज्वलद्भिः ।
तेजोभिरापूर्य जगत्समग्रं भासस्तवोग्राः प्रतपन्ति विष्णो ॥

Vocabulary

√लिह् 2U, to lick
√ग्रस् 1U, to swallow, devour
समग्र mfn. all, entire, whole
√ज्वल् 1P, to burn brightly, blaze
आ√पॄ 9U, to fill up
भासः m. brightness, light, luster
उग्र mfn. powerful, mighty, formidable
प्र√तप् 1P, to give forth heat, shine, set on fire

### G. *Chāndogyopaniṣat* 6.11.1–3

Uddalāka Āruṇi is speaking to his son Śvetaketu. Note that the first segment can be divided into three sentences, the first and second both ending with the word स्रवेद्यः.

अस्य सोम्य महतो वृक्षस्य यो मूलेऽभ्याहन्याज्जीवन्स्रवेद्यो मध्येऽभ्याहन्याज्जीवन्स्रवेद्योऽग्रेऽभ्याहन्याज्जीवन्स्रवेत्। स एष जीवेनात्मनानुप्रभूतः पेपीयमानो मोदमानस्तिष्ठति ॥ १ ॥

अस्य यदेकाँ शाखां जीवो जहात्यथ सा शुष्यति। द्वितीयां जहात्यथ सा शुष्यति। तृतीयां जहात्यथ सा शुष्यति। सर्वँ जहाति सर्वः शुष्यति ॥ २ ॥

एवमेव खलु सोम्य विद्धीति होवाच। जीवापेतं वाव किलेदं म्रियते न जीवो म्रियत इति। स य एषोऽणिमैतदात्म्यमिदँ सर्वम्। तत्सत्यम्। स आत्मा। तत्त्वमसि श्वेतकेतो इति। भूय एव मा भगवान्विज्ञापयत्विति। तथा सोम्येति होवाच ॥ ३ ॥

Vocabulary

सोम्य used for सौम्य mfn. gentle, soft, moonlike, here meaning "son" or "my dear son"
अभ्या√हन् 2P, to strike
जीवः m. living essence, sap
√स्रु 1P, to flow
अनुप्रभूत mfn. penetrated

The *Chāndogyopaniṣat* is one of the earliest *upaniṣads*, dating to around the sixth to seventh century B.C.E. Contained within the *Chāndogya Brāhmaṇa*, it is associated with the songs of the *Sāma Veda*. It is considered a foundational text of Vedanta philosophy, made popular through the commentary of Ādi Śaṅkarācārya.

अपेत mfn. escaped, departed, gone
वाव ind. just, indeed, even
किल ind. as they say, reportedly
इदम् this (n. nom. sg.)
अणिमन् n. the smallest particle, finest essence
ऐतदात्म्यम् n. the state of having the nature or property of this, having the same nature

The word *aṇima* is cognate with the words anima and animus, used by Carl Jung to denote archetypes of the feminine collective unconscious within the male and the masculine collective unconscious within the female, respectively.

## DENOMINATIVE VERBS

Denominative verbs are derived from nouns and adjectives in a variety of ways, turning them into actions. Similarly to causative verbs, denominatives are usually conjugated as tenth class verbs.

1. The suffix -(अ)ाय is added to a noun/adjective before adding *ātmanepada* endings, with the meaning "to be," "to become," or "to act like X."

   शुक्ल white ⇒ शुक्लायते to be or become white
   तरुण young ⇒ तरुणायते to be, become, or act young
   आनन्दः happiness ⇒ आनन्दयते to become happy

2. The suffix -य is added to a noun/adjective before *parasmaipada* endings, with the meaning "to turn into," "make," "treat," or "desire as X."

   शुक्ल white ⇒ शुक्लयति to make white
   नमः bow, salutation ⇒ नमस्यति to make a salutation

3. If the noun/adjective ends in अ, आ, अन्, or इ it may be changed to ई, and if it ends in उ it may become ऊ.

   पुत्रः son ⇒ पुत्रीयति to treat as or desire a son
   महा great ⇒ महीयते to be glad, happy, joyous

4. The suffix -य is added to a noun/adjective before *parasmaipada* or *ātmanepada* endings, with varied meanings.

   काम desire ⇒ कामयते to feel desires

5. A few denominatives are formed with no suffix and *parasmaipada* endings.

   कृष्ण the god Kṛṣṇa, black ⇒ कृष्णाति to act like Kṛṣṇa, to become black

## Example: *Aṣṭāṅga Yoga Mantra*

Note that चरणारविन्दे and all of the adjectives that follow it are neuter dual.

वन्दे गुरूणां चरणारविन्दे सन्दर्शितस्वात्मसुखावबोधे ।
निःश्रेयसे जाङ्गलिकायमाने संसारहालाहलमोहशान्त्यै ॥
आबाहुपुरुषाकारं शङ्खचक्रासिधारिणम् ।
सहस्रशिरसं श्वेतं प्रणमामि पतञ्जलिम् ॥

Many years ago, Viṣṇu advised the *devas* (gods) to work together with the *asuras* (demons) to churn the Ocean of Milk, in order to obtain the *amṛta* (nectar) of immortality. They used the snake Vasuki as a churning rope and Mount Mandara, placed on the back of the great tortoise *kūrma*, the *avatāra* (incarnation) of Viṣṇu, as the churning pole. In the process, the *hālāhala*, a terrible deadly poison, emerged, threatening to engulf the universe. Śiva, in his great compassion, swallowed the poison, which, thanks to his wife, Pārvatī, was contained in his throat, causing it to turn blue and giving him the name Nīlakaṇṭha. Many treasures then emerged from the ocean, including the *amṛta*, which eventually made its way into the hands of the *devas*.

Vocabulary

चरण mn. foot
सन्दर्शित mfn. shown, manifested, revealed
स्वात्मन् m. one's own self, Soul
अवबोधः m. awakening, knowledge, understanding
निःश्रेयसम् mn. ultimate refuge, final beatitude, having no better, best, most excellent
जाङ्गलिकायते denom. to act like a snake doctor (जाङ्गलिकः = जाङ्गुलिकः m. snake doctor)
हालाहलमोहः m. delusions [caused by/from] the poison, delusion [which is] the poison
हालाहलम् n. a deadly poison, produced in the churning of the ocean
मोहः m. delusion
आबाहु mf. up to the arms
चक्रम् n. wheel, discus
असिः m. sword

I bow (वन्दे) to the two lotus feet (चरणारविन्दे) of the gurus (गुरूणाम्),
Through which the understanding (अवबोधे) of the happiness (सुख) in my own Soul (स्वात्म) has been revealed (सन्दर्शित).
My ultimate refuge (निःश्रेयसे), **acting like a snake doctor** (जाङ्गलिकायमाने),
For the pacifying (शान्त्यै) of the delusions (मोह) caused by the poison (हालाहल) of cyclic existence (संसार).

Who has the form (आकारम्) of a human (पुरुष) up to the arms (आबाहु),
Bearing (धारिणम्) a conch (शङ्ख), a discus (चक्र), and a sword (असि).
White (श्वेतम्), with a thousand (सहस्र) heads (शिरसम्),
I bow (प्रणमामि) to Patañjali (पतञ्जलिम्).

## Translate

### H. *Haṭhapradīpikā* 3.58

उड्डीयानं तु सहजं गुरुणा कथितं सदा ।
अभ्यसेत्सततं यस्तु वृद्धोऽपि तरुणायते ॥

Vocabulary
सहज mfn. natural

### I. *Bṛhadāraṇyakopaniṣat* 3.2.7–9

Yājñavalkya is answering the questions "What are the eight organs of apprehension? What are the eight objects of the organs of apprehension?" These are three of the eight.

मनो वै ग्रहः । स कामेनातिग्राहेण गृहीतः । मनसा हि कामान्कामयते ॥ ७ ॥
हस्तौ वै ग्रहः । स कर्मणातिग्राहेण गृहीतः । हस्ताभ्याँ हि कर्म करोति ॥ ८ ॥
त्वग्वै ग्रहः । स स्पर्शेनातिग्राहेण गृहीतः । त्वचा हि स्पर्शान्वेदयते ।

Vocabulary
ग्रहः m. grasper, organ of apprehension
अतिग्राहः m. overgrasper, object of an organ of apprehension
हस्तः m. the hand
√विद् 2P, to know, feel, consider; caus. to feel, experience

### J. *Kaṭhopaniṣat* 2.17

The foundation being spoken of here is Oṃ.

एतदालम्बनँ श्रेष्ठमेतदालम्बनं परम् ।
एतदालम्बनं ज्ञात्वा ब्रह्मलोके महीयते ॥

Vocabulary
आलम्बनम् n. foundation, support

## Review Exercises

### K. *Aparokṣānubhūti* 121

विषयेष्वात्मतां दृष्ट्वा मनसश्चितिमज्जनम् ।
प्रत्याहारः स विज्ञेयोऽभ्यसनीयो मुमुक्षुभिः ॥

Vocabulary

आत्मता f. Soul, Soul-ness, Selfhood
चित् f. understanding, true knowledge, consciousness
मज्जनम् n. immersion, bathing
विज्ञेय mfn. to be known

### L. *Chāndogyopaniṣat* 7.5.1

चित्तं वाव सङ्कल्पाद्भूयः । यदा वै चेतयतेऽथ सङ्कल्पयते । अथ मनस्यति । अथ वाचमीरयति ।
तामु नाम्नीरयति । नाम्नि मन्त्रा एकं भवन्ति । मन्त्रेषु कर्माणि ॥ १ ॥

Vocabulary

चित्तम् n. thought, thinking
√ईर् 10U, utter, pronounce, proclaim

### M. *Kathopaniṣat* 2.4–5

Death is speaking to Naciketas.

दूरमेते विपरीते विषूची
अविद्या या च विद्येति ज्ञाता ।
विद्याभीप्सिनं नचिकेतसं मन्ये
न त्वा कामा बहवोऽलोलुपन्त ॥ ४ ॥

अविद्यायामन्तरे वर्तमानाः
स्वयंधीराः पण्डितं मन्यमानाः ।
दन्द्रम्यमाणाः परियन्ति मूढा
अन्धेनैव नीयमाना यथान्धाः ॥ ५ ॥

Vocabulary

दूरम् ind. far from
विपरीत mfn. turned around, reversed, contrary
विषूची going in different directions (f. du. विष्वञ्च्)
अभीप्सिन् mfn. wishing for, desirous of obtaining (desid. form of अभ्य√आप् 5P, to reach)
√लुप् 4P, to disturb, bewilder, perplex, confound
स्वयंधीर mfn. wise in one's own mind
धीर mfn. intelligent, wise
√द्रम् 1P, to wander about
परि√इ 2P, to go around, move in a circle
मूढः m. a fool
अन्ध mfn. blind

# 18

# Demonstrative Pronouns इदम् and अदस्; Past Active Participles; Neuter Nouns Ending in इ and उ; Irregular Declensions

**द्रष्टृदृश्योपरक्तं चित्तं सर्वार्थम् ॥ ४.२३ ॥**
**draṣṭṛ-dṛśyoparaktaṃ cittaṃ sarvārtham**
The mind, colored by both the seer and the seen, is capable of understanding all things.
॥ *Yogasūtra* 4.23 ॥

## DEMONSTRATIVE PRONOUNS इदम् AND अदस्

In addition to the demonstrative pronouns we have learned—तत् and एतत्—there are two others that are far less common—इदम् and अदस्. We have already encountered them in a few verses, the former being used more frequently. इदम् refers to relatively nearby objects, while एतत् refers to objects that are very near; अदस् refers to objects that are relatively far away, while तत् refers to objects that are distant.

**इदम् m. this**

| | Singular | Dual | Plural |
|---|---|---|---|
| **Nominative** | अयम् | इमौ | इमे |
| **Accusative** | इमम् | इमौ | इमान् |
| **Instrumental** | अनेन | आभ्याम् | एभिः |
| **Dative** | अस्मै | आभ्याम् | एभ्यः |
| **Ablative** | अस्मात् | आभ्याम् | एभ्यः |
| **Genitive** | अस्य | अनयोः | एषाम् |
| **Locative** | अस्मिन् | अनयोः | एषु |

**इदम् n. this**

| | Singular | Dual | Plural |
|---|---|---|---|
| **Nom./Acc.** | इदम् | इमे | इमानि |

**इदम् f. this**

| | Singular | Dual | Plural |
|---|---|---|---|
| **Nominative** | इयम् | इमे | इमाः |
| **Accusative** | इमाम् | इमे | इमाः |
| **Instrumental** | अनया | आभ्याम् | आभिः |
| **Dative** | अस्यै | आभ्याम् | आभ्यः |
| **Ablative** | अस्याः | आभ्याम् | आभ्यः |
| **Genitive** | अस्याः | अनयोः | आसाम् |
| **Locative** | अस्याम् | अनयोः | आसु |

**अदस् m. that**

| | Singular | Dual | Plural |
|---|---|---|---|
| **Nominative** | असौ | अमू | अमी |
| **Accusative** | अमुम् | अमू | अमून् |
| **Instrumental** | अमुना | अमूभ्याम् | अमीभिः |
| **Dative** | अमुष्मै | अमूभ्याम् | अमीभ्यः |
| **Ablative** | अमुष्मात् | अमूभ्याम् | अमीभ्यः |
| **Genitive** | अमुष्य | अमुयोः | अमीषाम् |
| **Locative** | अमुष्मिन् | अमुयोः | अमीषु |

**अदस् n. that**

| | Singular | Dual | Plural |
|---|---|---|---|
| **Nom./Acc.** | अदः | अमू | अमूनि |

**अदस् f. that**

| | Singular | Dual | Plural |
|---|---|---|---|
| **Nominative** | असौ | अमू | अमूः |
| **Accusative** | अमूम् | अमू | अमूः |
| **Instrumental** | अमुया | अमूभ्याम् | अमूभिः |
| **Dative** | अमुष्यै | अमूभ्याम् | अमूभ्यः |
| **Ablative** | अमुष्याः | अमूभ्याम् | अमूभ्यः |
| **Genitive** | अमुष्याः | अमुयोः | अमूषाम् |
| **Locative** | अमुष्याम् | अमुयोः | अमूषु |

## Translate

### A. *Aparokṣānubhūti* 14

अज्ञानप्रभवं सर्वं ज्ञानेन प्रविलीयते ।
संकल्पो विविधः कर्ता विचारः सोऽयमीदृशः ॥

Vocabulary
प्रभवः m. production, source (in compound, produced by, derived from)
प्रवि√ली 1P, to melt away, disappear

In the *Aparokṣānubhūti*, an *advaitavedānta* text, मूलबन्धः (*mūlabandha*), the root lock, refers to a subtle, metaphysical awareness. In *haṭhayoga* texts, it refers to an actual physical engagement, practiced in order to access the subtle energy. Whether it is subtle or gross, awareness and engaging of this point can serve as an anchor for both *āsana* practice and meditation.

### B. *Aparokṣānubhūti* 114

यन्मूलं सर्वभुतानां यन्मूलं चित्तबन्धनम् ।
मूलबन्धः सदा सेव्यो योग्योऽसौ राजयोगिनाम् ॥

Vocabulary
सेव्य mfn. to be resorted to, practiced
योग्य mfn. useful, proper (takes the genitive)

### C. *Bhagavadgītā* 3.24

उत्सीदेयुरिमे लोका न कुर्यां कर्म चेदहम् ।
संकरस्य च कर्ता स्यामुपहन्यामिमाः प्रजाः ॥

Vocabulary
उत्√सद् 1P, to sink down, fall into ruin or decay
संकरः m. mixing together, confusion
उप√हन् 2P, to destroy

### D. *Bhagavadgītā* 7.13

त्रिभिर्गुणमयैर्भावैरेभिः सर्वमिदं जगत् ।
मोहितं नाभिजानाति मामेभ्यः परमव्ययम् ॥

Vocabulary
भावः m. state of being
मोहित mfn. deluded
अभि√ज्ञा 9P, to recognize

## PAST ACTIVE PARTICIPLES (PAP)

The past active participle is used to replace a past active verb, although it is not seen as commonly as the past passive participle. It is formed by adding the suffix -वत् (ई) to the past passive participle. It is declined as masculine/neuter nouns ending in -वत् or feminine nouns ending in -ई and agrees with the subject in case, number, and gender.

### Translate

> The word *prasāda* is also used for the food presented to a deity, which, after the ritual *pūjā*, is considered to be blessed by the god and is distributed among the devotees.

#### E. *Bhagavadgītā* 18.75

व्यासप्रसादाच्छ्रुतवानेतद् गुह्यमहं परम्।
योगं योगेश्वरात्कृष्णात्साक्षात्कथयतः स्वयम्॥

Vocabulary
प्रसादः m. graciousness, kindness, favor

#### F. *Dattātreyayogaśāstra* 2

सांकृतिर्मुनिवर्योऽसौ भूतलं योगलिप्सया।
सकलं च परिभ्रम्य नैमिषारण्यमाप्तवान्॥

Vocabulary
वर्य mfn. excellent, eminent, best of
लिप्सा f. the desire to gain, wish to obtain, longing for
परि√भ्रम् 1, 4P to rove, ramble, wander about
नैमिषम् n. name of a sacred forest

#### G. *Dattātreyayogaśāstra* 6

In the Naimiṣa forest, Sāṃkṛti saw Dattātreya seated in *padmāsana*, gazing at the tip of his nose, radiant, on a platform under a mango tree.

ततः प्रणम्य तमृषिं दत्तात्रेयं स सांकृतिः।
तच्छिष्यैः सह तत्रैव सम्मुखश्चोपविष्टवान्॥

Vocabulary
शिष्यः m. a pupil, scholar, disciple, student
सम्मुख mfn. facing, being in front of

## NEUTER NOUNS ENDING IN इ AND उ

Neuter nouns ending in इ and उ have parallel declensions.

**स्वस्ति n. well-being, fortune**

| | Singular | Dual | Plural |
|---|---|---|---|
| **Nominative** | स्वस्ति | स्वस्तिनी | स्वस्तीनि |
| **Accusative** | स्वस्ति | स्वस्तिनी | स्वस्तीनि |
| **Instrumental** | स्वस्तिना | स्वस्तिभ्याम् | स्वस्तिभिः |
| **Dative** | स्वस्तिने | स्वस्तिभ्याम् | स्वस्तिभ्यः |
| **Ablative** | स्वस्तिनः | स्वस्तिभ्याम् | स्वस्तिभ्यः |
| **Genitive** | स्वस्तिनः | स्वस्तिनोः | स्वस्तीनाम् |
| **Locative** | स्वस्तिनि | स्वस्तिनोः | स्वस्तिषु |
| **Vocative** | स्वस्ति | स्वस्तिनी | स्वस्तीनि |

**मधु n. honey**

| | Singular | Dual | Plural |
|---|---|---|---|
| **Nominative** | मधु | मधुनी | मधूनि |
| **Accusative** | मधु | मधुनी | मधूनि |
| **Instrumental** | मधुना | मधुभ्याम् | मधुभिः |
| **Dative** | मधुने | मधुभ्याम् | मधुभ्यः |
| **Ablative** | मधुनः | मधुभ्याम् | मधुभ्यः |
| **Genitive** | मधुनः | मधुनोः | मधूनाम् |
| **Locative** | मधुनि | मधुनोः | मधुषु |
| **Vocative** | मधु | मधुनी | मधूनि |

Vocabulary

वारि n. water
अश्रु n. tears
अम्बु n. water
वस्तु n. thing

### Decline

वारि, वस्तु

## Translate

### H. *Gheraṇḍasaṃhitā* 7.19

भूचराः खेचराश्चामी यावन्तो जीवजन्तवः ।
वृक्षगुल्मलतावल्लीतृणाद्या वारि पर्वताः ।
सर्वं ब्रह्म विजानीयात्सर्वं पश्यति चात्मनि ॥

Vocabulary
भूचर mfn. moving on the earth, creature of the earth
खेचर mfn. moving in the air, creature of the air
जीवजन्तुः m. living creature
गुल्म mn. cluster of trees, thicket, bush
लता f. creeper
वल्ली f. vine
पर्वतः m. mountain

The *Aruṇapraśna*, the first chapter of the *Taittirīya Āraṇyaka* of the *Yajur Veda*, is the most significant Vedic mantra for worshipping the Sun God. It is often called *sūryanamaskāra*, and recited in conjunction with practicing *sūryanamaskāra*, "salutations to the sun."

### I. *Aruṇapraśna*

भद्रं कर्णेभिः शृणुयाम देवाः । भद्रं पश्येमाक्षभिर्यजत्राः ।
स्थिरैरङ्गैस्तुष्टुवांसस्तनूभिः । व्यशेम देवहितं यदायुः ।
स्वस्ति न इन्द्रो वृद्धश्रवाः । स्वस्ति नः पूषा विश्ववेदाः ।
स्वस्ति नस्तार्क्ष्यो अरिष्टनेमिः । स्वस्ति नो बृहस्पतिर्दधातु ॥

Vocabulary
भद्रम् n. auspiciousness, welfare, good fortune
अक्षन् mfn. the eye
यजत्र mfn. worthy of worship or sacrifice
तुष्टुवांसः we have praised, celebrated (m. nom. pl. perfect active participle of √स्तु 2P, to praise, celebrate)
व्यु√अश् 1Ā, to attain
वृद्ध mfn. great
श्रवस् n. glory, fame, renown
पूषन् m. a Vedic deity connected with the sun, and therefore the surveyor of all things
विश्ववेदस् mfn. all-knowing, omniscient
तार्क्ष्यः m. Garuḍa
अरिष्टनेमिः m. the protector

## IRREGULAR DECLENSIONS ENDING IN VOWELS

**सखि: m. friend**

| | Singular | Dual | Plural |
|---|---|---|---|
| **Nominative** | सखा | सखायौ | सखायः |
| **Accusative** | सखायम् | सखायौ | सखीन् |
| **Instrumental** | सख्या | सखिभ्याम् | सखिभिः |
| **Dative** | सख्ये | सखिभ्याम् | सखिभ्यः |
| **Ablative** | सख्युः | सखिभ्याम् | सखिभ्यः |
| **Genitive** | सख्युः | सख्योः | सखीनाम् |
| **Locative** | सख्यौ | सख्योः | सखिषु |
| **Vocative** | सखे | सखायौ | सकायः |

**पतिः m. husband (declined regularly when the last member of a compound)**

| | Singular | Dual | Plural |
|---|---|---|---|
| **Nominative** | पतिः | पती | पतयः |
| **Accusative** | पतिम् | पती | पतीन् |
| **Instrumental** | पत्या | पतिभ्याम् | पतिभिः |
| **Dative** | पत्ये | पतिभ्याम् | पतिभ्यः |
| **Ablative** | पत्युः | पतिभ्याम् | पतिभ्यः |
| **Genitive** | पत्युः | पत्योः | पतीनाम् |
| **Locative** | पत्यौ | पत्योः | पतिषु |
| **Vocative** | पते | पती | पतयः |

**गो mf. bull, cow**

| | Singular | Dual | Plural |
|---|---|---|---|
| **Nominative** | गौः | गावौ | गावः |
| **Accusative** | गाम् | गावौ | गाः |
| **Instrumental** | गवा | गोभ्याम् | गोभिः |
| **Dative** | गवे | गोभ्याम् | गोभ्यः |
| **Ablative** | गोः | गोभ्याम् | गोभ्यः |
| **Genitive** | गोः | गवोः | गवाम् |
| **Locative** | गवि | गवोः | गोषु |
| **Vocative** | गौः | गावौ | गावः |

### स्त्री f. woman

| | Singular | Dual | Plural |
|---|---|---|---|
| **Nominative** | स्त्री | स्त्रियौ | स्त्रियः |
| **Accusative** | स्त्रियम् / स्त्रीम् | स्त्रियौ | स्त्रियः / स्त्रीः |
| **Instrumental** | स्त्रिया | स्त्रीभ्याम् | स्त्रीभिः |
| **Dative** | स्त्रियै | स्त्रीभ्याम् | स्त्रीभ्यः |
| **Ablative** | स्त्रियाः | स्त्रीभ्याम् | स्त्रीभ्यः |
| **Genitive** | स्त्रियाः | स्त्रियोः | स्त्रीणाम् |
| **Locative** | स्त्रियाम् | स्त्रियोः | स्त्रीषु |
| **Vocative** | स्त्रि | स्त्रियौ | स्त्रियः |

### धी f. thought, understanding, intelligence, mind

| | Singular | Dual | Plural |
|---|---|---|---|
| **Nominative** | धीः | धियौ | धियः |
| **Accusative** | धियम् | धियौ | धियः |
| **Instrumental** | धिया | धीभ्याम् | धीभिः |
| **Dative** | धिये / धियै | धीभ्याम् | धीभ्यः |
| **Ablative** | धियः / धियाः | धीभ्याम् | धीभ्यः |
| **Genitive** | धियः / धियाः | धियोः | धियाम् / धीनाम् |
| **Locative** | धियि / धियाम् | धियोः | धीषु |
| **Vocative** | धीः | धियौ | धियः |

### अक्षि n. eye

| | Singular | Dual | Plural |
|---|---|---|---|
| **Nominative** | अक्षि | अक्षिणी | अक्षीणि |
| **Accusative** | अक्षि | अक्षिणी | अक्षीणि |
| **Instrumental** | अक्ष्णा | अक्षिभ्याम् | अक्षिभिः |
| **Dative** | अक्ष्णे | अक्षिभ्याम् | अक्षिभ्यः |
| **Ablative** | अक्ष्णः | अक्षिभ्याम् | अक्षिभ्यः |
| **Genitive** | अक्ष्णः | अक्ष्णोः | अक्ष्णाम् |
| **Locative** | अक्ष्णि / अक्षणि | अक्ष्णोः | अक्षिषु |
| **Vocative** | अक्षे / अक्षि | अक्षिणी | अक्षीणि |

## IRREGULAR DECLENSIONS ENDING IN CONSONANTS

### पथिन् m. path

| | Singular | Dual | Plural |
|---|---|---|---|
| **Nominative** | पन्थाः | पन्थानौ | पन्थानः |
| **Accusative** | पन्थानम् | पन्थानौ | पथः |
| **Instrumental** | पथा | पथिभ्याम् | पथिभिः |
| **Dative** | पथे | पथिभ्याम् | पथिभ्यः |
| **Ablative** | पथः | पथिभ्याम् | पथिभ्यः |
| **Genitive** | पथः | पथोः | पथाम् |
| **Locative** | पथि | पथोः | पथिषु |
| **Vocative** | पन्थाः | पन्थानौ | पन्थानः |

### अप् f. water (only pl.)

| | Plural |
|---|---|
| **Nominative** | आपः |
| **Accusative** | अपः |
| **Instrumental** | अद्भिः |
| **Dative** | अद्भ्यः |
| **Ablative** | अद्भ्यः |
| **Genitive** | अपाम् |
| **Locative** | अप्सु |
| **Vocative** | आपः |

### अहन् n. day

| | Singular | Dual | Plural |
|---|---|---|---|
| **Nominative** | अहः | अह्नी / अहनी | अहानि |
| **Accusative** | अहः | अह्नी / अहनी | अहानि |
| **Instrumental** | अह्ना | अहोभ्याम् | अहोभिः |
| **Dative** | अह्ने | अहोभ्याम् | अहोभ्यः |
| **Ablative** | अह्नः | अहोभ्याम् | अहोभ्यः |
| **Genitive** | अह्नः | अह्नोः | अह्नाम् |
| **Locative** | अह्नि / अहनि | अह्नोः | अहस्सु |
| **Vocative** | अहः | अह्नी / अहनी | अहानि |

### J. *Haṭhapradīpikā* 2.6

प्राणायामं ततः कुर्यान्नित्यं सात्त्विकया धिया ।
यथा सुषुम्नानाडीस्था मलाः शुद्धिं प्रयान्ति च ॥

Vocabulary
सात्त्विक mfn. endowed with clarity and calmness

In Āyurvedic medicine, there are thought to be 72,000 *nāḍīs*, or subtle channels, running through the body, analogous to the meridians of Chinese medicine. On either side of the *suṣumṇā* are the *iḍā* and *piṅgalā nāḍīs*, the lunar and solar channels, which are purified through *haṭhayoga*.

### K. *Bhagavadgītā* 5.18

The subject is in the fourth *pāda*.

विद्याविनयसंपन्ने ब्राह्मणे गवि हस्तिनि ।
शुनि चैव श्वपाके च पण्डिताः समदर्शिनः ॥

Vocabulary
विनयः m. education, moral training, decency
संपन्न mfn. endowed with, possessed of
श्वन् m. a dog
श्वपाकः m. "dog cooker," untouchable

### L. *Yogayājñavalkya* 1.20

Yājñavalkya is speaking to his wife, Gārgī, and telling her the story of his meeting with Brahmā, who taught him yoga. The subject is Brahmā.

मामालोक्य प्रसन्नात्मा ज्ञानकर्माण्यभाषत ।
ज्ञानस्य द्विविधौ ज्ञेयौ पन्थानौ वेदचोदितौ ॥

Vocabulary
आ√लोक् 1Ā, to look at
प्रसन्न mfn. gracious, propitious, kindly disposed
ज्ञेय mfn. to be known, investigated
चोदित mfn. put forward, taught

**M. *Bhāgavatapurāṇa* 10.20.41**

तत् in the fourth *pāda* refers to the mind.

केदारेभ्यस्त्वपोऽगृह्णन् कर्षका दृढसेतुभिः ।
यथा प्राणैः स्रवज्ज्ञानं तन्निरोधेन योगिनः ॥

Vocabulary

केदारः m. a field or meadow, especially one underwater
कर्षकः m. one who plows, farmer
सेतुः m. embankment

## Review Exercises

### N. *Bhagavadgītā* 4.1

Kṛṣṇa is speaking to Arjuna about the lineage of yoga.

इमं विवस्वते योगं प्रोक्तवानहमव्ययम् ।
विवस्वान्मनवे प्राह मनुरिक्ष्वाकवेऽब्रवीत् ॥

> Vivasvat, "the Brilliant One," was the Sun God and father of Manu Vaivasvata. Manu was the progenitor of the present race of living beings, saved from a great flood by Viṣṇu in the form of a fish, *matsyāvatāra*. He was also the founder and first king of the solar race of kings who ruled at Ayodhyā, and the father of Ikṣvāku.

### O. *Bhagavadgītā* 11.52–53

सुदुर्दर्शमिदं रूपं दृष्टवानसि यन्मम ।
देवा अप्यस्य रूपस्य नित्यं दर्शनकाङ्क्षिणः ॥

नाहं वेदैर्न तपसा न दानेन न चेज्यया ।
शक्य एवंविधो द्रष्टुं दृष्टवानसि मां यथा ॥

Vocabulary

सुदुर्दर्श mfn. very difficult to be discerned or seen
काङ्क्षिन् mfn. desiring, longing for
इज्या f. sacrifice, ritual
द्रष्टुम् ind. to be seen (note that the infinitive can have passive meaning when used with an auxiliary verb that is in the passive, i.e., शक्ये)

### P. *Chāndogyopaniṣat* 6.8.3–4

Uddalāka Āruṇi is speaking to his son Śvetaketu. He is explaining that every शुङ्गम् or "bud" must have a मूलम् or "root," or in other words, that every "effect" must have a "cause."

तत्रैतदेव शुङ्गमुत्पतितँ सोम्य विजानीहि । नेदममूलं भविष्यतीति ॥ तस्य क्व मूलँ स्यादन्यत्राद्भ्यः । अद्भिः सोम्य शुङ्गेन तेजोमूलमन्विच्छ । तेजसा सोम्य शुङ्गेन सन्मूलमन्विच्छ । सन्मूलाः सोम्येमाः सर्वाः प्रजाः सदायतनाः सत्प्रतिष्ठाः ।

Vocabulary

शुङ्गम् n. sheath or calyx of a bud, effect
उत्पतित mfn. sprung up, arisen
वि√ज्ञा 9P, to discern, observe, know, understand
अमूलम् n. rootless, without a root

आयतनम् n. resting place, home
प्रतिष्ठम् n. support

Q. *Chāndogyopaniṣat* 6.9

Uddalāka Āruṇi is still speaking to Śvetaketu.

यथा सोम्य मधु मधुकृतो निस्तिष्ठन्ति नानात्ययानां वृक्षाणाँ रसान्समवहारमेकताँ रसं गमयन्ति ॥ १ ॥
ते यथा तत्र न विवेकं लभन्तेऽमुष्याहं वृक्षस्य रसोऽस्म्यमुष्याहं वृक्षस्य रसोऽस्मीति। एवमेव खलु सोम्येमाः सर्वाः प्रजाः सति संपद्य न विदुः सति संपद्यामह इति ॥ २ ॥
त इह व्याघ्रो वा सिँहा वा वृको वा वराहो वा कीटो वा पतङ्गो वा दँशो वा मशको वा यद्यद्भवन्ति तदाभवन्ति ॥ ३ ॥
स य एषोऽणिमैतदात्म्यमिदँ सर्वम्। तत्सत्यम्। स आत्मा। तत्त्वमसि। श्वेतकेतो इति।
भूय एव मा भगवान्विज्ञापयत्विति। तथा सोम्येति होवाच ॥ ४ ॥

Vocabulary
मधुकृत् m. making honey, a bee
नि√ष्ठा 1U, to fix in, give forth, emit, yield
नानात्यय mfn. various, manifold
समवहारम् ind. by gathering [the रसान्, nectars]
एकताँ रसम् one, unified nectar (acc. sg.)
तत्र ind. there [in that unified nectar]
सं√पद् 1Ā, meet or unite with, enter into, come together, attain, arrive, become complete
वृकः m. wolf
वराहः m. boar
कीटः m. worm
पतङ्गः m. moth
दँशः m. gadfly, gnat
मशकः m. mosquito

# 19
# Nominal Derivation: कृत् and तद्धित Suffixes; Pronoun: एनम्

परिणामैकत्वाद्वस्तुतत्त्वम् ॥ ४.१४ ॥
**pariṇāmaikatvād vastu-tattvam**
The tangibility of things exists due to the single origin of transformation.
॥ *Yogasūtra* 4.14 ॥

## NOMINAL DERIVATION

One of the reasons for the richness of Sanskrit vocabulary is the derivation of nouns from verbs and other nouns by the addition of various suffixes (प्रत्यय). These can be divided into two major categories—कृत् and तद्धित. The former are primary suffixes added directly to verbal roots to form nouns and adjectives. The latter are added to already existing nouns or adjectives to form more complex nouns and adjectives.

As an example of the usefulness and relevance of learning these suffixes, consider some of the possible derivations from the root √युज्, 7P, "to join, unite, yoke, concentrate one's attention."

**योगः** m. union, yoking, concentration of the mind, meditation, system of philosophy established by Patañjali
**योगिन्** / **-इनी** mf. practitioner of yoga
**युक्त** mfn. joined, united, yoked, engaged, absorbed in
**युक्तिः** f. method, reason
**योक्तव्य** mfn. to be joined, yoked, united
**योक्त्रम्** n. a cord, rope, the tie of the yoke of a plow
**योक्तृ** m. one who yokes, joins, unites
**युगम्** n. yoke, pair, age of the world
**योग्य** mfn. fit, proper, suitable

According to the Hindu view of cosmology, there are considered to be four *yugas*, or ages, of the world. The first is the *kṛta yuga*, the golden age, compared to a cow standing on four legs. The second is the *tretā yuga*, compared to a cow standing on three legs. The third is the *dvāpara yuga*, compared to a cow on two legs. The final age, in which we live now, is the *kali yuga*, the dark age, in which the cow is teetering on one leg. At the end of the cycle, the world dissolves and the cycle starts again anew.

योग्यता f. fitness, propriety
यौक्तिक mfn. suitable, fit, proper
यौगः m. a follower of the yoga system of philosophy
योजनम् n. joining, uniting, a measure of distance
योजनीय mfn. to be joined, united

## कृत् SUFFIXES

The following are some of the most commonly encountered कृत् suffixes (primary suffixes added directly to verbal roots to form nouns and adjectives).

1. The suffix -अन can be added to verbal roots to form neuter nouns expressing action, or the location or means of action. The root vowel takes गुण if possible.

   आ√यत् ⇒ आयतनम्
   to arrive, rest on ⇒ resting place, support

   √आस् ⇒ आसनम्
   to sit ⇒ seat, posture

   √दा ⇒ दानम्
   to give ⇒ giving, gift

   निर्√वा ⇒ निर्वाणम्
   to blow out, be extinguished ⇒ extinction, dissolution, final liberation

   √नी ⇒ नयनम्
   to lead ⇒ leader, eye

   √बध् ⇒ बन्धनम्
   to bind ⇒ binding, bond

   √भुज् ⇒ भोजनम्
   to eat ⇒ eating, food

   √युज् ⇒ योजनम्
   to yoke, join ⇒ joining, uniting, a measure of distance

   √वच् ⇒ वचनम्
   to speak ⇒ speech, saying

   √श्रु ⇒ श्रवनम्
   to hear ⇒ hearing, ear

2. The suffix -अ can also be added to verbal roots to form masculine nouns expressing action. A medial root vowel is subject to गुण, except for medial अ, which can take वृद्धि. Final palatals च् / ज् become gutturals क् / ग्.

√जि ⇒ जयः
to conquer ⇒ conquest, victory

√त्यज् ⇒ त्यागः
to abandon ⇒ renunciation

√भुज् ⇒ भोगः
to enjoy ⇒ enjoyment

√युज् ⇒ योगः
to yoke, join ⇒ union

√विद् ⇒ वेदः
to know ⇒ knowledge, the Vedas

वि√शिष् ⇒ विशेषः
to distinguish ⇒ distinction

√शुच् ⇒ शोकः
to grieve ⇒ grief

3. The suffix -ति can be added to verbal roots to form feminine action nouns. The root vowel is generally unchanged, although final palatals च् / ज् again become gutturals क् / ग्.

√दृश् ⇒ दृष्टिः
to see ⇒ sight, vision, gaze

√बुध् ⇒ बुद्धिः
to wake ⇒ intellect, discernment, understanding

√भज् ⇒ भक्तिः
to share, distribute, divide ⇒ division, devotion

√मुच् ⇒ मुक्तिः
to liberate ⇒ liberation

√युज् ⇒ युक्तिः
to yoke, join ⇒ junction, application, plan

√शक् ⇒ शक्तिः
to be able ⇒ power

√श्रु ⇒ श्रुतिः
to hear ⇒ heard, revealed texts, for example, the Vedas

√स्मृ ⇒ स्मृतिः
to remember ⇒ remembered, traditional texts with human authors, e.g., the *Vedāṅgas*, *sūtras*, epics

4. The suffix -त्र can be added to verbal roots to form nouns expressing an instrument or means of action of that verbal root. These nouns are mostly neuter, and root vowels are subject to गुण.

√तन् ⇒ तन्त्रम्
to extend, stretch ⇒ loom, instrument of stretching

√नी ⇒ नेत्रम्
to lead ⇒ eye, instrument of leading

√मन् ⇒ मन्त्रम्
to think of (in prayer) ⇒ instrument of thought, sacred prayer

√यम् ⇒ यन्त्रम्
to hold, restrain ⇒ instrument for holding or restraining

√युज् ⇒ योक्त्रम्
to yoke ⇒ a cord, rope, the tie of the yoke of a plow

√शास् ⇒ शास्त्रम्
to rule, teach ⇒ an instrument of teaching, religious or scientific treatise

√श्रु ⇒ श्रोत्रम्
to hear ⇒ ear, instrument of hearing

## Translate

### A. *Bhagavadgītā* 5.24

योऽन्तःसुखोऽन्तरारामस्तथान्तर्ज्योतिरेव यः ।
स योगी ब्रह्मनिर्वाणं ब्रह्मभूतोऽधिगच्छति ॥

#### Vocabulary

अन्तर् ind. within, inside
आरामः m. delight, pleasure
अधि√गम् 1P, to attain

### B. *Rāmāyaṇa* 2.17

This verse is considered to be the origin of poetry. The sage Vālmīki, author of the *Rāmāyaṇa*, saw a hunter shoot two *krauñca* birds in the act of mating. He cried out in sorrow and his utterance came out spontaneously in the form of a verse.

पादबद्धोऽक्षरसमस्तन्त्रीलयसमन्वितः ।
शोकार्तस्य प्रवृत्तो मे श्लोको भवतु नान्यथा ॥

Vocabulary
तन्त्री f. wire or string of a lute, strings of the heart, stringed instruments
लयः m. melting, dissolution, absorption in, percussion instruments
समन्वित mfn. connected with, endowed with, capable of
आर्त mfn. afflicted, pained, disturbed
प्रवृत्त mfn. came forth, occurred
श्लोकः m. verse, poetry

### C. *Chāndogyopaniṣat* 6.8.2

स यथा शकुनिः सूत्रेण प्रबद्धो दिशं दिशं पतित्वान्यत्रायतनमलब्ध्वा बन्धनमेवोपश्रयते। एवमेव खलु सोम्य तन्मनो दिशं दिशं पतित्वान्यत्रायतनमलब्ध्वा प्राणमेवोपश्रयते । प्राणबन्धनँ हि सोम्य मन इति ॥

Vocabulary
शकुनिः m. a bird
सूत्रम् n. thread, string
प्रबद्ध mfn. bound, tied, fettered
√पत् 1P, to fly
उप√श्रि 1P, to lean against, go toward

## तद्धित SUFFIXES

These suffixes are added to already existing nouns or adjectives to form more complex nouns and adjectives. The following are some of the most common examples.

1. Abstract Nouns
   An abstract noun is formed by adding the suffixes -त्व, -ता, or -इमन् or by a combination of वृद्धि strengthening of the root vowel, dropping the final vowel, and adding

the suffix -य. When these suffixes are added to the end of a noun or adjective, they are equivalent to the English -ness or -hood.

लघु ⇒ लाघव / लघुत्व / लघुता / लघिमन्
light ⇒ lightness

स्थिर ⇒ स्थैर्य / स्थिरत्व / स्थिरता
steady ⇒ steadiness

Abstract nouns are usually used in conjunction with a word in the genitive case (e.g., the X-ness of Y). Abstract nouns are often used in the instrumental or ablative cases.

The word तत्त्व (*tattva*) is a perfect example of an abstract noun, literally meaning "that-ness." It then comes to mean a true state or principle. The *tattvas* are enumerated as twenty-five, according to *Sāṃkhya* philosophy. They begin with *prakṛti* (Nature), from which evolves *mahat* (intellect), *ahaṃkāra* (ego), *manas* (mind), the five *tanmātras* (objects), the five sense organs, the five organs of action, and the five elements.

### Example: *Yogasūtra* 2.53

The previous *sūtras* speak about the practice of *prāṇāyāma* and what happens as a result.

धारणासु च योग्यता मनसः ।

And (च), of the mind (मनसः), there is **fitness** (योग्यता) for concentration (धारणासु). ⇒ And the mind is then fit for concentration.

2. Patronymics and other relationship terms
   पर्वतः mountain ⇒ पार्वती Śiva's wife, daughter of the mountain
   पुत्रः son ⇒ पौत्रः grandchild
   विष्णुः Viṣṇu ⇒ वैष्णव relating or belonging to Viṣṇu, worshipper of Viṣṇu
   शिवः Śiva ⇒ शैवः relating or belonging to Śiva, worshipper of Śiva

3. Derivatives formed with the suffixes -य, -इय, -ईय, -एय
   अदितिः Aditi ⇒ आदित्यः descendant of Aditi, the sun
   कविः poet ⇒ काव्यः poetry
   कुन्ती mother of Arjuna ⇒ कौन्तेय son of Kuntī, Arjuna
   क्षत्र ruling class ⇒ क्षत्रिय member of the ruling class
   सत् existence ⇒ सत्य truth

4. Diminutives formed with the suffix -क
   अध्यात्मः Self ⇒ अध्यात्मिकः relating to the Self

धर्मः law, justice ⇒ धार्मिकः virtuous
पुत्रः son ⇒ पुत्रकः little son
मम my ⇒ मामक mine

## Translate

### D. *Bhagavadgītā* 7.8

रसोऽहमप्सु कौन्तेय प्रभास्मि शशिसूर्ययोः ।
प्रणवः सर्ववेदेषु शब्दः खे पौरुषं नृषु ॥

Vocabulary
प्रभा f. light, splendor, radiance
पौरुषम् n. manhood

### E. *Bhagavadgītā* 18.37

यत्तदग्रे विषमिव परिणामेऽमृतोपमम् ।
तत्सुखं सात्त्विकं प्रोक्तमात्मबुद्धिप्रसादजम् ॥

Vocabulary
विषम् n. poison
परिणामः m. change, transformation

The word परिणाम (*pariṇāma*), or transformation, is the most frequently used word in the *Yogasūtra*. It is a constant reminder of our natural state of change and evolution.

### F. *Haṭhapradīpikā* 1.17

Note that तदासनम् in the third *pāda* refers to "these postures" that will be described in the subsequent verses, which give the qualities listed in the third and fourth *pādas*. The yoga described here is *ṣaḍaṅgayoga*, or six-limbed yoga, beginning with *āsana*.

हठस्य प्रथमाङ्गत्वादासनं पूर्वमुच्यते ।
कुर्यात्तदासनं स्थैर्यमारोग्यं चाङ्गलाघवम् ॥

Vocabulary
आरोग्यम् n. absence of disease, health

### G. *Gheraṇḍasaṃhitā* 1.9–11

शोधनं दृढता चैव स्थैर्यं धैर्यं च लाघवम् ।
प्रत्यक्षं च निर्लिप्तं च घटस्य सप्तसाधनम् ॥

The घटः (*ghata*), or vessel, referred to here is the body.

षट्कर्मणा शोधनं च आसनेन भवेदृढम् ।
मुद्रया <u>स्थिरता</u> चैव प्रत्याहारेण <u>धीरता</u> ॥

प्राणायामाल्लाघवं च ध्यानात्प्रत्यक्षमात्मनः ।
समाधिना निर्लिप्तं च मुक्तिरेव न संशयः ॥

Vocabulary

**शोधनम्** n. purifying, purification
**निर्लिप्तः** m. untaintedness, unsmeared, indifference, unobscured awareness
**घटः** m. large earthen water jar, pot, the body
**मुद्रा** f. seal, various bodily actions such as the *bandhas*, described as tenfold in the *Haṭhapradīpikā*

## THE PRONOUN एनम्

**एनम्** is another third-person pronoun, meaning "him, it, her, this." It is enclitic and has only a limited number of forms.

| | Masculine | | |
|---|---|---|---|
| | Singular | Dual | Plural |
| **Accusative** | एनम् | एनौ | एनान् |
| **Instrumental** | एनेन | | |
| **Genitive/Locative** | | एनयोः | |

| | Neuter | | |
|---|---|---|---|
| | Singular | Dual | Plural |
| **Accusative** | एनत् | एने | एनानि |
| **Instrumental** | एनेन | | |
| **Genitive/Locative** | | एनयोः | |

| | Feminine | | |
|---|---|---|---|
| | Singular | Dual | Plural |
| **Accusative** | एनाम् | एने | एनाः |
| **Instrumental** | एनया | | |
| **Genitive/Locative** | | एनयोः | |

## Translate

### H. *Bhagavadgītā* 4.42

In the previous verse, Kṛṣṇa advises Arjuna to renounce action through yoga so that he is not bound by his actions. Note that आत्मनः here just means "of yourself," or "your."

तस्मादज्ञानसंभूतं हृत्स्थं ज्ञानासिनात्मनः ।
छित्त्वैनं संशयं योगमातिष्ठोत्तिष्ठ भारत ॥

Vocabulary
आ√स्था 1P, to undertake, perform, practice
उद्√स्था 1P, to stand up, arise

### I. *Ādityahṛdayam* 25

एनम् here is referring to the Sun God.

एनमापत्सु कृच्छ्रेषु कान्तारेषु भयेषु च ।
कीर्तयन्पुरुषः कश्चिन्नावसीदति राघव ॥

Vocabulary
आपद् f. calamity, misfortune, danger
कृच्छ्र mn. difficulty, trouble, hardship
कान्तार mn. large or dreary forest
√कृत् 10U, to praise
राघवः m. descendant of Raghu

### J. *Bhagavadgītā* 15.11

एनम् refers to the Soul.

यतन्तो योगिनश्चैनं पश्यन्त्यात्मन्यवस्थितम् ।
यतन्तोऽप्यकृतात्मनो नैनं पश्यन्त्यचेतसः ॥

Vocabulary
√यत् 1Ā, to persevere
अकृतात्मन् mfn. ignorant, foolish, having an uncontrolled mind
अचेतस mfn. unconscious, unthinking, insensible

## Review Exercises

### K. *Bhagavadgītā* 13.32

यथा सर्वगतं सौक्ष्म्यादाकाशं नोपलिप्यते ।
सर्वत्रावस्थितो देहे तथात्मा नोपलिप्यते ॥

Vocabulary
सर्वगत mfn. all-pervading, omnipresent
सौक्ष्म्यम् n. subtlety
उप√लिप् 6P, to defile, besmear

### L. *Aparokṣānubhūti* 32

अयम् in the third *pāda* means "this [body]."

अहं द्रष्टृतया सिद्धो देहो दृश्यतया स्थितः ।
ममायमिति निर्देशात्कथं स्याद्देहकः पुमान् ॥ ३२ ॥

Vocabulary
सिद्ध mfn. established
निर्देशः m. description, statement

### M. *Aparokṣānubhūti* 129

In the fourth *pāda*, infer "thinking of."

भाववृत्त्या हि भावत्वं शून्यवृत्त्या हि शून्यता ।
ब्रह्मवृत्त्या हि पूर्णत्वं तथा पूर्णत्वमभ्यसेत् ॥

Vocabulary
भावः m. being, existence, object, thing
शून्यम् n. a void, empty place, vacuity, nonentity

### N. *Bhagavadgītā* 2.29

एनम् refers to the Soul.

आश्चर्यवत्पश्यति कश्चिदेनमाश्चर्यवद्वदति तथैव चान्यः ।
आश्चर्यवच्चैनमन्यः शृणोति श्रुत्वाप्येनं वेद न चैव कश्चित् ॥

Vocabulary
आश्चर्यवत् ind. wondrously, as a wonder

# 20
# The Aorist

**न चैकचित्ततन्त्रं वस्तु तदप्रमाणकं तदा किं स्यात् ॥ ४.१६ ॥**
**na caika-citta-tantraṃ vastu tad apramāṇakaṃ tadā kiṃ syāt**
An object is not dependent upon one mind for its existence, for if it were,
when it is not cognized by that mind, then what would it be?
|| *Yogasūtra* 4.16 ||

## THE AORIST

The aorist is the last past tense we will learn; its name, अद्यतन, means "of today." In the classical language, the aorist is undistinguished in meaning from the other past tenses; but in the Vedic language, where it is much more common, it refers to a recent past action still relevant to the speaker. Unlike the imperfect, which is formed from the present stem, the aorist is formed by adding the augment अ directly to the **root**, adding the tense sign and then the imperfect endings, with some minor changes. There are seven types of aorists, differentiated by the tense sign added. Four of them are sigmatic, meaning that the tense sign contains a sibilant. Some roots can be seen in more than one category of aorist. Don't worry too much about memorizing the specific categorizations, just learn to recognize the aorist when you see it.

## SIGMATIC AORIST

### -स् Aorist

This form of the aorist consists of the augment अ + root + स् + athematic imperfect endings. Note, however, the variant *parasmaipada* endings—third-person singular -ईत्, second-person singular -ईः, and third-person plural -उः. The -स् aorist is used for roots ending in consonants or vowels other than -आ. *Parasmaipada* roots take *vṛddhi* strengthening; *ātmanepada* roots take *guṇa*.

**√श्रु to hear**

| | Singular | Dual | Plural | Singular | Dual | Plural |
|---|---|---|---|---|---|---|
| 3 | अश्रौषीत् | अश्रौष्टाम् | अश्रौषुः | अश्रोष्ट | अश्रोषाताम् | अश्रोषत |
| 2 | अश्रौषीः | अश्रौष्टम् | अश्रौष्ट | अश्रोष्ठाः | अश्रोषाथाम् | अश्रोढ्वम् |
| 1 | अश्रौषम् | अश्रौष्व | अश्रौष्म | अश्रोषि | अश्रोष्वहि | अश्रोष्महि |

### Common Roots

√कृ to do ⇒ अकार्षीत् he/she did
√दृश् to see ⇒ अद्राक्षीत् he/she saw
√नी to lead ⇒ अनैषीत् he/she led
√वस् to live ⇒ अवात्सीत् he/she lived

## Translate

### A. *Bhagavadgītā* 18.74

Sañjaya, Dhṛtarāṣṭra's minister, who narrated the *Bhagavadgītā*, speaks the concluding verses. Translate the two lines together.

इत्यहं वासुदेवस्य पार्थस्य च महात्मनः ।
संवादमिममश्रौषमद्भुतं रोमहर्षणम् ॥

#### Vocabulary

संवादः m. speaking together, conversation, dialogue
अद्भुत mfn. extraordinary, supernatural, wonderful, marvelous
रोमहर्षण mfn. causing the hair to stand on end or bristle (through joy or terror)

### B. *Kaṭhopaniṣat* 1.27

For his third wish, Naciketas asks Death to explain to him about death. Death doesn't want to comply and tries to dissuade him, but Naciketas is insistent. The "we" refers to human beings. Note that the second *pāda* is a question.

न वित्तेन तर्पणीयो मनुष्यो
लप्स्यामहे वित्तमद्राक्ष्म चेत्त्वा ।
जीविष्यामो यावदीशिष्यसि त्वं
वरस्तु मे वरणीयः स एव ॥

Vocabulary

तर्पणीय mfn. to be satisfied
√ईश् 2Ā, to command, allow
वरः m. wish, request, boon
वरणीय mfn. to be chosen

## -इष् Aorist

This form of the aorist consists of the augment अ + root + इष् + athematic imperfect endings. The variant endings are the same as for the -स् aorist above; however, in the second- and third-person singular forms, the sibilant tense marker is dropped. The -इष् aorist is used for roots ending in consonants and vowels other than -आ. *Parasmaipada* roots take *vṛddhi* or *guṇa* strengthening; *ātmanepada* roots take *guṇa*.

**√बुध् to awaken**

| | Parasmaipada | | | Ātmanepada | | |
|---|---|---|---|---|---|---|
| | Singular | Dual | Plural | Singular | Dual | Plural |
| 3 | अबोधीत् | अबोधिष्टाम् | अबोधिषुः | अबोधिष्ट | अबोधिषाताम् | अबोधिषत |
| 2 | अबोधीः | अबोधिष्टम् | अबोधिष्ट | अबोधिष्ठाः | अबोधिषाथाम् | अबोधिढ्वम् |
| 1 | अबोधिषम् | अबोधिष्व | अबोधिष्म | अबोधिषि | अबोधिष्वहि | अबोधिष्महि |

### Common Roots

√तॄ to cross ⇒ अतारीत् he/she crossed
√वद् to speak ⇒ अवादीत् he/she spoke
√विद् to know ⇒ अवेदीत् he/she knew

## Translate

### C. *Taittirīyopaniṣat* 1.12

शं नो मित्रः शं वरुणः । शं नो भवत्वर्यमा ।
शं न इन्द्रो बृहस्पतिः । शं नो विष्णुरुरुक्रमः ।
नमो ब्रह्मणे । नमस्ते वायो । त्वमेव प्रत्यक्षं ब्रह्मासि ।
त्वामेव प्रत्यक्षं ब्रह्मावादिषम् । ऋतमवादिषम् । सत्यमवादिषम् ।
तन्मामावीत् । तद्वक्तारमावीत् । आवीन्माम् । आवीद्वक्तारम् ।
ॐ शान्तिः शान्तिः शान्तिः ॥

### Vocabulary

See Exercise 7D.

## -सिष् Aorist

This is a pretty rare form of the aorist, used only for a few roots ending in -आ or -अम् and only found in *parasmaipada* forms. It consists of the augment अ + root + सिष् + athematic imperfect endings, with the same exceptions noted earlier.

**√ज्ञा to know**

| | Singular | Dual | Plural |
|---|---|---|---|
| 3 | अज्ञासीत् | अज्ञासिष्टाम् | अज्ञासिषुः |
| 2 | अज्ञासीः | अज्ञासिष्टम् | अज्ञासिष्ट |
| 1 | अज्ञासिषम् | अज्ञासिष्व | अज्ञासिष्म |

### Common Roots

√नम् to bow ⇒ अनंसीत् he/she bowed
√या to go ⇒ अयासीत् he/she went
√स्था to stand ⇒ अस्थासीत् he/she stood

## Translate

### D. *Bṛhadāraṇyakopaniṣat* 5.2.1–3

त्रयाः प्राजापत्याः प्रजापतौ पितरि ब्रह्मचर्यमूषुर्देवा मनुष्या असुराः।
उषित्वा ब्रह्मचर्यं देवा ऊचुर्ब्रवीतु नो भवानिति। तेभ्यो हैतदेवाक्षरमुवाच द इति।
व्यज्ञासिष्टा३ इति। व्यज्ञासिष्मेति होचुः। दाम्यतेति न आत्थेति।
ओमिति होवाच व्यज्ञासिष्टेति ॥ १ ॥
अथ हैनं मनुष्या ऊचुर्ब्रवीतु नो भवानिति। तेभ्यो हैतदेवाक्षरमुवाच द इति।
व्यज्ञासिष्टा३ इति। व्यज्ञासिष्मेति होचुः। दत्तेति न आत्थेति।
ओमिति होवाच व्यज्ञासिष्टेति ॥ २ ॥
अथ हैनमसुरा ऊचुर्ब्रवीतु नो भवानिति। तेभ्यो हैतदेवाक्षरमुवाच द इति।
व्यज्ञासिष्टा३ इति। व्यज्ञासिष्मेति होचुः। दयध्वमिति न आत्थेति।
ओमिति होवाच व्यज्ञासिष्टेति। तदेतदेवैषा दैवी वागनुवदति स्तनयित्नुर्द द द इति।

दाम्यत दत्त दयध्वमिति। तदेतत्त्रयँ शिक्षेद्दमं दानं दयामिति ॥ ३ ॥

Vocabulary

प्राजापत्यः m. descendant of Prajāpati
ब्रह्मचर्यम् n. religious studentship, the first stage of life for a Brahmin boy, spent in celibacy, studying the Vedas
असुरः m. demon
√दम् 4P, to be tamed, subdued, self-controlled
√दय् 1Ā, to be compassionate
अनु√वद् 1P, to repeat
स्तनयित्नुः m. thunder
√शिक्ष् 1Ā, to learn, study, practice
दमः m. self-control

ओम् can simply be a particle of assent, meaning "yes, verily, so be it."

This passage was made famous by T. S. Eliot in his long poem *The Waste Land*, in the fifth section, "What the Thunder Said."

## -स Aorist

This form of the aorist consists of the augment अ + root + स + thematic imperfect endings. Note, however, the variant *ātmanepada* endings—first-person singular -इ, second-person dual -आथाम्, and third-person dual -आताम्. The -स aorist is very rare and is only used for a few roots ending in -श् or -ह्. *Parasmaipada* roots take *vṛddhi* strengthening; *ātmanepada* roots take *guṇa*.

**√दिश् to show**

| | Parasmaipada | | | Ātmanepada | | |
|---|---|---|---|---|---|---|
| | Singular | Dual | Plural | Singular | Dual | Plural |
| 3 | अदिक्षत् | अदिक्षताम् | अदिक्षन् | अदिक्षत | अदिक्षाताम् | अदिक्षन्त |
| 2 | अदिक्षः | अदिक्षतम् | अदिक्षत | अदिक्षथाः | अदिक्षाथाम् | अदिक्षध्वम् |
| 1 | अदिक्षम् | अदिक्षाव | अदिक्षाम | अदिक्षि | अदिक्षावहि | अदिक्षामहि |

Common Roots

√दुह् to milk ⇒ अदुक्षत् he/she milked

# NONSIGMATIC AORIST

## Root Aorist

This form of the aorist is found only in *parasmaipada*. It consists of the augment अ + root + athematic imperfect endings, with no intervening tense sign. It is used for roots ending in -आ and the root √भू. Note that in general, the third-person plural ending is -उः; however, the third-person plural form of √भू is अभूवन्. Also note the first-person singular form of √भू, अभूवम्.

| | √दा to give | | | √भू to be | | |
|---|---|---|---|---|---|---|
| | Singular | Dual | Plural | Singular | Dual | Plural |
| 3 | अदात् | अदाताम् | अदुः | अभूत् | अभूताम् | अभूवन् |
| 2 | अदाः | अदातम् | अदात | अभूः | अभूतम् | अभूत |
| 1 | अदाम् | अदाव | अदाम | अभूवम् | अभूव | अभूम |

#### Common Roots

√धा to place ⇒ अधात् he/she placed
√पा to protect ⇒ अपात् he/she protected

## Translate

### E. *Īśopaniṣat* 7

Note that here यस्मिन् and तत्र are referring to the आत्मन् as it was described in previous verses.

यस्मिन्सर्वाणि भूतान्यात्मैवाभूद्विजानतः ।
तत्र को मोहः कः शोक एकत्वमनुपश्यतः ॥

Vocabulary
विजानत् m. wise man, sage, one who knows

The *Īśopaniṣat*, also known as the *Īśāvāsyopaniṣat*, is named after its first words, *īśā-vāsya*, enveloped by the Lord, and consists of eighteen verses describing and praising this Lord. From the *Śukla* (white) *Yajur Veda*, it is dated to roughly 500–100 B.C.E.

## अ Aorist

This form of the aorist is usually only *parasmaipada* as well. It consists of the augment अ + root + अ + thematic imperfect endings. It can be formed from a variety of roots. The root vowel does not take *guṇa* or *vṛddhi*. Note that √वच् uses the irregular stem वोच्.

**√गम् to go**

| | Parasmaipada | | | Ātmanepada | | |
|---|---|---|---|---|---|---|
| | Singular | Dual | Plural | Singular | Dual | Plural |
| 3 | अगमत् | अगमताम् | अगमन् | अगमत | अगमेताम् | अगमन्त |
| 2 | अगमः | अगमतम् | अगमत | अगमथाः | अगमेथाम् | अगमध्वम् |
| 1 | अगमम् | अगमाव | अगमाम | अगमे | अगमावहि | अगमामहि |

**√वच् to speak**

| | Parasmaipada | | | Ātmanepada | | |
|---|---|---|---|---|---|---|
| | Singular | Dual | Plural | Singular | Dual | Plural |
| 3 | अवोचत् | अवोचताम् | अवोचन् | अवोचत | अवोचेताम् | अवोचन्त |
| 2 | अवोचः | अवोचतम् | अवोचत | अवोचथाः | अवोचेथाम् | अवोचध्वम् |
| 1 | अवोचम् | अवोचाव | अवोचाम | अवोचे | अवोचावहि | अवोचामहि |

### Common Roots

√आप् to obtain ⇒ आपत् he/she obtained
√पत् to fall⇒ अपप्तत् he/she fell (irregular)
√शास् to rule⇒ अशिषत् he/she ruled (irregular)

## Translate

### F. *Kathopaniṣat* 2.9

नैषा तर्केण मतिरापनेया
प्रोक्तान्येनैव सुज्ञानाय प्रेष्ठ ।
यां त्वमापः सत्यधृतिर्बतासि
त्वादृङ् नो भूयान्नचिकेतः प्रष्टा ॥

Vocabulary
तर्कः m. reasoning, speculation, inquiry
मतिः f. idea
आपनेय mfn. to be obtained, reached
सुज्ञान mfn. easy to be known or understood
प्रेष्ठ mfn. dearest, most beloved
बत ind. particle expressing astonishment

त्वादृश् mfn. like you
भूयात् may there be (3rd p. sg. benedictive)
प्रष्टृ m. one who asks or inquires, questioner

## Reduplicated Aorist

The reduplicated aorist is used mainly for tenth class verbs, causatives, and denominatives, and is relatively rare. It consists of the augment अ + reduplicated root + अ + thematic imperfect endings. Most reduplicated aorists consist of the metrical pattern of alternating light and heavy syllables, which means that the reduplicating syllable will be heavy.

**√मुच् to liberate (caus. मोचय)**

| | Parasmaipada | | | Ātmanepada | | |
|---|---|---|---|---|---|---|
| | Singular | Dual | Plural | Singular | Dual | Plural |
| 3 | अमूमुचत् | अमूमुचताम् | अमूमुचन् | अमूमुचत | अमूमुचेताम् | अमूमुचन्त |
| 2 | अमूमुचः | अमूमुचतम् | अमूमुचत | अमूमुचथाः | अमूमुचेथाम् | अमूमुचध्वम् |
| 1 | अमूमुचम् | अमूमुचाव | अमूमुचाम | अमूमुचे | अमूमुचावहि | अमूमुचामहि |

### Common Roots

√कृ to do (caus. करय) ⇒ अचीकरत् he/she caused to do
√जन् to be born (caus. जनय) ⇒ अजीजनत् he/she gave birth to
√दृश् to see (caus. दर्शय) ⇒ अदीदृशत् he/she showed
√पत् to fall (caus. पातय) ⇒ अपीपतत् he/she caused to fall

## Translate

### G. *Bṛhadāraṇyakopaniṣat* 4.5.14

Maitreyī once asked her husband, Yājñavalkya, to tell her everything he knows. He then gave a long discourse on *ātman*. This is Maitreyī's reply and Yājñavalkya's response to it.

सा होवाच मैत्रेयी । अत्रैव मा भगवान्मोहान्तमापीपतत् । न वा अहमिमं विजानामीति ।
स होवाच न वा अरेऽहं मोहं ब्रवीमि । अविनाशी वा अरेऽयमात्मानुच्छित्तिधर्मा ॥

Vocabulary
मोहान्तः m. deep bewilderment of mind
अरे ind. interjection of calling

अविनाशिन् mfn. imperishable
अनुच्छित्तिः f. indestructibility
धर्मः m. nature

### Passive Aorist

The aorist can be made passive by using *ātmanepada* endings. However, there is also a special passive aorist that occurs only in the third-person singular. It is formed by adding the ending -इ to the strengthened root.

#### Examples

√कृ to do ⇒ अकारि it was done
√दा to give ⇒ अदायि it was given
√बुध् to know ⇒ अबोधि it was known
√विद् to know ⇒ अवेदि it was known

### Translate

#### H. *Bṛhadāraṇyakopaniṣat* 4.4.14

तद् refers to आत्मन्. Translate each *pāda* separately; note that each *pāda* has eleven syllables.

इहैव सन्तोऽथ विद्मस्तद्वयं न चेदवेदि महती विनष्टिः ।
ये तद्विदुरमृतास्ते भवन्त्यथेतरे दुःखमेवापियन्ति ॥

Vocabulary
विनष्टिः f. loss, ruin, destruction
अपि√इ 2P, to go to, enter into

### Injunctive Aorist

Augmentless forms of the aorist can be used as injunctives in conjunction with मा, the particle of negation.

#### Examples

मा गमः You must not go.
मा भूत् Let it not be.
मा शुचः Do not grieve.

## Translate

### I. *Bhagavadgītā* 2.3

क्लैब्यं मा स्म गमः पार्थ नैतत्त्वय्युपपद्यते ।
क्षुद्रं हृदयदौर्बल्यं त्यक्त्वोत्तिष्ठ परंतप ॥

Vocabulary
क्लैब्यम् n. cowardice
स्म ind. indeed
उप√पद् 1Ā, to be suitable, possible, fit
क्षुद्र mfn. minute, small, low, base
दौर्बल्यम् n. weakness, impotence

### J. *Bhagavadgītā* 11.49

The रूपम् being referred to in the fourth *pāda* is Kṛṣṇa's [familiar] "form."

मा ते व्यथा मा च विमूढभावो दृष्ट्वा रूपं घोरमीदृङ्ममेदम् ।
व्यपेतभीः प्रीतमनाः पुनस्त्वं तदेव मे रूपमिदं प्रपश्य ॥

Vocabulary
√व्यथ् 1Ā, to tremble, waver
विमूढ mfn. deluded, confused, foolish
घोर mfn. terrific, frightful, terrible
व्यपेत mfn. gone away, disappeared, freed from
भीः f. fear, apprehension
प्रीत mfn. pleased, delighted
पुनः ind. again
प्र√दृश् 1P, to see, behold

### K. *Bhagavadgītā* 18.66

सर्वधर्मान्परित्यज्य मामेकं शरणं व्रज ।
अहं त्वा सर्वपापेभ्यो मोक्षयिष्यामि मा शुचः ॥

Vocabulary
परि√त्यज् 1P, to leave, abandon, give up
√व्रज् 1P, to take

## Review Exercises

### L. *Kathopaniṣat* 6.18

This is the final verse of the *Kathopaniṣat*.

मृत्युप्रोक्तां नचिकेतोऽथ लब्ध्वा
विद्यामेतां योगविधिं च कृत्स्नम् ।
ब्रह्मप्राप्तो विरजोऽभूद्विमृत्युर्
अन्योऽप्येवं यो विदध्यात्ममेव ॥

Vocabulary
कृत्स्न mfn. all, whole, entire
विमृत्यु mfn. free from death, immortal

### M. *Chāndogyopaniṣat* 6.13.1–3

This is a continuation of the dialogue between Uddalāka Āruṇi and his son, Śvetaketu.

लवणमेतदुदकेऽवधायाथ मा प्रातरुपसीदथा इति । स ह तथा चकार । तँ होवाच ।
यद्दोषा लवणमुदकेऽवाधा अङ्ग तदाहरेति । तद्धावमृश्य न विवेद ॥ १ ॥
यथा विलीनमेव । अङ्गास्यान्तादाचामेति । कथमिति । लवणमिति । मध्यादाचामेति ।
कथमिति । लवणमिति । अन्तादाचामेति । कथमिति । लवणमिति । अभिप्रास्यैतदथ मोपसीदथा इति ।
तद्ध तथा चकार । तच्छश्वत्संवर्तते । तँ होवाचात्र वाव किल तत्सोम्य न निभालयसेऽत्रैव किलेति ॥ २ ॥
स य एषोऽणिमैतदात्म्यमिदँ सर्वम् । तत्सत्यम् । स आत्मा । तत्त्वमसि । श्वेतकेतो इति ।
भूय एव मा भगवान्विज्ञापयत्विति । तथा सोम्येति होवाच ॥ ३ ॥

Vocabulary
अव√धा 3P, to place down, plunge into, deposit
प्रातर् ind. in the early morning, at daybreak, at dawn, tomorrow
उपसीदथाः approach (2nd p. sg. unaugmented injunctive imperfect उप√सद्)
दोषा f. darkness, night
अङ्ग ind. a particle implying attention, assent, or desire, and sometimes impatience, "Now, come on . . ."
अव√मृश् 6P, to touch, reach for
√विद् 6P, to find

विलीन mfn. immersed, dissolved
अभिप्र√अस् 4P, to throw
शश्वत् ind. perpetually, continually, always
नि√भल् 10U, to see, perceive

N. *Taittirīyopaniṣat* 1.11

This is a set of instructions given by the teacher to the student upon having completed Vedic study.

वेदमनूच्याचार्योऽन्तेवासिनमनुशास्ति। सत्यं वद। धर्मं चर। स्वाध्यायान्मा प्रमदः। आचार्याय प्रियं धनमाहृत्य प्रजातन्तुं मा व्यवच्छेत्सीः। सत्यान्न प्रमदितव्यम्। धर्मान्न प्रमदितव्यम्। कुशलान्न प्रमदितव्यम्। भूत्यै न प्रमदितव्यम्। स्वाध्यायप्रवचनाभ्यां न प्रमदितव्यम्॥ १॥ देवपितृकार्याभ्यां न प्रमदितव्यम्। मातृदेवो भव। पितृदेवो भव। आचार्यदेवो भव। अतिथिदेवो भव। यान्यनवद्यानि कर्माणि। तानि सेवितव्यानि। नो इतरानि। यान्यस्माकँ सुचरितानि। तानि त्वयोपास्यानि॥ २॥ नो इतराणि। ये के चास्मच्छ्रेयाँसो ब्राह्मणाः। तेषां त्वयासनेन प्रश्वसितव्यम्। श्रद्धया देयम्। अश्रद्धयादेयम्। श्रिया देयम्। ह्रिया देयम्। भिया देयम्। संविदा देयम्। अथ यदि ते कर्मविचिकित्सा वा वृत्तविचिकित्सा वा स्यात्॥ ३॥ ये तत्र ब्राह्मणाः संमर्शिनः। युक्ता आयुक्ताः। अलूक्षा धर्मकामाः स्युः। यथा ये तत्र वर्तेरन्। तथा तत्र वर्तेरन्। अथाभ्याख्यातेषु। ये तत्र ब्राह्मणाः संमर्शिणः। युक्ता आयुक्ताः। अलूक्षा धर्मकामाः स्युः। यथा ते तेषु वर्तेरन्। तथा तेषु वर्तेथाः। एष आदेशः। एष उपदेशः। एषा वेदोपनिषत्। एतदनुशासनम्। एवमुपासितव्यम्। एवमु चैतदुपास्यम् ॥ ४॥

Vocabulary
अनु√वच् 2P, to cause to repeat/recite, teach
अन्तेवासिन् m. a pupil who dwells near or in the house of his teacher
अनु√शास् 2P, to teach, advise
प्र√मद् 4P, to neglect
प्रजातन्तु m. a line of descendants
व्यव√च्छिद् 7P, to cut off, separate
कुशलम् n. welfare, well-being
भूतिः f. wealth, fortune, prosperity
प्रवचनम् n. teaching
अनवद्य mfn. irreproachable, faultless
सेवितव्य mfn. to be followed or practiced

सुचरितम् n. virtuous actions
उपास्य mfn. to be revered, honored, esteemed
प्रश्वसितव्य mfn. to be comforted
श्री f. dignity
ह्री f. modesty
संविद् f. understanding
विचिकित्सा f. doubt, uncertainty
संमर्शिन् mfn. able to judge
युक्त mfn. experienced
आयुक्त mfn. accredited
अलूक्ष mfn. not hard, soft, gentle
अभ्याख्यात mfn. accused falsely
आदेशः m. rule, symbolic rule, instruction
उपदेशः m. teaching
उपनिषद् f. sitting down at the feet of another to listen to their words, secret knowledge, hidden meaning
उपासितव्य mfn. to be revered, honored, respected

# 21
# Conditional and Benedictive Mode; Composite Verbs and च्वि Formation; Directional Words with the Suffix -अञ्च्

क्षणप्रतियोगी परिणामापरान्तनिर्ग्राह्यः क्रमः ॥ ४· ३३ ॥
**kṣaṇa-pratiyogī pariṇāmāparānta-nirgrāhyaḥ kramaḥ**
As the progression of time is dependent upon a series of moments, it is perceivable only at the final moment of transformation.
॥ *Yogasūtra* 4.33 ॥

## CONDITIONAL MOOD

The conditional mood is used (on rare occasions) to express a hypothetical and counterfactual situation, meaning "had X happened, Y would have happened." It is formed by adding the augment अ to the future stem + past imperfect endings.

| | √गम् to go | | | √भाष् to speak | | |
|---|---|---|---|---|---|---|
| | Parasmaipada | | | Ātmanepada | | |
| | Singular | Dual | Plural | Singular | Dual | Plural |
| 3 | अगमिष्यत् | अगमिष्यताम् | अगमिष्यन् | अभाषिष्यत | अभाषिष्येताम् | अभाषिष्यन्त |
| 2 | अगमिष्यः | अगमिष्यतम् | अगमिष्यत | अभाषिष्यथाः | अभाषिष्येथाम् | अभाषिष्यध्वम् |
| 1 | अगमिष्यम् | अगमिष्याव | अगमिष्याम | अभाषिष्ये | अभाषिष्यावहि | अभाषिष्यामहि |

### Example: *Tantrāloka*, 3.100cd–101ab

अस्थास्यदेकरूपेण वपुषा चेन्महेश्वरः ।
महेश्वरत्वं संवित्त्वमत्यक्ष्यद् घटादिवत् ॥

Vocabulary
संवित्त्वम् n. consciousness

> Written by Abhinavagupta in the eleventh century C.E., the *Tantrāloka* is considered the masterwork of Kashmiri Shaivism.

If (चेत्) Śiva (महेश्वरः) **had remained** (अस्थास्यद्) in only one (एकरूपेण) form (वपुषा),
**He would have abandoned** (अत्यक्ष्यद्) his divinity (महेश्वरत्वम्),
Which is consciousness (संवित्त्वम्),
Like a pot and other objects (घटादिवत्).

## Translate

### A. *Chāndogyopaniṣat* 6.1.3–7

Śvetaketu's father, Āruṇi, told him to become a *brahmacarin*, or a celibate student, for everyone in their family was a Brahmin because of study, not just from birth. So Śvetaketu went away and became a student from the ages of twelve to twenty-four years. After learning all of the Vedas, he returned, arrogant and thinking himself knowledgeable.

तँ ह पितोवाच। श्वेतकेतो यन्नु सोम्येदं महामना अनूचानमानी स्तब्धोऽसि।
उत तमादेशमप्राक्ष्यो येनाश्रुतँ श्रुतं भवत्यमतं मतमविज्ञातं विज्ञातमिति।
कथं नु भगवः स आदेशो भवतीति॥ ३॥
यथा सोम्यैकेन मृत्पिण्डेन सर्वं मृन्मयं विज्ञातँ स्यात्।
वाचारम्भणं विकारो नामधेयं मृत्तिकेत्येव सत्यम्॥ ४॥
यथा सोम्यैकेन लोहमणिना सर्वं लोहमयं विज्ञातँ स्यात्।
वाचारम्भणं विकारो नामधेयं लोहमित्येव सत्यम्॥ ५॥
यथा सोम्यैकेन नखनिकृन्तनेन सर्वं कार्ष्णायसं विज्ञात स्यात्।
वाचारम्भणं विकारो नामधेयं कृष्णायसमित्येव सत्यम्। एवँ सोम्य स आदेशो भवतीति॥ ६॥
न वै नूनं भगवन्तस्त एतदवेदिषुः। यद्ध्येतदवेदिष्यन्कथं मे नावक्ष्यन्निति भगवाँस्त्वेव मे ब्रवीत्विति।
तथा सोम्येति होवाच॥ ७॥

#### Vocabulary

महामनस् mfn. arrogant, swollen-headed
अनूचान mfn. well versed in the Vedas, knowledgeable
मानिन् mfn. thinking oneself to be
स्तब्ध mfn. puffed up, proud, arrogant
उत ind. could it be that . . . (interrogative particle)
मृद् f. earth, clay
पिण्डः m. roundish mass or heap, lump
वाचारम्भण = वागालम्बन mfn. dependent on just words
नामधेयम् n. a name, title, appellation
मृत्तिका f. earth
लोह mfn. made of copper

मणिः m. jewel, gem, pearl
नख mn. fingernail, toenail
निकृन्तनम् n. an instrument for cutting
कार्ष्णायस mfn. made of black iron
कृष्णायसम् n. black iron
भगवन्तः m. nom. pl. those venerable teachers

## BENEDICTIVE MOOD

The benedictive or precative is a rare optative form of the aorist, used in blessings and prayers. It is formed from the root, often in its weak form + the optative sign या + स्. The third-person singular *parasmaipada* ending loses this स् and is simply -यात्.

**√मुच् 6U, to free, let loose, liberate**

| | Parasmaipada | | | Ātmanepada | | |
|---|---|---|---|---|---|---|
| | Singular | Dual | Plural | Singular | Dual | Plural |
| 3 | मुच्यात् | मुच्यास्ताम् | मुच्यासुः | मुक्षीष्ट | मुक्षीयास्ताम् | मुक्षीरन् |
| 2 | मुच्याः | मुच्यास्तम् | मुच्यास्त | मुक्षीष्ठाः | मुक्षीयास्थाम् | मुक्षीढ्वम् |
| 1 | मुच्यासम् | मुच्यास्व | मुच्यास्म | मुक्षीय | मुक्षीवहि | मुक्षीमहि |

**√भू 1P, to be**

| | Parasmaipada | | |
|---|---|---|---|
| | Singular | Dual | Plural |
| 3 | भूयात् | भूयास्ताम् | भूयासुः |
| 2 | भूयाः | भूयास्तम् | भूयास्त |
| 1 | भूयासम् | भूयास्व | भूयास्म |

### Example: *Kaṭhopaniṣat* 2.9d

त्वादृङ् नो भूयान्नचिकेतः प्रष्टा ।

**May there be** for us a questioner like you, Naciketas.

### Translate

#### B. *Ṛg Veda*, 7.59.2, *Mahāmṛtyuṃjaya Mantra*

The three-eyed one is Śiva. Note that the मा in the fourth *pāda* means "not" or "don't [keep me]."

त्र्यम्बकं यजामहे सुगन्धिं पुष्टिवर्धनम्।
उर्वारुकमिव बन्धनान्मृत्योर्मुक्षीय मामृतात्॥

Vocabulary
अम्बकम् n. an eye
उर्वारुकम् n. cucumber, gourd
बन्धनम् n. the act of binding, bondage, stalk, stem

The *Ṛg Veda* is the oldest Vedic text, composed sometime between 1700 and 1100 B.C.E. It is a collection of hymns describing the origins of the world and contains prayers to various deities and for attaining various aspirations.

### C. *Gāyatrī Mantra*

ॐ भूर्भुवः स्वः। तत्सवितुर्वरेण्यम्।
भर्गो देवस्य धीमहि। धियो यो नः प्रचोदयात्॥

Vocabulary
भुवः m. the air, atmosphere, place between heaven and earth
स्वर् ind. heaven
सवितृ m. the Sun God, the divine influence and vivifying power of the sun
वरेण्य mfn. desirable, excellent
भर्गस् n. radiance, splendor
प्र√चुद् 1P, to set in motion, impel, inspire

The *Gāyatrī Mantra* is a chant to the three worlds, and to everything encompassed within them. It is traditionally taught to young boys at the *upanayana*, or thread ceremony, which is the rite of passage into adulthood and marks the beginning of their Vedic studies.

### D. *Taittirīyopaniṣat* 1.4.1

यश्छन्दसामृषभो विश्वरूपः
छन्दोभ्योऽध्यमृतात्सम्बभूव।
स मेन्द्रो मेधया स्पृणोतु
अमृतस्य देव धारणो भूयासम्।
शरीरं मे विचर्षणम्। जिह्वा मे मधुमत्तमा।
कर्णाभ्यां भूरि विश्रुवम्॥
ब्रह्मणः कोशोऽसि
मेधया पिहितः।
श्रुतं मे गोपाय॥

Vocabulary

विश्वरूप mfn. manifold, with various forms
अधि ind. above, over, besides
मेधा f. intelligence, mental vigor
धारण mfn. keep in remembrance, memory
विचर्षण mfn. very active or busy
मधुमत् mfn. sweet, rich in honey
भूरि ind. much, abundantly
कोशः m. sheath
पिहित mfn. covered
√गुप् 4P, to protect, preserve

## COMPOSITE VERBS AND च्वि FORMATION

A composite verb can be formed by adding the verb √भू or √कृ, in any form, to a nominal element or adverb. It indicates that something either becomes or is made into something it is not, either literally or figuratively.

नमस् √कृ to do homage
अलं √कृ to adorn

These verbs can also be the basis for nouns:

नमस्कारः m. salutation
अलंकारः m. ornament

Composite verbs with √भू are intransitive and with √कृ are transitive.

### Translate

**E. *Bhagavadgītā* 18.65**

मन्मना भव मद्भक्तो मद्याजी मां नमस्कुरु ।
मामेवैष्यसि सत्यं ते प्रतिजाने प्रियोऽसि मे ॥

Vocabulary

याजिन् mfn. worshipping, sacrificing
प्रति√ज्ञा 9P, to acknowledge, promise

### F. *Yogavāsiṣṭha* 2.14.22

The subject in the first two *pādas* is ज्योतिस्, "the light."

विवेकितोदिता देहे सर्वं शीतलयत्यलम्।
अलंकरोति चात्यन्तं ज्योत्स्नेव भुवनं यथा॥

Vocabulary
विवेकित mfn. that which has been discerned
उदित mfn. born, produced
√शीतलय denom. to cool
अलम् ind. able
अत्यन्तम् ind. absolutely, completely
ज्योत्स्ना f. moonlight

### G. *Vivekamārtaṇḍa* 108

बद्धपद्मासनो योगी नमस्कृत्य गुरुं शिवम्।
नासाग्रदृष्टिरेकाकी प्राणायामं समभ्यसेत्॥

Vocabulary
एकाकिन् mfn. alone, solitary

The च्वि formation changes the final vowel of a noun or adjective to ई before joining it with √भू or √कृ:

स्थिर steady
स्थिरी √कृ to make steady
स्थिरी √भू to become steady

As an example of how verses are passed from text to text, with slight variation, consider the following two verses:

### H. *Haṭhapradīpikā* 2.14

अभ्यासकाले प्रथमे शस्तं क्षीराज्यभोजनम्।
ततोऽभ्यासे दृढीभूते न तादृङ्नियमग्रहः॥

Vocabulary
शस्त mfn. praised, recommended
क्षीरम् n. milk
आज्यम् n. clarified butter, ghee
तादृक् ind. in such a manner

I. *Śivasaṃhitā* 3.43

अभ्यासकाले प्रथमं कुर्यात्क्षीराज्यभोजनम्।
ततोऽभ्यासे स्थिरीभूते न तादृङ्नियमग्रहः॥

## DIRECTIONAL WORDS WITH THE SUFFIX -अञ्च्

प्राञ्च् eastern, ahead, in front
प्रत्यञ्च् western, behind
उदञ्च् northern, above
अदारञ्च् southern, below
विश्वञ्च् facing in all directions, pervading
तिर्यञ्च् horizontal, diagonal
संयञ्च् turned together or in one direction, proper, in one line, straight
पराञ्च् turned away

The strong stem is -अञ्च्, the middle stem is -अच्, and the weak stem is either ईच् or ऊच्, depending on whether a य् or व् precedes -अञ्च् in the stem.

**प्रत्यञ्च् m. western, behind**

| | Singular | Dual | Plural |
|---|---|---|---|
| **Nominative** | प्रत्यङ् | प्रत्यञ्चौ | प्रत्यञ्चः |
| **Accusative** | प्रत्यञ्चम् | प्रत्यञ्चौ | प्रतीचः |
| **Instrumental** | प्रतीचा | प्रत्यग्भ्याम् | प्रत्यग्भिः |
| **Dative** | प्रतीचे | प्रत्यग्भ्याम् | प्रत्यग्भ्यः |
| **Ablative** | प्रतीचः | प्रत्यग्भ्याम् | प्रत्यग्भ्यः |
| **Genitive** | प्रतीचः | प्रतीचोः | प्रतीचाम् |
| **Locative** | प्रतीचि | प्रतीचोः | प्रत्यक्षु |
| **Vocative** | प्रत्यङ् | प्रत्यञ्चौ | प्रत्यञ्चः |

**प्रत्यञ्च् n. western, behind**

| | Singular | Dual | Plural |
|---|---|---|---|
| **Nom./Acc./Voc.** | प्रत्यक् | प्रतीची | प्रत्यञ्चि |

प्रतीची f. western, behind (same as नदी)

## Translate

### J. *Gheraṇḍasaṃhitā* 5.33

कुशासने मृगाजिने व्याघ्राजिने च कम्बले ।
स्थूलासने समासीनः प्राङ्मुखो वाप्युदङ्मुखः ।
नाडीशुद्धिं समासाद्य प्राणायामं समभ्यसेत् ॥

Vocabulary
अजिनम् n. skin (of an animal)
कम्बल mn. a woolen blanket
स्थूल mfn. large, thick
समासीन mfn. sitting

### K. *Chāndogyopaniṣat* 6.10.1–3

इमाः सोम्य नद्यः पुरस्तात्प्राच्यः स्यन्दन्ते पश्चात्प्रतीच्यः । ताः समुद्रात्समुद्रमेवापियन्ति । स समुद्र एव भवति । ता यथा तत्र न विदुरियमहमस्मीयमहमस्मीति ॥ १ ॥ एवमेव खलु सोम्येमाः सर्वाः प्रजाः सत आगम्य न विदुः सत आगच्छामह इति । त इह व्याघ्रो वा सिंहा वा वृको वा वराहो वा कीटो वा पतङ्गो वा दँशो वा मशको वा यद्यद्भवन्ति तदाभवन्ति ॥ २ ॥
स य एषोऽणिमैतदात्म्यमिदँ सर्वम् । तत्सत्यम् । स आत्मा । तत्त्वमसि । श्वेतकेतो इति ।
भूय एव मा भगवान्विज्ञापयत्विति । तथा सोम्येति होवाच ॥ ३ ॥

Vocabulary
पुरस्तात् ind. eastward
√स्यन्द् 1Ā, to flow
पश्चात् ind. westward
अपि√इ 2P, to enter into, join, merge

### L. *Chāndogyopaniṣat* 6.14.1–3

यथा सोम्य पुरुषं गन्धारेभ्योऽभिनद्धाक्षमानीय तं ततोऽतिजने विसृजेत् । स यथा तत्र प्राङ् वोदङ् वाधराङ् वा प्रध्मायीताभिनद्धाक्ष आनीतोऽभिनद्धाक्षो विसृष्टः ॥ १ ॥ तस्य यथाभिनहनं प्रमुच्य प्रब्रूयादेतां दिशं गन्धारा

एतां दिशं व्रजेति। स ग्रामाद् ग्रामं पृच्छन्पण्डितो मेधावी गन्धारानेवोपसंपद्येत। एवमेवेहाचार्यवान्पुरुषो वेद। तस्य तावदेव चिरं यावन्न विमोक्ष्येऽथ संपत्स्य इति ॥ २ ॥

स य एषोऽणिमैतदात्म्यमिदँ सर्वम्। तत्सत्यम्। स आत्मा। तत्त्वमसि। श्वेतकेतो इति।

भूय एव मा भगवान्विज्ञापयत्विति। तथा सोम्येति होवाच ॥ ३ ॥

Vocabulary

गन्धारः m. ancient kingdom
अभिनद्धाक्ष mfn. blindfold
अभिनद्ध mfn. tied round
आ√नी 1P, to lead toward or near, bring
अतिजन mfn. "beyond men," uninhabited
वि√सृज् 6P, to release
प्र√ध्मा 1P, to be tossed about, wander about
विसृष्ट mfn. left, let go
अभिनहनम् n. a bandage over the eyes, blindfold
प्र√मुच् 6P, to set free, liberate
प्र√ब्रू 2P, to say, tell, relate
ग्रामः m. village
√प्रछ् 6P, to ask
पण्डित mfn. learned, wise
मेधाविन् m. learned, wise man
उपसम्√पद् 1Ā, to come to, arrive at
चिरम् ind. for a long time, after a long time
सम्√पद् 1Ā, to come together, attain, arrive, become complete

## Review Exercises

### M. *Abhijñānaśākuntala*, by Kālidāsa, Verse 5.2

रम्याणि वीक्ष्य मधुरांश्च निशम्य शब्दान्
पर्युत्सुकीभवति यत्सुखितोऽपि जन्तुः ।
तच्चेतसा स्मरति नूनमबोधपूर्वं
भावस्थिराणि जननान्तरसौहृदानि ॥

Vocabulary

रम्य mfn. enjoyable, pleasing, delightful, beautiful
वि√ईक्ष् 1Ā, to look at, see, behold
नि√शम् 4P, to hear
पर्युत्सुकी√भू 1P, to become restless
सुखितः mfn. happy, contented
√स्मृ 1P, to remember
नूनम् ind. now, at present
अबोधपूर्वम् without his knowing
जननम् n. birth
सौहृदम् n. friendship, affection, love

*Abijñānaśākuntala*, or "Śakuntalā and the Token of Remembrance," is the story of love found, forgotten, and rediscovered. Kālidāsa's play is a dramatization of the story of Śakuntalā, told in the *Mahābhārata*. King Duṣyanta, while out hunting, meets and falls in love with Śakuntalā, the adopted daughter of a sage. He is summoned back to court, but he leaves her with a wedding ring and she promises to join him. Śakuntalā, then pregnant, goes to meet him, but because of the curse of the sage Durvāsas, she loses the ring and the king does not recognize her and sends her away. Eventually, the ring is restored, along with Duṣyanta's memory, and they are once again united in love.

### N. *Bṛhadāraṇyakopaniṣat* 4.2.4

Yājñavalkya is teaching Janaka, king of Videha. The first तस्य refers to पुरुषस्य.

तस्य प्राची दिक्प्राञ्चः प्राणा दक्षिणा दिग्दक्षिणे प्राणाः प्रतीची दिक्प्रत्यञ्चः प्राणा उदीची दिगुदञ्चः प्राणा ऊर्ध्वा दिगूर्ध्वाः प्राणा अवाची दिगवाञ्चः प्राणाः सर्वा दिशः सर्वे प्राणाः ।
स एष नेति नेत्यात्मा । अगृह्यो न हि गृह्यते । अशीर्यो न हि शीर्यते । असङ्गो न हि सज्यते ।
असितो न व्यथते । न रिष्यति । अभयं वै जनक प्राप्तोऽसीति होवाच याज्ञवल्क्यः ।

Kālidāsa, who lived sometime around the fourth to fifth century C.E., is considered to be the greatest Sanskrit poet and dramatist. As legend has it, he was once a simple-minded cowherd, married to a princess for his good looks. She constantly humiliated him for his lack of knowledge, leading him to pray every day to the goddess Kālī, who one day granted him immeasurable knowledge. Thus, his name means servant (*dāsa*) of Kālī.

स होवाच जनको वैदेहोऽभयं त्वा गच्छताद्याज्ञवल्क्य यो नो भगवन्नभयं वेदयसे ।
नमस्तेऽस्तु । इमे विदेहा अयमहमस्मि ॥ ४ ॥

Vocabulary
दक्षिण mfn. right, southern
अशीर्य mfn. indestructible
√शॄ 9P, to break; pass. to be worn out, decay
असित mfn. unbound
√रिष् 1,4P, to be hurt or injured
अभय mfn. fearless

## O. Patañjali Invocation

यस्त्यक्त्वा रूपमाद्यं प्रभवति जगतोऽनेकधानुग्रहाय ।
प्रक्षीणक्लेशराशिर्विषमविषधरोऽनेकवक्त्रः सुभोगी ।
सर्वज्ञानप्रसूतिर्भुजगपरिकरः प्रीतये यस्य नित्यम् ।
देवोऽहीशः स वोऽव्यात्सितविमलतनुर्योगदो योगयुक्तः ॥

Vocabulary
अनेकधा ind. in various ways
अनुग्रहः m. favor, kindness
प्रक्षीण mfn. destroyed, diminished
राशिः m. a heap, mass
विषम mfn. dangerous
विषधरः m. containing poison, venomous, a snake
अनेक mfn. not one, many
वक्त्रम् n. mouth, face, head
सुभोगिन् mfn. beautifully ringed
प्रसूतिः f. bringing forth
परिकरः m. attendants, retinue
प्रीतिः f. pleasure, joy
अहिः m. snake
सित mfn. white, pure
विमल mfn. spotless

# Part III Review: *Chāndogyopaniṣat* 4.4–9

This is the story of Satyakāma Jābāla, his mother, Jabālā, his teacher, Hāridrumata Gautama, and his unusual path to knowledge.

सत्यकामो ह जाबालो जबालां मातरमामन्त्रयांचक्रे। ब्रह्मचर्यं भवति विवत्स्यामि किंगोत्रो न्वहमस्मीति ॥ १ ॥
सा हैनमुवाच। नाहमेतद्वेद तात यद्गोत्रस्त्वमसि। बह्वहं चरन्ती परिचारिणी यौवने त्वामलभे। साहमेतन्न वेद यद्गोत्रस्त्वमसि। जबाला तु नामाहमस्मि। सत्यकामो नाम त्वमसि । स सत्यकाम एव जाबालो ब्रुवीथा इति ॥ २ ॥

स ह हारिद्रुमतं गौतममेत्योवाच। ब्रह्मचर्यं भगवति वत्स्यामि। उपेयां भगवन्तमिति ॥ ३ ॥ तँ होवाच किंगोत्रो नु सोम्यासीति। स होवाच। नाहमेतद्वेद भो यद्गोत्रोऽहमस्मि। अपृच्छं मातरम्। सा मा प्रत्यब्रवीत् बह्वहं चरन्ती परिचारिणी यौवने त्वामलभे। साहमेतन्न वेद यद्गोत्रस्त्वमसि। जबाला तु नामाहमस्मि। सत्यकामो नाम त्वमसीति। सोऽहँ सत्यकामो जाबालोऽस्मि भो इति ॥ ४ ॥

तँ होवाच। नैतदब्राह्मणो विवक्तुमर्हति। समिधँ सोम्याहर। उप त्वा नेष्ये न सत्यादगा इति। तमुपनीय कृशानामबलानां चतुःशता गा निराकृत्योवाचेमाः सोम्यानुसंव्रजेति। ता अभिप्रस्थापयन्नुवाच। नासहस्रेणावर्तयेति। स ह वर्षगणं प्रोवास। ता यदा सहस्रँ संपेदुः ॥ ५ ॥

अथ हैनमृषभोऽभ्युवाद सत्यकाम३ इति। भगव इति ह प्रतिशुश्राव। प्राप्ताः सोम्य सहस्रँ स्मः। प्रापय न आचार्यकुलम् ॥ १ ॥

ब्रह्मणश्च ते पादं ब्रवाणीति। ब्रवीतु मे भगवानिति। तस्मै होवाच। प्राची दिक्कला। प्रातीची दिक्कला। दक्षिणा दिक्कला। उदीची दिक्कला। एष वै सोम्य चतुष्कलः पादो ब्रह्मणः प्रकाशवान्नाम ॥ २ ॥

स य एतमेवं विद्वाँश्चतुष्कलं पादं ब्रह्मणः प्रकाशवानित्युपास्ते प्रकाशवानस्मिँल्लोके भवति। प्रकाशवतो ह लोकाञ्जयति य एतमेवं विद्वाँश्चतुष्कलं पादं ब्रह्मणः प्रकाशवानित्युपास्ते ॥ ३ ॥

अग्निष्टे पादं वक्तेति। स ह श्वो भूते गा अभिप्रस्थापयांचकार। ता यत्राभिसायं बभूवुस्तत्राग्निमुपसमाधाय गा उपरुध्य समिधमाधाय पश्चादग्नेः प्राङुपोपविवेश ॥ १ ॥

तमग्निरभ्युवाद सत्यकाम३ इति। भगव इति ह प्रतिशुश्राव ॥ २ ॥ ब्रह्मणः सोम्य ते पादं ब्रवाणीति। ब्रवीतु मे भगवानिति। तस्मै होवाच। पृथिवी कला। अन्तरिक्षं कला। द्यौः कला। समुद्रः कला। एष वै सोम्य चतुष्कलः पादो ब्रह्मणोऽनन्तवान्नाम ॥ ३ ॥ स य एतमेवं विद्वाँश्चतुष्कलं पादं ब्रह्मणोऽनन्तवानित्युपास्तेऽनन्तवानस्मिँल्लोके भवति। अनन्तवतो ह लोकाञ्जयति य एतमेवं विद्वाँश्चतुष्कलं पादं ब्रह्मणोऽनन्तवानित्युपास्ते ॥ ४ ॥

हँसस्ते पादं वक्तेति। स ह श्वो भूते गा अभिप्रस्थापयांचकार। ता यत्राभिसायं बभूवुस्तत्राग्निमुपसमाधाय गा उपरुध्य समिधमाधाय पश्चादग्नेः प्राङुपोपविवेश ॥ १॥ तँ हँस उपनिपत्याभ्युवाद सत्यकाम३ इति। भगव इति ह प्रतिशुश्राव ॥ २॥ ब्रह्मणः सोम्य ते पादं ब्रवाणीति। ब्रवीतु मे भगवानिति। तस्मै होवाच। अग्निः कला। सूर्यः कला। चन्द्रः कला। विद्युत्कला। एष वै सोम्य चतुष्कलः पादो ब्रह्मणो ज्योतिष्मान्नाम ॥ ३॥ स य एतमेवं विद्वाँश्चतुष्कलं पादं ब्रह्मणो ज्योतिष्मानित्युपास्ते ज्योतिष्मानस्मिँल्लोके भवति। ज्योतिष्मतो ह लोकाञ्जयति य एतमेवं विद्वाँश्चतुष्कलं पादं ब्रह्मणो ज्योतिष्मानित्युपास्ते ॥ ४॥

मद्गुष्टे पादं वक्तेति। स ह श्वो भूते गा अभिप्रस्थापयांचकार। ता यत्राभिसायं बभूवुस्तत्राग्निमुपसमाधाय गा उपरुध्य समिधमाधाय पश्चादग्नेः प्राङुपोपविवेश ॥ १॥

तं मद्गुरुपनिपत्याभ्युवाद सत्यकाम३ इति। भगव इति ह प्रतिशुश्राव ॥ २॥ ब्रह्मणः सोम्य ते पादं ब्रवाणीति। ब्रवीतु मे भगवानिति। तस्मै होवाच। प्राणः कला। चक्षुः कला। श्रोत्रं कला। मनः कला। एष वै सोम्य चतुष्कलः पादो ब्रह्मण आयतनवान्नाम ॥ ३॥

स य एतमेवं विद्वाँश्चतुष्कलं पादं ब्रह्मण आयतनवानित्युपास्त आयतनवानस्मिँल्लोके भवति। आयतनवतो ह लोकाञ्जयति य एतमेवं विद्वाँश्चतुष्कलं पादं ब्रह्मण आयतनवानित्युपास्ते ॥ ४॥

प्राप हाचार्यकुलम्। तमाचार्योऽभ्युवाद सत्यकाम३ इति। भगव इति ह प्रतिशुश्राव ॥ १॥ ब्रह्मविदिव वै सोम्य भासि। को नु त्वानुशशासेति। अन्ये मनुष्येभ्य इति ह प्रतिजज्ञे। भगवाँस्त्वेव मे कामे ब्रूयात् ॥ २॥ श्रुतँ ह्येव मे भगवद्दृशेभ्य आचार्याद्धैव विद्या विदिता साधिष्ठं प्रापतीति। तस्मै हैतदेवोवाच। अत्र ह न किंचन वीयायेति वीयायेति ॥ ३॥

Vocabulary (in Sanskrit Alphabetical Order)

अनन्तवत् mfn. eternal, infinite
अनुसं√व्रज् 1P, to look after, attend to
अभिप्र√स्था 1P, to start or advance toward; caus. to drive (as the cattle to pasture)
अभिसायम् ind. about evening, at sunset
आ√मन्त्र् 10Ā, to speak, say
आयतनवत् mfn. having a seat or home or support
उप√निपत् 1P, to fly down
उप√नी 1P, to initiate
उप√रुध् 7P, to lock in, shut up
उपसमा√धा 3P, to kindle (a fire)
√उपे = उप√इ 2P, to approach a teacher, become a student
कला f. one-sixteenth
कृश mfn. lean, emaciated, feeble
गोत्रम् n. lineage, family name
परिचारिणी f. a maid moving about, attending on, serving
प्रकाशवत् mfn. bright, brilliant, shining, renowned, celebrated

मद्गुः m. a diver bird
यौवनम् n. youth
वर्षगणः m. a long series of years
वि√वस् 1P, to live, spend time, enter into an apprenticeship
श्वस् ind. tomorrow, on the following day
समिधः m. fuel, wood

# Notes on the Translations

My intention in translating is always to bring the reader closer to the original text. In my translations, I have attempted to be, simultaneously, faithful to meaning and to the poetry and rhythm of the texts. I have kept words and phrases as close to their original order as possible. One of the biggest decisions a translator has to make is which words (if any) are untranslatable. Are some words better understood if they are left in Sanskrit? I have chosen not to translate words that are technical terms specific to the yoga tradition, words that my own teachers would not translate, such as the limbs of yoga. These words, whose definitions you will find in the glossary, are:

> *yoga, yogī, guru, yama, niyama, āsana, prāṇāyāma, pratyāhāra, dhāraṇā, dhyāna, samādhi, saṃyama, Brahman, mudrā, bandha, kriyā, prāṇa, nāḍī, prakṛti, guṇa, sattva, rajas, tamas.*

I have chosen to translate words such as *dharma* and *karma* because they have such a wide spectrum of definitions and associations that it seems too ambiguous to leave them untranslated. I have tried to use the same translation for keywords throughout my translations. A few in particular I would like to note:

*Ātman*: Soul
*buddhi*: understanding
*dharma*: justice, duty
*karma*: action
*siddhi*: fulfillment

These words are particularly problematic because of the connotations and associations we have with the possible English definitions. For example, *siddhi* is often translated as "success," "accomplishment," "attainment," or "perfection," but these words can imply that one has achieved an external goal, rather than reaching an internal state, so I have chosen to translate it as "fulfillment," although this has its own potential problems. Note that *siddhi* is also the word used for the superpowers that one can attain through practice. Similarly, I have chosen to translate *buddhi* as "understanding," because of the scholarly associations we have with "intelligence" and "intellect."

A recent convention is to use brackets for any words that are not "literally" part of the text, a method I have chosen not to adopt in most of my own translations. Because Sanskrit words have so many different meanings, I do not think it is possible, or even desirable, to have a definitive literal translation. The reason so many translations exist is precisely that there are things left unsaid and that there is a wide realm of possibility for each verse. Additionally, I think that brackets tend to separate readers from the text and to compartmentalize the way in which they interact with it. Both what is within the brackets and what is without are treated with a heightened awareness, which does not allow the reader the experience of immersion in the text. It is important to remember that this was once, and in many places still is, an oral tradition, which means that poetry, sound, and rhythm are of primary importance. However, for the sake of clarity, I have used brackets in the examples, in verse introductions, and in vocabulary lists when a word or words need to be inferred.

Although most verses use masculine pronouns when not speaking of a specific person, whenever possible I have translated these into the gender-neutral "one" or "that person" in order for the verses to feel more relevant to modern yogīs, the majority of whom are female.

All of these are choices I have made after much deliberation; however, there are no absolute answers. As you approach these texts yourself, it is important that you sit with these questions and issues, for that process of contemplation will bring you closer to the texts. I have tried to provide a wide selection of texts in order to give a sense of the rich fabric of the yoga tradition, while giving enough verses from key texts to provide an experience of the philosophy and traditions contained within them. Obviously, within the framework of this textbook, it is a limited and subjective selection; however, I hope it will provide an entry point and pique readers' curiosity for further inquiry.

# Answer Key: Translations

## Chapter 1

A.

1. *āsana* = posture, seat
2. *yama* = restraint, first limb of *aṣṭāṅgayoga*
3. *atha* = now (i.e., at this auspicious moment), the first word of the *Yogasūtra*
4. *haṭha* = force (as in *haṭhayoga*, "the yoga of force")
5. *hala* = plow
6. *japa* = muttering, mantra recitation
7. *baka* = crow
8. *pada* = foot
9. *jaya* = victory
10. *jana* = person
11. *kapha* = one of the three *doṣas*, or psychophysical components of the body, according to *Āyurveda*, comprised of water + earth
12. *rasa* = taste, flavor, essence

B.

1. *sat* = existence, being
2. *asat* = nonexistence, nonbeing
3. *tapas* = discipline, heat, austerity, one of the *niyamas* or disciplines (second limb of *aṣṭāṅgayoga*)
4. *tamas* = inertia, one of the three *guṇas*, or qualities of mind
5. *rajas* = activity, one of the three *guṇas*, or qualities of mind
6. *namas* = bow, salutation
7. *manas* = mind
8. *ekam* = one

C.

1. *sādhana* = practice
2. *pāda* = foot, chapter
3. *sādhanapāda* = chapter on practice, the second chapter of the *Yogasūtra*
4. *dhāraṇā* = concentration, the sixth limb of *aṣṭāṅgayoga*

5. *vāta* = one of the three *doṣas* of *Āyurveda*, comprised of space + air
6. *apāna* = the downward breath
7. *ākāśa* = ether
8. *mālā* = garland
9. *hālāhala* = the poison of cyclic existence
10. *halāsana* = plow pose
11. *pāśāsana* = noose pose
12. *śalabhāsana* = locust pose
13. *bakāsana* = crow pose
14. *rāga* = attraction
15. *rāja* = king
16. *Rāma* = Rāma, an incarnation of the god Viṣṇu, hero of the *Rāmāyaṇa*
17. *Rāmāyaṇa* = one of the great epics, by Vālmīki, the story of Rāma
18. *Mahābhārata* = one of the great epics, by Vyāsa, the great story of the Bhāratas
19. *rādhā* = Rādhā, name of a *gopī* or cowherdess, loved by Kṛṣṇa
20. *anāhata* = "unstruck," the heart *cakra*, or psychoenergetic center

D.

1. *yoga* = union, yoking, deep meditation, contemplation, absorption, method, means
2. *niyama* = discipline, second limb of *aṣṭāṅgayoga*
3. *samādhi* = meditative absorption, eighth and final limb of *aṣṭāṅgayoga*
4. *anuśāsanam* = teaching, instruction
5. *guru* = teacher, heavy
6. *vīra* = hero
7. *Sītā* = a furrow, heroine of the *Rāmāyaṇa*
8. *sukha* = happiness
9. *duḥkha* = suffering
10. *śauca* = cleanliness, first *niyama*
11. *doṣa* = the three psychophysical components of the body, according to *Āyurveda*; in the context of yoga, it can mean fault, deficiency, and disease
12. *loka* = world, people of the world
13. *śoka* = grief
14. *veda* = sacred knowledge, the *Vedas*, divided into three or four works, known as the *Ṛg-veda*, *Yajur-veda*, *Sāma-veda*, and *Atharva-veda*
15. *mūla* = root
16. *ahiṃsā* = nonviolence, first *yama*
17. *guṇa* = the three qualities of mind

18. *Śiva* = "the auspicious one," god of death and destruction (within the triad of gods, the other two being Brahmā, the creator, and Viṣṇu, the preserver)
19. *daivata* = divine
20. *amṛta* = nectar, immortality
21. *vibhūti* = superhuman power, name of the third chapter of the *Yogasūtra*
22. *pṛthivī* = earth
23. *hṛdaya* = heart
24. *Bhagavad Gītā* = song of the Beloved Lord, famous dialogue between Kṛṣṇa and Arjuna on the battlefield of Kurukṣetra
25. *asato mā sad gamaya* = From the unreal to the real, lead me!
26. *heyaṃ duḥkam anāgatam* = Suffering that has not yet come is to be avoided.
27. *vīra* + *āsana* = *vīrāsana* = hero pose
28. *kapota* + *āsana* = *kapotāsana* = pigeon pose
29. *māyura* + *āsana* = *māyurāsana* = peacock pose
30. *bhujapīḍa* + *āsana* = *bhujapīḍāsana* = arm-pressure pose
31. *yoga* + *anuśāsanam* = *yogānuśāsanam* = teaching of yoga
32. *atha yogānuśāsanam* = Now, there is the teaching of yoga.

E.

1. *namaste* = I bow to you
2. *abhyāsa* = practice
3. *vairāgya* = detachment
4. *dhyāna* = meditation, seventh limb of *aṣṭāṅgayoga*
5. *satya* = truthfulness, second *yama*
6. *asteya* = nonstealing, third *yama*
7. *santoṣa* = contentment, second *niyama*
8. *svādhyāya* = self-study, fourth *niyama*
9. *śānti* = peace
10. *samasthiti* = equal standing position, standing evenly
11. *pādahastāsana* = pose in which the hands are under the feet
12. *utkaṭāsana* = awkward pose
13. *bandha* = binding, bond
14. *vande* = I honor, I bow
15. *aravinda* = lotus
16. *vande gurūṇāṃ caranāravinde* = I bow to the two lotus feet of the *gurus* . . .
17. *sthira-sukham āsanam* = The *āsana* should be steady and comfortable.

F.

1. *aṣṭāṅga* = eight limbs/aspects
2. *padma* = lotus
3. *sahasra* = a thousand
4. *Īśvara* = Lord
5. *śveta* = white
6. *bhakti* = devotion, love
7. *mantra* = chant
8. *citta* = mind, consciousness
9. *pitta* = one of the three *doṣas* of *Āyurveda*, comprised of fire + water
10. *sattva* = equilibrium, one of the three *guṇas*, or qualities of mind
11. *jñāna* = knowledge
12. *mokṣa* = liberation
13. *sūtra* = thread
14. *Patañjali* = author of the *Yogasūtra*
15. *śaṅkha* = conch shell
16. *vighna* = obstacle
17. *yuddha* = battle
18. *kṣetra* = field

G.

1. *karma* = action
2. *dharma* = duty, justice
3. *sarva* = all
4. *carya* = act
5. *śirṣāsana* = headstand
6. *prāṇa* = breath, life force
7. *pramāṇa* = testimony, evidence
8. *praṇidhāna* = surrender
9. *cakra* = psychospiritual center
10. *kriyā* = action
11. *aparigraha* = nongrasping, fifth *yama*
12. *vīrabhadrāsana* = Vīrabhadra's pose (Vīrabhadra was an incarnation or form of Śiva)
13. *nāsāgra* = tip of the nose
14. *brahmacarya* = celibacy, chastity, fourth *yama*, stage of religious studentship
15. *dharma-kṣetre kuru-kṣetre samavetā yuyutsavaḥ* = In the field of justice, in the field of the Kurus, come together, desiring to fight . . .

### Review Exercises

1.
*vidyā dadāti vinayaṃ vinayād yāti pātratām |*
*pātratvād dhanam āpnoti dhanād dharmas tataḥ sukham ||*

2.
*santy atra bahavo vighnāḥ dāruṇā durnivāraṇāḥ |*
*tathāpi sādhayed yogī prāṇaiḥ kaṇṭha-gatair api ||*

3.
*ahiṃsā-pratiṣṭhāyāṃ tat-sannidhau vaira-tyāgaḥ |*
*satya-pratiṣṭhāyāṃ kriyā-phalāśrayatvam |*

4.
*yatroparamate cittaṃ niruddhaṃ yoga-sevayā |*
*yatra caivātmanātmānaṃ paśyann ātmani tuṣyati ||*

*sukham ātyantikaṃ yat tad buddhi-grāhyam atīndriyam |*
*vetti yatra na caivāyaṃ sthitaś calati tattvataḥ ||*

*yaṃ labdhvā cāparaṃ lābhaṃ manyate nādhikaṃ tataḥ |*
*yasmin sthito na duḥkhena guruṇāpi vicālyate ||*

## Chapter 2

A.
1. I see.
2. She goes.
3. You study.
4. They (m.) know.
5. You both fall.
6. We sit.

B.
1. I see and bow.
2. She goes and eats.
3. You don't study.
4. They (m.) know and speak.

5. You both don't fall.
6. We don't sit.

D.

1. They both (f.) dance.
2. He plays and throws.
3. They (n.) are not lost.
4. You all think and tell.
5. They both (m.) don't touch.
6. We are both content.

## Chapter 3

### Translation I

1. Yoga is practice.
2. Yoga conquers.
3. Rāma sees.
4. Arjuna knows.
5. The people study.
6. The two feet go.
7. The two hearts know.
8. The lotuses bow.

### Translation II

1. Yoga conquers doubt.
2. Rāma sees the worlds.
3. Arjuna knows yoga and justice.
4. The people study words.
5. The two hearts know truth.
6. The two people eat food.

### Translation III

1. I conquer doubt by means of yoga.
2. Yoga conquers impurities by means of *āsana.*
3. Rāma sees the worlds with his heart.
4. Arjuna knows justice with his mind.

5. The people study words through practice.
6. The two people eat food with their mouths.

### Translation IV

1. You speak the truth for the sake of yoga.
2. Rāma conquers Rāvaṇa for the sake of the worlds.
3. Arjuna studies yoga for the sake of justice.
4. She reads the book to the two boys.
5. He abandons wealth for the sake of liberation.

### Translation V

1. I know happiness because of yoga.
2. People know happiness because of suffering.
3. You stand up from the seat and go.
4. Arjuna conquers because of justice.
5. The boy falls from the tree.
6. I eat fruit from the tree.

### Translation VI

1. The purpose of yoga is liberation.
2. The food of the mind is knowledge.
3. The food of the heart is happiness.
4. People abandon the impurities of the body through yoga.

### Translation VII

1. In yoga, Arjuna conquers the impurities of the mind.
2. In the heart, there is both truth and happiness.
3. In the ocean, you abandon anger.
4. In the worlds, yoga is victorious.

### Translation VIII

1. O Yoga, you are happiness.
2. O Gods, you abandon anger.
3. O Rāma, you speak the truth.

## INVOCATIONS, MANTRAS, AND *SUBHĀṢITĀNI*

### "A Generous Person" (6M)

Among hundreds, one hero is born,
And among thousands, one wise person.
In tens of thousands, one eloquent speaker,
But a generous person may or may not exist.

### Bathing Mantra (4D)

O Gaṅgā and O Yamunā,
O Godāvarī, O Sarasvatī,
O Narmadā, O Sindu, O Kāverī,
In this water I invoke your presence.

### Dawn Prayer (15N)

Seven seas and seven mountain ranges,
Seven seers, seven islands, and forests.
Having considered the seven worlds beginning with earth,
May all of these render my daybreak beautiful.

### "For the Sake of Others" (3D)

For the sake of helping others, trees bear fruit,
For the sake of helping others, rivers flow.
For the sake of helping others, cows give milk,
This body is for the purpose of helping others.

### *Gaṇeśa Mantra* (3H)

O Gaṇeśa, god with a curved trunk, of great stature,
Whose brilliance is equal to ten million suns.
Grant me freedom from obstacles,
In all things, at all times.

### *Gāyatrī Mantra* (21C)

Earth, Heaven, the Whole Between.
The excellent divine power of the Sun.
May we contemplate the radiance of that god,
May this inspire our understanding.

### *Guru Stotram* I (5A)

The guru is Brahmā, God of Creation.
The guru is Viṣṇu, God of Preservation.
The guru is Śiva, God of Destruction.
The guru is clearly the Supreme Spirit.
I bow to that sacred guru.

### *Guru Stotram* III (7E)

I bow to that sacred guru,
By whom the eyes,
Of one who was blind because of the darkness of ignorance,
Were opened, with the collyrium pencil of knowledge.

### *Maṅgala Mantra* (3J)

May the rulers of the earth protect the well-being of the people,
With justice, by means of the right path.
May there always be good fortune for cows, Brahmins, and all living beings.
May all the inhabitants of the world be full of happiness.

### Morning Mantra (4C)

At the tip of the hand lives Lakṣmī,
In the middle of the hand, Sarasvatī.
At the root of the hand, Parvatī resides,
Looking at the hand at daybreak.

## "No Equal" (2E)

There is no eye equal to knowledge,
There is no discipline equal to truth.
There is no suffering equal to attachment,
There is no happiness equal to renunciation.

## Patañjali Invocation (21O)

Patañjali, abandoning his previous form, incarnates in various ways,
For the sake of bestowing favor to this world.
By whom the mass of afflictions is destroyed, who possesses dangerous poison,
Who has many heads, is beautifully ringed and brings forth all knowledge.
Whose retinue of snakes is always for his happiness.
May that Lord of snakes protect you,
Whose body is pure white and spotless,
Who transmits yoga, while absorbed in yoga.

## "Relatives" (6B)

Truth is my mother, my father is knowledge,
Justice is my brother, compassion is my friend.
Peace is my wife, patience is my son,
These six are my relatives.

## *Śānti Mantra* I (5H)

May the rain cloud rain down in the proper season,
May the earth be abounding in crops.
May this country be free from disturbance,
May those with divine knowledge be free from fear.

## *Śānti Mantra* II (5I)

May the childless become parents,
May parents become grandparents.
May the poor become wealthy,
May they live for a hundred autumns.

## *Śānti Mantra* III (5O)

May all be happy,
May all be free from disease.
May all see good fortune,
May no one have bad luck.

## *Śānti Mantra* IV (7I)

May there be well-being for all,
May there be peace for all.
May there be wholeness for all,
May there be happiness for all.

## "Truth" (8D)

Speak the truth, speak what is pleasant,
Don't speak the truth that is unkind.
But never tell a lie, even if pleasant,
This is the eternal law.

## Viṣṇu Mantra I (3K)

Just as water that has fallen from the sky,
Goes to the ocean.
Salutations to all the gods,
Go toward Lord Viṣṇu.

## Viṣṇu Mantra II (13A)

One should meditate upon Lord Viṣṇu, wearing a white garment,
All-pervading, with the appearance of the moon, four armed,
With a bright, kind face,
For the pacifying of all obstacles.

## Viṣṇu Mantra III (13B)

I bow to Viṣṇu, whose form is tranquil, whose bed is a serpent,
Whose navel sprouts a lotus, Lord of the gods.

Support of the whole world, resembling the sky,
Whose appearance is like a cloud, with beautiful limbs.

Beloved of Lakṣmī, with eyes like lotuses,
Who can be approached through meditation by yogīs.
Who removes the fear of existence,
The one Lord of all the worlds.

### "You Alone" (6A)

You, alone, are my mother, and you, alone, are my father,
You, alone, are my relative, and you, alone, are my friend.
You, alone, are my knowledge, you, alone, are my wealth,
You are truly my everything, O God, O God.

## TEXTS

### *Abhijñānaśākuntala*

5.2 (21M)

Seeing beautiful things,
Hearing sweet sounds,
Even a happy person,
Becomes restless.

For he remembers with his heart,
Loves from former lives,
Fixed in his heart,
Without his knowing.

### *Ādityahṛdayam*

2 (6L)

And having come, together with the gods,
To see the imminent battle.
Approaching Rāma,
The divine sage Agastya said:

16 (5B)

Salutations to the eastern mountain,
Salutations to the western mountain.
To the Lord of the heavenly bodies,
To the ruler of the day, salutations!

25 (19I)

In the midst of calamities and hardships,
In the dreary forest and in times of fear.
A person singing praises to that Sun God,
Will not sink down, O descendant of Raghu!

26 (7B)

Worship this Lord of the universe, the God of gods,
With one-pointed attention.
Chanting this prayer three times,
You will succeed in conflict.

27 (14A)

In this moment, O Mighty-Armed Rāma,
You will kill Rāvaṇa.
And thus having said this, Agastya then left,
In the same manner as he had arrived.

29–30 (6G)

Looking at the sun and chanting,
He attained the highest joy.
Sipping water thrice and becoming radiant,
The valorous hero, taking hold of his bow . . .

Seeing Rāvaṇa, the delighted-minded Rāma,
Approached for battle.
With a great and all-encompassing effort,
He was resolved in his intent to kill.

## *Amaruśataka*

105 (8C)

She is in the palace and she is in all the directions,
She is behind and she is in front,
She is on the sofa and she is on every path,
For one who is tortured by separation from her.
Oh! My heart! There is no other woman
For me but she, she,
She, she, she, she.
In this entire world,
What is this talk of nonduality?

## *Aparokṣānubhūti*

12 (7M)

Who am I? How is this world created?
And who, indeed, is the creator of this?
What is the material cause here in this world?
Such is this reflection.

14 (18A)

Everything is produced by ignorance,
It melts away through knowledge.
Our various intentions are the creator,
Such is this reflection.

32 (19L)

"I" am established as the seer,
The body is considered the seen.
From that description, "This body belongs to me,"
How could this body be the Soul?

33 (13G)

I, the Soul, am without change,
But the body is perpetually changing.

This is recognized with one's own eyes.
How could this body be the Soul?

112 (12B)

In which, comfortably, there might be,
Meditation on *Brahman* forever.
One should know that to be *āsana*,
And not any other posture that destroys happiness.

114 (18B)

That which is the root of all beings,
That which is the root of focusing the mind.
That *mūlabandha* is always to be practiced,
As useful for *rājayogīs*.

116 (12G)

Having made one's vision full of insight,
One might see the world full of *Brahman*.
That gaze is the most noble,
Not that which looks at the tip of the nose.

121 (17K)

Seeing Soul in all objects,
The mind is immersed in understanding.
That is to be known as *pratyāhāra*,
To be practiced by those desiring freedom.

129 (19M)

By the thought of an object, there is objecthood.
By the thought of a void, there is emptiness.
By the thought of *Brahman*, there is fullness.
Therefore, one should practice thinking of fullness.

## *Aruṇapraśna* (18I)

May we hear with our ears what is auspicious, O Gods!
May we see with our eyes what is auspicious, O you who are worthy of worship!
With a body with steady limbs, we have celebrated you,
May we attain a long life, which is beneficial to the gods.
May Indra of great fame, grant us well-being and good fortune.
May the omniscient Pūṣā grant us well-being and good fortune.
May Garuḍa, the protector, grant us well-being and good fortune.
May Bṛhaspati, lord of prayer and devotion, grant us well-being and good fortune.
*Oṃ* Peace, Peace, Peace!

## *Bhagavadgītā*

### Chapter 1

13 (6E)

Then the conch shells and kettledrums,
Cymbals, drums, and "cow-faced" trumpets,
Suddenly were all struck.
The noise was tumultuous!

14 (16C)

Then, standing in the great chariot,
Yoked with white horses.
Kṛṣṇa, descendant of Madhu, and Arjuna, son of Pāṇḍu,
Blew into their divine conch shells.

26 (6F)

Arjuna, son of Pṛthā, saw standing there,
Fathers and also grandfathers.
Teachers, maternal uncles, brothers,
Sons, grandsons, and friends as well.

29 (2G)

My limbs sink down,
And my mouth becomes dry.

In my body there is trembling,
And my hair stands on end.

30 (6I)

Gāṇḍīva falls down from my hand,
And even my skin burns.
I am not able to remain standing,
And my mind is as if wandering about.

31 (2H)

And I see adverse omens,
O Handsome-haired Kṛṣṇa.
And I do not perceive good fortune,
Having killed my own people in battle.

47 (6K)

Thus, Arjuna, having spoken in the midst of the battle,
Sat down upon the chariot seat.
Throwing down his bow and arrow,
With a heart overcome by sorrow.

### Chapter 2

3 (20I)

You must not go toward cowardice, O Son of Pṛthā,
This is not suitable for you.
Abandoning small weakness of heart,
Stand up, O Enemy-Scorcher!

6 (17A)

And this we do not know, which of the two for us is preferable—
Whether we should conquer them or whether they should conquer us.
Having killed them, we would not desire to live—
These sons of Dhṛtarāṣṭra who are standing here before us.

14 (17B)

Indeed, O son of Kuntī, material sensations,
Producing cold, heat, happiness, and suffering,
Are transient, always coming and going.
You must desire to bear them with courage, O descendant of Bharata!

16 (13L)

There is no existence of the unreal,
There is no nonexistence of the real.
Indeed, the certainty of these two is surely seen,
By seers of true nature.

19 (8E)

One who considers this Soul to be a slayer,
And one who thinks this Soul has been slain.
Both of these do not understand.
This Soul does not slay, nor is it slain.

22 (10N)

Just as, casting away old, worn-out clothes,
A person acquires new ones.
In the same way, casting away old, worn-out bodies,
The Soul comes into new ones.

23 (10J)

Weapons do not pierce this Soul,
Fire does not burn it.
Water does not make it wet,
Nor does the wind cause it to dry.

24–25 (14H)

This Soul is not to be pierced, it is not to be burned,
Not to be wetted and surely not to be dried.
It is eternal, all-pervading, fixed.
It is unmoving, everlasting.

This Soul is unmanifest, it is unthinkable,
It is unchanging, so it is said.
Therefore, knowing this Soul to be so,
You should not grieve.

27 (6J)

Indeed, for one who has been born, death is certain,
And for one who has died, there is certainly birth.
Therefore, in this unavoidable concern,
You should not grieve.

29 (19N)

Someone sees this Soul as a wonder.
And another, similarly, speaks of this Soul as a wonder.
And yet another, hears of this Soul as a wonder,
But someone else, even having heard about this Soul, does not know it.

38 (11A)

Considering happiness and suffering equal,
Likewise gain and loss, victory and defeat.
Then absorb yourself in battle,
Thus you shall not attain misfortune.

39 (11M)

This understanding has been explained to you in *Sāṃkhya* philosophy,
But hear this in regard to yoga practice.
Absorbed in this understanding, O Son of Pṛthā,
You shall avoid the bondage of action.

46 (7O)

As much value as there is in a well,
When water is overflowing in every direction.
There is that much value in all the Vedas,
For a Brahmin who understands.

47 (9A)

In action alone is your right,
Not in its fruits, at any time.
The motive of fruits of action should never arise,
Never may you have attachment to inaction.

48 (11O)

Established in yoga, perform actions,
Abandoning attachment, O Conqueror of Wealth.
Becoming equal in success or failure,
That equanimity is said to be yoga.

49 (5J)

Indeed, action is by far inferior,
To the yoga of understanding, O Conqueror of Wealth.
Seek refuge in understanding!
Miserable are those whose motives are the fruits of action.

50 (8J)

One who is absorbed in understanding, casts off here in this world,
Both good and evil actions.
Therefore, absorb yourself in yoga,
Yoga is skillfulness in action.

52 (16H)

When your understanding completely crosses over,
The thicket of delusion.
Then you shall reach complete indifference to
That which is yet to be heard and that which has already been heard.

53 (7L)

When your understanding, which is perplexed by hearing sacred texts,
Will remain steady,
Unmoving, in *samādhi*,
Then you will attain yoga.

54 (5M)

What is the description of one whose wisdom is steady,
Who is established in *samādhi*, O Kṛṣṇa?
How might one who has a steady mind speak?
How might he sit? How might he move?

58 (11N)

And when one draws together completely,
Like a tortoise its limbs,
The senses from the objects of the senses,
One's true wisdom is firmly established.

65 (4H)

In tranquillity, the disappearance,
Of all of one's suffering occurs.
For, the understanding of one whose mind is tranquil,
Quickly becomes steady.

66 (5D)

There is no understanding for one who is not concentrated,
And for one who is not concentrated, there is no meditation.
And for one who is not meditating there is no peace,
For one who is not peaceful, how can there be happiness?

69 (8G)

In that which is night for all beings,
One who is absorbed in *saṃyama* is awake.
In the time when all beings are awake,
That is night for the sage who sees.

### Chapter 3

4 (9E)

Not from not undertaking actions,
Does a person obtain exemption from acts and their consequences.

And not from renunciation alone,
Does one approach fulfillment.

21 (15J)

Whatever the most brilliant person does,
Other people will try to do too.
Whatever standard that person creates,
The world follows that.

24 (18C)

These worlds would fall into ruin,
If I should not perform action.
And I would be the creator of confusion,
I would destroy these creatures.

25 (16K)

Just as those who are unwise act,
Attached to action, O descendant of Bharata.
So the wise should act, unattached,
Desiring to hold together the world.

27 (13R)

Actions are universally being performed,
By the three *guṇas* of *prakṛti*.
One who is perplexed by egotism,
Thinks, "I am the doer."

28 (9I)

But one who knows the truth, O Mighty-Armed One,
Of the role of the three *guṇas* and their actions.
Thinking, "The *guṇas* act among the *guṇas*,"
That person is not attached.

35 (15H)

Better one's own duty, even if imperfect,
Than someone else's duty, performed well.
Better death in following one's own duty,
Someone else's duty brings danger.

## Chapter 4

1 (18N)

I declared this imperishable yoga,
To Vivasvat, the Sun God.
Vivasvat taught it to Manu,
And Manu related it to Ikṣvāku.

2 (12K)

Thus received by oral tradition,
The royal seers knew this.
But through a long time here on earth,
That yoga was lost, O Scorcher of Enemies.

24 (9C)

*Brahman* is the act of offering, *Brahman* is the offering,
Offered by *Brahman* into the fire of *Brahman.*
*Brahman*, alone, is to be attained by one,
Who is absorbed in the action of *Brahman.*

26 (15L)

Others offer the senses—hearing and so forth,
Into the fires of restraint.
And others offer the objects of the senses—sound, et cetera,
Into the fires of the senses.

27 (12N)

Others offer all actions of the senses,
And all actions of the breath.

Into the fire of the yoga of *saṃyama* on the Soul,
Which is kindled by knowledge.

29 (8H)

Others, offer the inhalation into the exhalation,
And likewise, the exhalation into the inhalation.
Restraining the movement of the inhalation and exhalation,
Completely focused on control of the breath.

42 (19H)

Therefore, with the sword of knowledge,
Having cut away this doubt of yours,
Which is born from ignorance and resides in the heart.
Practice yoga! Arise O descendant of Bharata!

### Chapter 5

5 (11I)

That state which is attained by followers of Sāṃkhya,
Is also reached by practitioners of yoga.
Sāṃkhya and yoga are one,
Who sees this, truly sees.

8–9 (13J)

"I do not actually do anything,"
Thus, absorbed in yoga, the knower of true nature thinks—
While seeing, hearing, touching, smelling,
Eating, walking, sleeping, breathing.

Talking, eliminating, grasping,
Opening eyes, shutting eyes too.
Bearing in mind that,
"The senses are acting among the sense objects."

11 (10A)

With the body, with the mind, with understanding,
Or even with the senses alone.
Yogīs perform action, having abandoned attachment,
For true knowledge of the Soul.

18 (18K)

In a Brahmin, endowed with knowledge and education,
In a cow, in an elephant,
And even in a dog or an untouchable,
The wise see the same.

24 (19A)

One whose happiness is within, whose delight is within,
And likewise whose light is only within.
That yogī, having become *Brahman*,
Attains the liberation of *Brahman*.

### Chapter 6

3 (17C)

For an inspired person, desirous of ascending to yoga,
Action is said to be the means.
Only for one who has already ascended to yoga,
Tranquillity is said to be the means.

5 (9B)

One should uplift the Soul by means of the Soul,
One should not let the Soul become disheartened.
For the Soul, alone, is the friend of the Soul,
And the Soul, alone, can be an enemy of the Soul.

11–12 (10M)

Establishing, in a clean place,
A steady seat for oneself.

Not too high, not too low,
With a covering of cloth, antelope skin, and *kuśa* grass.

There, making the mind one pointed,
With activity of mind and senses controlled.
Sitting on that seat, one should practice yoga,
For true knowledge of the Soul.

13 (11F)

Holding the body, head, and neck straight,
Unmoving and steady.
Gazing at the tip of one's nose,
And not looking in any direction.

16 (13K)

But yoga is not for one who eats too much,
Nor for one who does not eat at all.
And not for one with the habit of sleeping too much,
Nor, surely, for one who is always awake, O Arjuna.

19 (13Q)

Just as a lamp standing sheltered from the wind does not tremble,
So the comparison is remembered,
To the yogī, whose mind is controlled,
Being absorbed in the yoga of the Soul.

23 (14I)

It should be known that the disjunction,
From union with suffering, is called yoga.
That yoga is to be practiced with determination,
With an undepressed mind.

35 (3C)

Without doubt, O Mighty-Armed One,
The mind is difficult to control and unsteady.

But through practice and detachment,
O Son of Kuntī, it is restrained.

44 (17D)

By that very previous practice,
One is carried on, even against one's will.
One who even desires to know of yoga,
Goes beyond the recitation of Vedic texts.

46 (14G)

The yogī is superior to the ascetics,
And also thought to be superior to the learned.
And the yogī is superior to those engaged in ritual actions,
Therefore, be a yogī, O Arjuna.

**Chapter 7**

7 (12L)

Higher than me, there is nothing else whatsoever,
O Conqueror of Wealth.
On me, this whole universe is strung,
Like pearls on a thread.

8 (19D)

I am the taste in water, O son of Kuntī,
I am the radiance of the moon and the sun.
The sacred syllable *Oṃ* in all the Vedas,
The sound in space, the manhood in men.

13 (18D)

By these three states of being, composed of the three *guṇas*,
This whole universe,
Deluded, does not recognize me,
Higher than these, eternal.

## Chapter 8

7 (7N)

Therefore at all times,
Remember me and engage in battle.
With your mind and understanding fixed on me,
You will come toward me, alone, undoubtedly.

## Chapter 9

1 (15O)

And this greatest secret,
I will teach to you, who are not envious.
It is knowledge combined together with experience,
Knowing which, you will be free from misfortune.

17 (6C)

I am the father of this world,
The mother, the supporter, the grandfather.
That which is to be known, the purifier, the syllable *Oṃ*,
And the *Ṛg*, *Sāma*, and *Yajur Vedas.*

19 (10H)

I give out heat,
I hold back and pour forth the rain.
I am immortality and death,
Existence and nonexistence, O Arjuna.

27 (9G)

Whatever you do, whatever you eat,
Whatever you offer, whatever you give.
Whatever austerities you undertake, O son of Kuntī,
Do that as an offering to me.

### Chapter 10

22 (3F)

Among the Vedas, I am the *Sāmaveda*,
Among the gods, I am Indra.
Of the senses, I am the mind,
And among living beings, I am consciousness.

37 (5C)

Among the Vṛṣṇis, I am Kṛṣṇa, son of Vasudeva,
Of the Pāṇḍavas, I am Arjuna, Conqueror of Wealth.
And among the sages, I am Vyāsa,
Of the poets, I am the poet Uśanas.

### Chapter 11

8 (8I)

But you are not able to see me,
With only this, your own eye.
I give to you a divine eye,
Behold my powerful yoga!

30 (17F)

You lick vigorously, devouring on all sides,
All the worlds, with your blazing mouths.
Filling the entire universe with brilliance,
Your powerful radiance sets the world on fire, O Viṣṇu!

34 (16I)

Droṇa and Bhīṣma and Jayadratha and Karṇa,
And other heroes in battle, too,
Have been killed by me. Kill! Do not waver! Fight!
You shall conquer your enemies in battle.

37 (15I)

And why might they not bow to you, O Great-Souled One,
To the original Creator, greater even than Brahmā.
O Infinite Lord of gods, the dwelling place of the universe,
You are imperishable, existence, and nonexistence and that which is beyond.

49 (20J)

You should not tremble and do not be in a confused state,
Having seen this terrible form of mine.
With your fear departed and your mind pleased,
Behold this, my familiar form again.

50 (16F)

Having spoken in that way to Arjuna,
Kṛṣṇa Vāsudeva revealed his own form again.
And the great-souled Kṛṣṇa calmed the frightened Arjuna,
Becoming again his gentle form.

52–53 (18O)

This form of mine that you have seen,
Is very difficult to behold.
Even the gods, are constantly desiring,
A vision of this form.

Not by study of the Vedas, not by austerities,
Not by charity and not by sacrifice,
Am I able to be seen,
In such a form as you have beheld me.

### Chapter 12 (Part II Review)

Arjuna said:

1.
Thus, those devotees, who constantly absorbed in yoga,
Meditate on you, Lord Kṛṣṇa.

And those who meditate on the imperishable unmanifest,
Among these, which has the best knowledge of yoga?

The Beloved Lord said:

2.
Those who, causing their mind to enter into me,
Constantly absorbed in yoga, meditate on me.
Endowed with the highest faith,
They are considered by me to be the most absorbed in yoga.

3.
But those who meditate on the imperishable,
The undefinable, unmanifest.
The omnipresent, and unthinkable,
Unchangeable, immovable, eternal.

4.
Controlling the multitude of senses,
With the same understanding everywhere.
They attain me too,
Delighting in the welfare of all creatures.

5.
The afflictions of those whose minds,
Are attached to the unmanifest are greater.
For the path of the unmanifest is attained,
With difficulty by those who identify themselves with the body.

6.
But those who, placing together all actions in me,
Holding me as the highest.
They meditate, contemplating me,
Through yoga, with no other object.

7.
For those whose minds have entered into me,
I soon become the uplifter,

From the ocean of worldly existence and death,
O Son of Pṛthā.

8.
Place your mind in me alone,
Cause your understanding to enter into me.
You shall dwell in me alone,
From then forward there is no doubt.

9.
But if you are not able,
To keep your mind steadily on me.
Then by the practice of yoga,
Endeavor to attain me, O Conqueror of Wealth.

10.
If you are incapable even of practice,
Hold my work as the highest object.
Even performing actions for my sake,
You shall attain fulfillment.

11.
But if you are even unable to do this,
Then, resorting to my yoga,
Abandoning all the fruits of actions,
Act with self-restraint.

12.
Knowledge is indeed better than practice,
Meditation is better than knowledge.
Abandoning attachment to the fruits of action is better than meditation.
From this surrender, peace immediately follows.

13.
One who has no hatred for any living creatures,
Friendly and compassionate.
Unselfish, free from egotism,
Equal in suffering and happiness, patient.

14.
The yogī, who is always content,
Self-controlled, with firm resolve.
Whose mind and understanding are fixed on me, devoted to me,
He is beloved to me.

15.
From whom the world does not shrink,
And who does not shrink from the world.
Who is freed from lustfulness, impatience, fear, and agitation,
He is beloved to me.

16.
Impartial, radiant, and dexterous,
Open-minded, with anguish gone.
Unattached in all undertakings, devoted to me,
He is beloved to me.

17.
Who does not gloat nor hate,
Who does not mourn nor lust.
Unattached to what is pleasant or unpleasant, filled with devotion,
He is beloved to me.

18 (11B)
Equal toward enemy and friend,
Likewise in honor and disgrace.
In cold and heat, happiness and suffering,
Equal, freed from attachment.

19.
Equal in blame or praise, reserved in speech,
Content with anything.
Having no fixed abode, steady minded, filled with devotion,
He is beloved to me.

20.
Those who meditate on this nectar of justice,
As declared above.
Holding faith, intent on me, devoted,
They are exceedingly beloved to me.

## Chapter 13

32 (19K)

Just as the all-pervading ether,
Because of its subtlety, is not defiled.
In the same way, the Soul,
Present everywhere in the body, is not defiled.

## Chapter 14

5–8 (10I)

*Sattva*, *rajas*, and *tamas*:
The three *guṇas*, whose origins are in *prakṛti*.
These threads bind in the body, O Mighty-Armed One,
The eternal embodied Soul.

Among these, *sattva*, because of its stainlessness,
Is bright and shining and free from disease.
It binds the Soul by attachment to happiness,
And by attachment to knowledge, O Sinless One.

Know that *rajas* has the nature of passion,
Arising from thirst and attachment.
This binds the Soul to the body,
By attachment to action, O son of Kuntī.

And know that *tamas* is born from ignorance,
Confusing all embodied beings.
By intoxication, laziness, and sleepiness,
This binds the Soul to the body, O descendant of Bharata.

### Chapter 15

1 (13E)

They say the sacred fig tree is eternal,
Whose roots are above and branches below,
Whose leaves are sacred hymns.
One who knows this is a knower of the Vedas.

11 (19J)

And the yogīs, who are persevering,
See this Soul, situated in their Soul.
But the foolish, unthinking ones,
Even though persevering, do not see this Soul.

20 (9J)

Thus this most secret sacred text,
Has been taught by me, O Faultless One.
Understanding this, one may become endowed with understanding,
And attain one's purpose, O descendant of Bharata.

### Chapter 16

5 (8B)

Divine destiny leads to liberation,
Demonic to bondage, it is thought.
Don't grieve. To a divine destiny,
You are born, O son of Pāṇḍu.

### Chapter 18

37 (19E)

That which at the beginning is like poison,
But when transformed, resembles nectar.
That happiness is said to have the quality of *sattva*,
Born from the tranquillity of the understanding of Soul.

48 (5P)

One should not abandon the action to which one is born,
Even if it has faults, O son of Kuntī.
For all undertakings are enveloped with deficiency,
Like fire is by smoke.

65 (21E)

Let your mind be on me, devoted to me,
Sacrificing to me, do homage to me.
Truly, you shall come to me,
I promise you, for you are dear to me.

66 (20K)

Abandoning all duties,
Take me as your one refuge.
I will free you from all misfortune,
Do not grieve.

69 (16J)

And no one among humans will be giving me more delight,
Than one who teaches this secret knowledge.
And there shall be no other on earth,
Dearer to me than that person.

71 (13F)

Even the person who might hear this,
Full of faith and free from spite.
He too, liberated, shall attain the happy worlds,
Of those whose actions are virtuous.

74 (20A)

Thus I have heard this extraordinary conversation,
Between Kṛṣṇa, the son of Vasudeva,
And the great-souled Arjuna, the son of Pṛthā,
Which causes the hair to stand on end with joy.

75 (18E)

Through the grace of Vyāsa I have heard,
This secret, supreme yoga.
From Kṛṣṇa, the lord of yoga,
Speaking himself, right before my eyes.

## *Bhāgavatapurāṇa*

### Chapter 3

28.1 (8F)

I will explain the characteristics of yoga,
Whose aim is *samādhi*, O daughter of the king.
By this practice, alone, the mind is delighted,
And approaches the path of truth.

28.10 (13P)

The mind of the yogī whose breath is controlled,
May soon be free from dust.
Just as gold, fanned by air and fire,
Becomes free of impurities.

### Chapter 10

20.41 (18M)

Farmers preserved the water from flooded fields,
By means of firm embankments.
Just as yogīs keep knowledge from flowing out through the breath,
By means of stilling the mind.

24.6 (16L)

Knowing and not knowing,
People perform actions.
The wise might attain their goal,
While the foolish may not.

### Chapter 11

28.41 (10E)

Some persevering yogīs, by various means,
Making this body very skilled and fixed in youth.
Thus they engage in yoga,
For the purpose of physical perfections.

## *Bhajagovindam*

Refrain (14M)

Worship Govinda, worship Govinda,
Worship Govinda you foolish person!
When the time of death has arrived at hand,
Rules of grammar surely won't save you.

## *Bṛhadāraṇyakopaniṣat*

1.3.28 (10O)

From the unreal to the Real,
Lead me.
From darkness to Light,
Lead me.
From death to Immortality,
Lead me.

3.2.7–9 (17I)

The mind, indeed, is an organ of apprehension.
It is grasped by its object—desire.
For one feels desires by means of the mind.

The hands, indeed, are an organ of apprehension.
They are grasped by their object—action.
For one performs actions by means of the hands.

The skin, indeed, is an organ of apprehension.
It is grasped by its object—touch.
For one feels sensations by means of the skin.

3.9.1 (15D)

Then, truly, Vidagdha Śākalya, "the clever grammarian," questioned him.
"How many gods are there, Yājñavalkya?"
"It is said there are as many as are in the ritual invocation to all of the gods."
He answered in accordance with this very ritual injunction:
"Three and three hundred and three and three thousand."

"Yes, of course, so be it," he said. "But how many gods are there really, Yājñavalkya?"
"Thirty-three."

"Yes, of course, so be it," he said. "But how many gods are there really, Yājñavalkya?"
"Six."

"Yes, of course, so be it," he said. "But how many gods are there really, Yājñavalkya?"
"Two."

"Yes, of course, so be it," he said. "But how many gods are there really, Yājñavalkya?"
"One and a half."

"Yes, of course, so be it," he said. "But how many gods are there really, Yājñavalkya?"
"One."

4.2.4 (21N)

"Of this person, the vital winds in front are the eastern region,
The vital winds on the right side are the southern region.
The vital winds at the back are the western region.
The vital winds on the left side are the northern region.
The vital winds in the upper direction are the highest region.
The vital winds in the downward direction are the lowest region.
All the vital winds constitute all the regions.

About this Soul, one can only say, "Not this, not this."
It is ungraspable for it cannot be grasped.

It is indestructible for it does not decay.
It is independent for it does not stick to anything.
It is unbound, it does not tremble.
It does not suffer injury.
"Certainly, Janaka, you have attained fearlessness," Yājñavalkya said.
Janaka of Videha replied,
"May you be fearless too, Yājñavalkya, you sir, who have taught us fearlessness.
May there be homage to you.
These people of Videha and I, myself, are here for you."

4.4.14 (20H)

While we are here in this world, we have come to know this Soul,
If it has not been known, what a great loss!
Those who know it become immortal,
As for the others, they enter into suffering.

4.5.14 (20G)

Then Maitreyī said, "Sir, you have caused me to fall into deep bewilderment.
I do not understand this."
He replied, "I have not said anything confusing at all.
This Soul is imperishable; its nature is indestructibility."

5.1.1 (3I)

That is Whole. This is Whole.
The Whole arises from the Whole.
Having taken the Whole from the Whole,
Only the Whole remains.

5.2.1–3 (20D)

The three kinds of descendants of Prajāpati—gods, humans, and demons,
Lived with their father, Prajāpati, as students of the Vedas.

Having completed their studentship, the gods said, "Tell us something, sir."
Then he spoke to them this syllable, "*Da*."
"Have you understood?" he asked.

"We have understood," they said. "Be self-controlled," you told us.
"Yes," he said. "You have understood."

Then the humans said to him, "Tell us something, sir."
Then he spoke to them this syllable, "*Da*."
"Have you understood?" he asked.
"We have understood," they said. "Be generous," you told us.
"Yes," he said. "You have understood."

Then the demons said to him, "Tell us something, sir."
Then he spoke to them this syllable, "*Da*."
"Have you understood?" he asked.
"We have understood," they said. "Be compassionate," you told us.
"Yes," he said. "You have understood."

Thunder, that divine voice, repeats this very syllable, "*Da*, *Da*, *Da*."
"Be self-controlled." "Be generous." "Be compassionate."
One should practice this triad—self-control, generosity, and compassion.

## *Chāndogyopaniṣat*

### Chapter 4

4–9 (Part III Review)

One day, Satyakāma Jābāla said to his mother, Jabālā,
"Mother, I want to live as a Vedic student. So now, tell me, what lineage am I?"
She replied: "I do not know, my son, what lineage you are. I had you in my youth.
I was a maid and moved around a lot. So I do not know what lineage you are.
But my name is Jabālā. And your name is Satyakāma.
So you should just say that you are Satyakāma Jābāla."

Then he went to Hāridrumata Gautama and said,
"Sir, I want to live as a Vedic student. I approach you, sir, as your student."
Hāridrumata said to him, "What lineage are you, my dear boy?"
And Satyakāma replied, "I do not know, sir, what lineage I am.
When I asked my mother she answered, 'I had you in my youth.
I was a maid and moved around a lot. So I do not know what lineage you are.

But my name is Jabālā. And your name is Satyakāma.'
So I am Satyakāma Jābāla, sir."

Then Hāridrumata said to him, "A non-Brahmin would not be able to speak this way.
Bring me some firewood, my dear boy. I will invest you with the sacred thread.
You have not departed from the truth."
Hāridrumata initiated him and, separating out four hundred emaciated and weak cows, instructed, "My dear boy, attend to these cows."
While he was driving away the cows Satyakāma said,
"Without a thousand, I will not return." So he lived away for a long series of years.
When they reached a thousand . . .

The bull called out to him, "Satyakāma!!!"
"Sir," he replied.
The bull spoke: "My dear boy, we have reached a thousand.
Take us back to the house of our teacher and I will tell you one-quarter of *Brahman*."
"Tell me please, sir."
So the bull told him:
"One-sixteenth is the eastern direction. One-sixteenth is the western direction.
One-sixteenth is the southern direction, and one-sixteenth is the northern direction.
This quarter of *Brahman*, consisting of these four-sixteenths, is called 'Illustrious.'
Someone who knows this and honors this quarter of *Brahman*,
Consisting of these four-sixteenths, as 'Illustrious,' will become illustrious in this world.
One who knows this and honors this quarter of *Brahman*,
Consisting of these four-sixteenths, as 'Illustrious,' will win illustrious worlds."

The bull spoke: "The fire will tell you one-quarter."
When the following day arrived, Satyakāma drove the cows on.
At the place they reached at sunset, he built a fire, locked up the cows,
Added fuel to the fire, and sat down behind the fire, facing east.
The fire called out to him, "Satyakāma!!!"
"Sir," he replied.
The fire spoke: "My dear boy, I will tell you one-quarter of *Brahman*."
"Tell me please, sir."

So the fire told him:
"One-sixteenth is the earth. One-sixteenth is the space between heaven and earth.
One-sixteenth is heaven and one-sixteenth is the ocean.
This quarter of *Brahman*, consisting of these four-sixteenths, is called 'Infinite.'
Someone who knows this and honors this quarter of *Brahman*,
Consisting of these four-sixteenths, as 'Infinite,' will become infinite in this world.
One who knows this and honors this quarter of *Brahman*,
Consisting of these four-sixteenths, as 'Infinite,' will win infinite worlds."

The fire spoke: "A goose will tell you one-quarter."
When the following day arrived, Satyakāma drove the cows on.
At the place they reached at sunset, he built a fire, locked up the cows,
Added fuel to the fire, and sat down behind the fire, facing east.
A goose flew down and called out to him, "Satyakāma!!!"
"Sir," he replied.
The goose said, "My dear boy, I will tell you one-quarter of *Brahman*."
"Tell me please, sir."
So the goose told him:
"One-sixteenth is fire. One-sixteenth is the sun.
One-sixteenth is the moon and one-sixteenth is lightning.
This quarter of *Brahman*, consisting of these four-sixteenths, is called 'Luminous.'
Someone who knows this and honors this quarter of *Brahman*,
Consisting of these four-sixteenths, as 'Luminous,' will become luminous in this world. One who knows this and honors this quarter of *Brahman*,
Consisting of these four-sixteenths, as 'Luminous,' will win luminous worlds."

The goose said, "A diver bird will tell you one-quarter."
When the following day arrived, Satyakāma drove the cows on.
At the place they reached at sunset, he built a fire, locked up the cows,
Added fuel to the fire, and sat down behind the fire, facing east.
A diver bird flew down and called out to him, "Satyakāma!!!"
"Sir," he replied.
The diver bird said, "My dear boy, I will tell you one-quarter of *Brahman*."
"Tell me please, sir."
So the diver bird told him:
"One-sixteenth is breath. One-sixteenth is sight.
One-sixteenth is hearing, and one-sixteenth is the mind.

This quarter of *Brahman*, consisting of these four-sixteenths, is called 'Supported.'
Someone who knows this and honors this quarter of *Brahman*,
Consisting of these four-sixteenths, as 'Supported,' will have a support in this world.
One who knows this and honors this quarter of *Brahman*,
Consisting of these four-sixteenths, as 'Supported,' will win supported worlds."

Then he reached the house of his teacher. His teacher called out to him, "Satyakāma!!!"
"Sir," he replied.
"My dear boy, you are shining like one who knows *Brahman*. Who taught you?"
"Other than human beings," he admitted, "but if you desire, please tell me yourself,
For I have heard from people like yourself that knowledge that is learned from a teacher is best to reach *Brahman*."
So Hāridrumata told this to him, without omitting anything.

### Chapter 6

1.3–7 (21A)

His father then said to him, "Śvetaketu, since here you are my dear son,
Arrogant, puffed up, thinking yourself knowledgeable,
You must have asked about that symbolic rule, by which the unheard becomes heard,
The unthought becomes thought, and the unknown becomes known."

"How does that symbolic rule work, sir?" Śvetaketu asked.

"My dear son, just as by one lump of clay, everything made of clay might be known,
So that transformation is dependent on just words, an appellation.
The clay itself is indeed the reality."

"My dear son, just as by one copper jewel, everything made of copper might be known,
So that transformation is dependent on just words, an appellation.
The copper itself is indeed the reality."

"My dear son, just as by one nail clipper, everything made of black iron might be known, so that transformation is dependent on just words, an appellation.
The black iron itself is indeed the reality.
That, my dear son, is how that symbolic rule works."
"Certainly those venerable teachers did not know this. For if they had known,

How could they not have told me? Sir, you tell me yourself."
"All right, my dear son," he said.

8.2 (19C)

"Just as a bird, tied with a string, flying about in every direction,
But not finding another resting place,
Will go back to the very support to which it is tied.
In the same way, my dear boy, the mind, flying about in every direction,
And not finding another resting place,
Will go back to the breath itself.
For the mind is bound to the breath, my dear boy."

8.3–4 (18P)

"You should know this as a bud that has sprung up, my dear boy,
This cannot come to be without a root. And what might be its root other than water?
With water as the bud, my dear boy, you will find that the root is fire,
With fire as the bud, my dear boy, you will find that the root is existence.
Existence is the root, my dear boy, of all of these creatures,
Existence is their resting place, existence is their support."

9 (18Q)

"My dear son, just as bees create honey, gathering the nectars of various trees,
And making it into one nectar.
And just as there, in that unified nectar, the various nectars cannot discern,
'I am the nectar of this tree,' 'I am the nectar of that tree.'
In the same way, my dear son, all these creatures, converging into existence,
Do not know, 'We are converging into existence.'

Whatever they are here in this world—a tiger or a lion or a wolf or a boar or a worm,
Or a moth or a gnat or a mosquito—they become that."

"And this finest essence here has the same nature as this whole world.
That is the truth. That is Soul. You are that, Śvetaketu."

"Teach me more please, sir," Śvetaketu said.
"All right, my dear son," he answered.

10.1–3 (21K)

"My dear son, these easterly rivers flow eastward and the westerly rivers flow westward,
From the ocean those rivers merge into that very ocean. They become that very ocean.
There, they do not know 'I am this river,' 'I am that river.'
Thus, in the same way, my dear son, all these creatures,
Having come into existence, do not know, 'We have come into existence.'

Whatever they are here in this world—a tiger or a lion or a wolf or a boar or a worm,
Or a moth or a gnat or a mosquito—they become that."

"And this finest essence here has the same nature as this whole world.
That is the truth. That is Soul. You are that, Śvetaketu."

"Teach me more please, sir," Śvetaketu said.
"All right, my dear son," he answered.

11.1–3 (17G)

"My dear son, if someone were to strike at the root of this great tree,
Its living essence, its sap, would flow.
If one were to strike it in the middle,
Its living essence, its sap, would flow.
If one were to strike it at the top,
Its living essence, its sap, would flow.
Penetrated by this living essence, the tree stands,
Endlessly drinking and rejoicing.
But if the living essence of one branch leaves,
Then that branch withers.
If it leaves a second branch,
Then that branch withers.
If it leaves a third branch,
Then that branch withers.
If it leaves the whole tree,
Then the whole tree withers."

"Thus, certainly, in the very same way, my dear son," he said,
"Know that when this living essence has departed, indeed, as they say, this dies,
But the living essence does not die.

And this finest essence here has the same nature as this whole world.
That is the truth. That is Soul. You are that, Śvetaketu."

"Teach me more please, sir," Śvetaketu said.
"All right, my dear son," he answered.

13.1–3 (20M)

"Having placed this salt in water, approach me tomorrow morning,"
Uddalāka Āruṇi said to his son, Śvetaketu.
And Śvetaketu did just that.
His father said to him,
"The salt you placed in the water last night, now, come on, bring that here."
Reaching for it, Śvetaketu could not find it, since it had fully dissolved.
"Now, take a sip from the end," said his father. "How is it?"
"Salty."
"Take a sip from the middle. How is it?"
"Salty."
"Take a sip from the other end. How is it?"
"Salty."
"Now, having thrown this salt out, then come back to me."
He did just that but found that the salt existed perpetually.
His father said to him,
"My dear son, you did not see it, but the salt was always right here."

"And this finest essence here has the same nature as this whole world.
That is the truth. That is Soul. You are that, Śvetaketu."

"Teach me more please, sir," Śvetaketu said.
"All right, my dear son," he answered.

14.1–3 (21L)

"My dear son, as, for instance, a person having been brought here, blindfolded,
From Gandhāra, and then released in an uninhabited place,
Just as he might wander about there, to the east or north or south,
Since he was brought there blindfolded and left there blindfolded.
But if someone, freeing him from the blindfold, said,
'Gandhāra is in this direction, go in this direction,'
He, being learned and intelligent, asking from village to village,

Would eventually arrive in Gandhāra.
In the same way, here in this world, when a person has a teacher, he knows,
'There is only so long until I will be freed, and then I will arrive.' "

"And this finest essence here has the same nature as this whole world.
That is the truth. That is Soul. You are that, Śvetaketu."

"Teach me more please, sir," Śvetaketu said.
"All right, my dear son," he answered.

### Chapter 7

5.1 (17L)

Thinking is indeed greater than intention,
For it is only when one thinks about something,
That one forms an intention,
Then one has it in mind.
Then pronounces it through speech,
And articulates it in a name.
In the name there are unique *mantras*,
In the *mantras* are actions.

## *Dattātreyayogaśāstra*

2 (18F)

Sāṃkṛti, that most excellent of sages,
With a desire to learn yoga.
After wandering about the entire earth,
Reached the Naimiṣa forest.

6 (18G)

Then, having bowed to that sage, Dattātreya,
He, Sāṃkṛti, there,
Together with Dattātreya's students,
Sat down right in front of him.

25 (16E)

If one practices in a relaxed state, in a place without people,
One might attain fulfillment.
And thus Śiva taught many secret practices,
Of *layayoga*, the yoga of cosmic absorption.

37 (14B)

Drawing in the breath, according to one's capacity,
One should slowly inhale into the belly.
And after that, according to one's capacity, alone,
One should slowly exhale the breath.

39 (13M)

O Sāṃkṛti, listen resolutely,
To the sequence of yoga practice,
Being explained carefully by me,
For yogīs, with all its characteristics.

41–2ab (9F)

Whether Brahmin, ascetic, Buddhist, or Jain,
Śaiva skullbearer or Cārvāka materialist.
A wise person, accompanied by faith,
Constantly devoted to the practice of yoga,
May attain complete fulfillment.

58 (6H)

Having sat down there, the wise yogī,
Taking *padmāsana*, the lotus posture.
With an upright body and with his hands joined together in respect,
Bowing to his favorite deity.

76–77 (15E)

Trembling arises in the body,
Of the yogī, staying in an *āsana*.

Then, from further practice,
He certainly becomes frog-like.

Just as a frog might move,
Jumping on the ground,
In that way, the yogī seated in *padmāsana*,
Moves on the ground.

93 (14C)

Every day at one time,
One should practice *kevalakumbhaka*, pure breath retention.
Thus, *pratyāhāra* may arise,
For the yogī practicing in this way.

130cd–131 (15M)

This path of the poet-seer has been taught,
To you, O Sāṃkṛti, as the yoga with eight limbs.

Thereupon, I will teach the ideology,
Of the inspired seers, such as Kapila.
The difference is because of the difference in practice,
But the fruit is the very same.

145 (11C)

*Prāṇa* and *apāna*, *nāda* and *bindu*,
Attaining unity by means of *mūlabandha*.
These bestow complete fulfillment of yoga,
Here there is no doubt.

### *Dhyānabindūpaniṣat*

1 (12H)

Even if misfortune is equal to mountains,
Extending for many miles.
By the yoga of meditation it is broken,
Never at any time, will another breaking open occur.

7 (11P)

Just as sesame oil dwells in the seeds,
And as fragrance in a flower,
So, too, in the body of a person,
The Soul resides inside and outside.

## *Gheraṇḍasaṃhitā*

### Chapter 1

4 (2F)

There is no fetter equal to illusion,
There is no strength greater than yoga.
There is no relative greater than knowledge,
There is no enemy greater than ego.

8 (13N)

Like an unbaked jar in water,
The body is always decaying.
Baking it with the fire of yoga,
One should practice purification of the body.

9–11 (19G)

Purification and also strength,
Stability, calmness, and lightness,
Clear vision and unobscured awareness,
Are the seven practices for the body.

By means of the six *kriyās*, there is purification,
And by means of *āsana* there may be strength.
By means of *mudrā* there is stability,
And by *pratyāhāra* there is calmness.

From *prāṇāyāma* there is lightness,
And from *dhyāna* there is clear vision of Soul.

Through *samādhi*, there is unobscured awareness,
And liberation, itself, there is no doubt.

### Chapter 2

43 (4I)

The fire in the body steadily increases,
There is the destruction of all diseases.
The serpent goddess awakens,
From the practice of *bhujaṅgāsana*.

### Chapter 5

3 (9H)

In a remote place, or in a forest,
In a metropolis, or near people,
One should not begin yoga practice.
If this is done, it may be devoid of fulfillment.

6 (11G)

And a pond, a well, or a tank,
Should be situated in the middle of the enclosure.
Not too high and not too low,
The hut should be free from insects.

7 (12C)

And completely smeared with cow dung,
The hut should be free from holes.
And in this way, only in a hidden place,
One should practice *prāṇāyāma*.

9 (8A)

In spring or in autumn it is declared,
One should begin the practice of yoga.
Then yoga might be attained,
And one may surely be freed from diseases.

22 (15B)

With food one should fill half of the stomach,
And with water, the third part.
The fourth quarter one should keep,
For the movement of the breath.

33 (21J)

Sitting on a thick seat,
Made of *kuśa* grass, a deer skin,
A tiger skin or a woolen blanket,
Facing east or facing north.
Having attained purification of the *nāḍīs*,
One should practice *prāṇāyāma*.

7.19 (18H)

All of these creatures of the earth and creatures of the air,
Tree, bush, creeper, vine, grass, water, mountains.
Know that everything is *Brahman*,
And see everything in the Soul.

## *Gurvaṣṭakam* (Part I Review)

शरीरं सुरूपं तथा वा कलत्रं यशश्चारु चित्रं धनं मेरुतुल्यम् ।
मनश्चेन्न लग्नं गुरोरङ्घ्रिपद्मे ततः किं ततः किं ततः किं ततः किम् ॥ १ ॥

कलत्रं धनं पुत्रपौत्रादि सर्वं गृहं बान्धवाः सर्वमेतद्धि जातम् ।
मनश्चेन्न लग्नं गुरोरङ्घ्रिपद्मे ततः किं ततः किं ततः किं ततः किम् ॥ २ ॥

षडङ्गादिवेदो मुखे शास्त्रविद्या कवित्वादि गद्यं सुपद्यं करोति ।
मनश्चेन्न लग्नं गुरोरङ्घ्रिपद्मे ततः किं ततः किं ततः किं ततः किम् ॥ ३ ॥

विदेशेषु मान्यः स्वदेशेषु धन्यः सदाचारवृत्तेषु मत्तो न चान्यः ।
मनश्चेन्न लग्नं गुरोरङ्घ्रिपद्मे ततः किं ततः किं ततः किं ततः किम् ॥ ४ ॥

क्षमामण्डले भूपभूपालवृन्दैः सदा सेवितं यस्य पादारविन्दम्
मनश्चेन्न लग्नं गुरोरङ्घ्रिपद्मे ततः किं ततः किं ततः किं ततः किम् ॥ ५ ॥

यशो मे गतं दिक्षु दानाप्रतापाज्जगद्वस्तु सर्वं करे यत्प्रसादात्।
मनश्चेन्न लग्नं गुरोरङ्घ्रिपद्मे ततः किं ततः किं ततः किं ततः किम्॥ ६॥

न भोगे न योगे न वा वाजिराजौ न कान्तामुखे नैव वित्तेषु चित्तम्।
मनश्चेन्न लग्नं गुरोरङ्घ्रिपद्मे ततः किं ततः किं ततः किं ततः किम्॥ ७॥

अरण्ये न वा स्वस्य गेहे न कार्ये न देहे मनो वर्तते मे त्वनर्घ्ये।
मनश्चेन्न लग्नं गुरोरङ्घ्रिपद्मे ततः किं ततः किं ततः किं ततः किम्॥ ८॥

गुरोरष्टकं यः पठेत्पुण्यदेही यतिर्भूपतिर्ब्रह्मचारी च गेही।
लभेद्वाञ्छितार्थं पदं ब्रह्मसंज्ञं गुरोरुक्तवाक्ये मनो यस्य लग्नम्॥ ९॥

1.
A well-formed body, and a beautiful wife,
Excellent and manifold fame, and wealth equal to Mt. Meru . . .
But if one's mind is not attached to the lotus feet of the guru,
What then? What then? What then? What then?

2.
Wife, wealth, children, and grandchildren, all these,
Home, relatives, all of this might exist . . .
But if one's mind is not attached to the lotus feet of the guru,
What then? What then? What then? What then?

3.
The Vedas with their six limbs on one's lips and knowledge of other sacred texts,
One may have poetic skill, and so forth, and may compose beautiful poetry and prose . . .
But if one's mind is not attached to the lotus feet of the guru,
What then? What then? What then? What then?

4.
To be respected in other countries, fortunate in one's own country,
In ways of virtuous conduct, there is no other better than me . . .
But if one's mind is not attached to the lotus feet of the guru,
What then? What then? What then? What then?

5.
One's lotus feet may always be served,
By multitudes of princes and kings all around the world . . .
But if one's mind is not attached to the lotus feet of the guru,
What then? What then? What then? What then?

6.
My fame has spread in all the directions, because of my generosity and prowess,
All of the things of the world are in my hand, from the favor of the guru . . .
But if one's mind is not attached to the lotus feet of the guru,
What then? What then? What then? What then?

7.
Not in enjoyment, not in yoga, and not in the king's horses,
Not in the face of the beloved and not in wealth is the mind . . .
For if one's mind is not attached to the lotus feet of the guru,
What then? What then? What then? What then?

8.
Not in the forest and not in one's own house, nor in what is to be done,
Not in the body, nor in what is invaluable, does my mind dwell . . .
For if one's mind is not attached to the lotus feet of the guru,
What then? What then? What then? What then?

9.
The virtuous person who might read this octet of verses on the guru,
Whether one is an ascetic, a king, a student, or a householder.
Whose mind is attached to the sayings of the guru,
Might obtain the desired goal, the state called *Brahman.*

## *Haṭhapradīpikā*

### Chapter 1

3 (8K)
For those who are unaware of *rājayoga*,
Through wandering in the darkness of too many different opinions.

The very compassionate Svātmarāma,
Composes the *Haṭhapradīpikā*, a lamp on *haṭhayoga*.

11 (14N)

The knowledge of *haṭhayoga* is to be kept absolutely secret,
By the yogī desiring fulfillment.
It may become powerful when concealed,
But impotent when put on display.

15 (3A)

Eating too much and overexertion,
Talking too much and holding on to rules.
Excessive socializing and restlessness,
Yoga is utterly lost by means of these six.

16 (3E)

From perseverance, from courage, from patience,
From knowledge of truth and from fixed intention,
From abandoning excessive socializing,
Yoga succeeds by means of these six.

17 (19F)

Since *āsana* is the first limb of *haṭhayoga*,
It is described first.
One should practice these *āsanas*,
Which give stability, health, and lightness of limbs.

23 (10L)

And having established *padmāsana*, the lotus posture,
Placing the hands between the knees and thighs onto the ground,
Raising up into the sky,
Is *kukkuṭāsana*, rooster pose.

29 (9L)

Thus, *paścimatānāsana* is foremost among *āsanas*,
It causes the breath to flow in the back of the body.

It can make the abdominal fire rise up,
Create thinness in the belly and good health for human beings.

32 (5E)

Lying on the back, like a corpse on the ground,
That act of rest is called *śavāsana*.
*Śavāsana* removes fatigue,
Creating repose in the mind.

38 (3G)

Just as moderate diet among the *yamas*,
As nonviolence among the *niyamas*.
The inspired seers know that *siddhāsana* is,
The best, most special of all *āsanas*.

42 (14K)

Then, when the one and only *siddhāsana*,
Is steady and perfected.
The three *bandhas* arise,
Spontaneously, without exertion.

63 (3B)

The yogī should partake of food that is:
Nourishing, very sweet, and oily.
It should come from a cow and nourish the constituent elements of the body,
It should be desired by the mind and suitable.

64 (9D)

Whether young, old, or very old,
Sick or even weak.
From practice, fulfillment is attained in all yoga,
For one who is not lazy.

65–66 (5N)

For one who is absorbed in practice, there may be fulfillment,
For one who is without practice, how might there be?

Fulfillment in yoga is not born,
Merely by reading sacred texts.

The cause of fulfillment is not wearing particular clothes,
Nor is it talking about it.
Practice is the only cause of fulfillment,
This is the truth; there is no doubt.

## Chapter 2

1 (14O)

Now, when the yogī is steady in *āsana*,
Possessing self-control and eating a wholesome and moderate diet,
By means of the path taught by the guru,
He should practice *prāṇāyāma*.

2 (14L)

When the breath is unsteady, the mind is unsteady,
When the breath is steady, the mind may become steady.
The yogī attains stability,
Therefore, one should control the breath.

3 (7G)

As long as there is breath remaining in the body,
For that long, there is said to be life.
Death is the departure of this breath,
Therefore, one should control the breath.

6 (18J)

Therefore, one should always practice *prāṇāyāma*,
With a clear and calm mind.
So that the impurities situated in the *suṣumnā nāḍī*,
Will attain purity.

7 (14P)

The yogī, sitting in *baddhapadmāsana*,
Should inhale the breath through the *iḍā nāḍī*.

Holding it as long as possible, according to his capacity,
He should then exhale through the *piṅgalā nāḍī*.

12–13 (5K)

At the beginning there may be sweat,
In the middle there is shaking,
At the ultimate stage, one obtains stability,
Therefore, one should control the breath.

One should practice rubbing the limbs,
With the sweat born from exertion.
Indeed by that, steadiness,
And lightness of the limbs arise.

14 (21H)

In the initial period of practice,
Eating milk and ghee is recommended.
Then, when practice has become steady,
Grasping on to such a rule is not necessary.

15 (5L)

Just as a lion, elephant, or tiger
May gradually be tamed.
So, in that way, the breath should be attended to,
Otherwise, it destroys the practitioner.

16 (12M)

Through appropriate *prāṇāyāma*,
There may be the waning of all diseases.
But through the improper practice of yoga,
There is the arising of all diseases.

37 (9M)

"By *prāṇāyāma* alone,
All impurities dry up."
And saying thus, other cleansing actions,
Are not approved of by some teachers.

## Chapter 3

2 (7H)

When the sleeping Kuṇḍalinī,
Is awakened by the grace of the guru.
Then, all the lotuses and even the knots,
Are split open.

55 (11L)

By this practice, the breath is bound in the *suṣumnā nāḍī*,
From which it flies upward.
Therefore, by yogīs this *bandha* is called,
By the name *uḍḍīyana*, "to fly upward."

58 (17H)

*Uḍḍīyānabandha* is always natural,
When taught by a guru.
One who might practice constantly,
Even if old, becomes young.

82 (12E)

Wrinkles and even gray hair,
Are not seen after six months.
But one who may practice every day for three hours,
Surely conquers death.

## Chapter 4

2 (12F)

Now, at this moment, I will teach,
The best method for attaining *samādhi*.
It is the destroyer of death, the means to happiness,
And the best creator of the bliss of *Brahman*.

21 (11H)

By whom the breath is bound,
By that person, alone, the mind is bound.

And by whom the mind is bound,
By that person, the breath is bound.

## *Īśopaniṣat*

7 (20E)

When, in the Soul of one who knows,
His very Soul has become all beings.
What delusion, what sorrow can there be,
There, in the Soul, of one seeing this oneness?

## *Kaṭhopaniṣaṭ*

### Chapter 1

1–3 (16D)

Uśan, son of Vājaśravas, gave away all of his wealth. He had a son named Naciketas.
Being a youth, while the cows given as a donation to the priest were being led away,
Faith penetrated him. And he thought:

"Whose water has been drunk, whose grass has been eaten,
Whose milk has been milked, who are barren.
Those worlds are called joyless,
To which one goes, giving these cows."

So he asked his father, "Father, to whom will you give me?"
He asked a second time and a third time. His father finally answered, "I will give you to Death!"

11 (16N)

Just as before, in the future, he will be pleased,
Auḍḍālaki Āruṇi is set free by me.
He, your father, will rest comfortably at night, his anger departed,
Having seen you, released from the jaws of Death.

27 (20B)

Not by wealth can a person be satisfied,
Will we obtain wealth if we have seen you?
We shall live only as long as you allow,
So this, alone, is the wish to be chosen by me.

### Chapter 2

4–5 (17M)

Far apart, contrary, and going in different directions are these two,
Ignorance and what is known as knowledge.
I think Naciketas is one desiring knowledge,
Many desires do not bewilder you.

Dwelling in ignorance,
Wise in their own minds, considering themselves learned,
Fools go around, running in all directions.
Like a group of blind people, led by one who is blind.

9 (20F)

This idea cannot be obtained by reasoning,
But when taught by another, it is easy to understand, dearest one.
You have reached it! You who hold fast to truth.
May there be for us a questioner like you, Naciketas.

17 (17J)

This is the foundation that is best,
This is the highest foundation.
Knowing this foundation,
One is joyous in the world of *Brahman*.

### Chapter 3

5–6 (13H)

But one who lacks discernment,
With mind always disengaged.

That person's senses are disobedient,
Like bad horses of a charioteer.

But one who possesses discernment,
With mind always engaged.
That person's senses are obedient,
Like good horses of a charioteer.

### Chapter 6

5 (16O)

Just as in a mirror, so in the Soul,
Just as in a dream, so in the world of the ancestors.
Just as in water something is seen, so in the world of the celestial musicians,
As in shadows and light, so in the world of *Brahman*.

18 (20L)

Then, Naciketas, taught by Death,
Having received this knowledge and all the rules of yoga,
Attained *Brahman*, and became free from dust and death,
Thus will others, too, who have this understanding of Soul.

## *Kṛṣṇāṣṭakam*

1 (4A)

I bow to Lord Kṛṣṇa, son of Vasudeva,
Destroyer of Kaṃsa and Cāṇūra.
The greatest joy of Devakī,
The spiritual guru of the universe.

## *Mahābhārata*

### Chapter 12

289.12 (9N)

And just as big fish, cutting through a net,
Return to water again.

In that same way, yogīs, freed from impurities,
Reach that state of liberation.

### *Praśnopaniṣat*

2.12 (10B)

Your form that resides in speech,
Your form in hearing and in seeing,
Your form extended in the mind,
Make them auspicious! Do not go away!

### *Rāmāyaṇa*

#### Chapter 1

8–9 (13O)

Born in the lineage of Ikṣvāku,
By the name Rāma, he is celebrated by the people.
He is self-controlled and has great strength,
Resplendent, steadfast, and masterful.

He is wise and prudent,
Eloquent and charming, destroying his enemies.
Broad-shouldered and great-armed,
His neck is like a conch shell, his jaws are mighty.

41–42 (16B)

But not paying attention to Mārīca's words,
Rāvaṇa, impelled by Fate,
Then went together with Mārīca,
To the hermitage of Rāma.

With the help of that expert in illusion,
Leading the two sons of the king far away,
He carried away the wife of Rāma,
Having killed the vulture, Jaṭāyu.

56–59 (16M)

And that best of monkeys,
Assembling all the monkeys,
Sent them out in all directions,
With the desire to find the daughter of Janaka.

Then, following the advice of the vulture Sampāti,
The powerful Hanumān,
Leaped over the saltwater ocean,
A hundred leagues broad.

Arriving there at the city of Laṅkā,
Guarded by Rāvaṇa,
He saw Sītā, sadly contemplating,
In a grove of *aśoka* trees.

Presenting Sītā with a token of recognition,
And telling her all the news,
And after comforting Vaidehī,
He smashed the arched doorway.

64–65 (16G)

Then, going together with Sugrīva,
To the bank of the great ocean.
Rāma made the ocean tremble,
With arrows, shining like the sun.

And the ocean, lord of the rivers,
Revealed himself.
And listening to the advice of the ocean,
Rāma had Nala build him a bridge.

2.17 (19B)

Bound in quarters, with an equal number of syllables,
Capable of melting the strings of the heart.
This utterance that came forth when I was afflicted with sorrow,
Shall be called poetry, and nothing else.

## *Ṛg Veda*

### 7.59.2, *Mahāmṛtyuṃjaya Mantra* (21B)

We worship the three-eyed Śiva,
Whose sweet fragrance nourishes our growth.
Just like the cucumber is released from its stalk when it ripens,
Free me from attachment and death, don't keep me from immortality.

## *Śivapañcākṣarīstotram* 1 (12D)

Yogīs meditate on the eternal sacred syllable *Oṃ*,
Endowed with a mystical dot.
Fulfilling desires and bestowing freedom,
Salutations to the sacred syllable *Oṃ*.

## *Śivasaṃhitā*

### Chapter 1

4–5 (7J)

Some praise truth,
And others austerity and purity.
Some praise patience,
And others equanimity and honesty.

Some praise charity,
And others rites for the ancestors.
Some praise action,
Others absolute detachment.

15 (7K)

These and various other different conceptions,
Have been taught by sages,
In sacred texts.
Surely, they create confusion in people.

39–40 (12O)

Just as the illusory snake disappears,
Because of knowledge of the rope.
So the illusory perception of this world disappears,
Because of knowledge of the Soul.

Just as this mistaken perception of silver disappears,
Because of knowledge of the pearl oyster, indeed,
So this mistaken perception of the world always disappears,
Because of knowledge of the Soul.

61 (8L)

The exteriors of all living beings,
Go to destruction, in the course of time.
But the Soul, for which words do not exist,
Is free from duality.

75–76 (13C)

Space has the attribute of sound,
Air moves to and fro and has the attribute of touch.
Fire has the attribute of form,
Water has the attribute of taste.

Earth has the attribute of smell,
It is certainly not otherwise.
Certain qualities manifest,
For which reason it is a settled rule from sacred texts.

79 (11J)

Form is grasped by the eye,
Smell is grasped by the nose,
Taste is grasped by the tongue,
And touch by nothing but the skin.
Sound is grasped by the ear,
This is surely how it exists and not otherwise.

## Chapter 2

23 (4E)

There, in the form of a creeping vine of lightning,
Is the great goddess, Kuṇḍalinī.
Coiled three and a half times,
Subtle, resembling a snake.

25–26 (4G)

The *nāḍī* which is named Iḍā,
Is situated on the left-hand path.
Clinging to the central channel,
Connected to the left nostril.

The *nāḍī* which is named Piṅgalā,
Is situated on the right-hand path.
Clinging to the *suṣumṇā nāḍī*,
She is connected to the right nostril.

41 (10D)

Whatever is seen in the world,
That all arises from actions.
According to all of its actions,
A living being experiences the results.

## Chapter 3

8 (15P)

There are five winds, beginning with *nāga*,
And these create in the body:
Belching, opening the eyes, hunger, and thirst,
Yawning and hiccups is the fifth.

10 (7A)

Now I shall quickly teach some guidelines,
For the sake of fulfillment in yoga.

Yogīs, knowing this,
Do not become disheartened in the practice of yoga.

19–20 (15C)

The first sign of fulfillment,
Is the confidence that one's practice will bear fruit.
The second is being absorbed in faith,
The third is honoring one's guru.

The fourth is a state of equanimity,
The fifth is holding fast the sense organs.
And the sixth is a measured diet,
The seventh does not really exist.

30 (14D)

Signs in the body of the yogī,
Are seen from the purification of the *nāḍīs*.
These signs in the body will be explained by me,
Completely and concisely.
The yogī has straight posture, is sweet smelling, very beautiful,
And a vessel for the nectar of the gods.

33 (14E)

The yogī has strong digestive fire, eats well,
Is happy and beautiful in all the limbs.
With a heart that is completely full,
And endowed with great energy and strength.
All these signs will certainly arise,
In the body of a yogī.

34 (8N)

Now I shall explain what is to be avoided,
The greatest obstacles to yoga.
By means of which yogīs can proceed,
Crossing the ocean of the suffering of cyclic existence.

43 (21I)

At the time of practice, at first,
One should eat milk and ghee.
Then, when practice has become steady,
Grasping on to such a rule is not necessary.

101 (15F)

No *āsana* greater than this secret one,
Is to be found on earth.
By merely meditating on it,
The yogī is liberated from misfortune.

## Chapter 4

17 (4B)

From practice, one obtains understanding,
From practice, yoga happens.
From practice, there is fulfillment of *mantras*,
From practice, there is mastery of the breath.

## Chapter 5

41 (14J)

This yoga is to be protected with great care,
It immediately creates faith.
Bestowing liberation in the world,
Beloved to me.

213 (7F)

What is bondage? And whose is liberation?
Indeed, the yogī should always see unity.
One who does this constantly is set free,
Here there is no doubt.
That one, alone, is a yogī, devoted to me,
Honored in all the worlds.

## *Taittirīyopaniṣat*

### Chapter 1

1 (7D)

May Mitra, the Sun God, grant us happiness and well-being.
May Varuṇa, god of the oceans, grant us happiness and well-being.
May Aryaman, who presides over the Milky Way, grant us happiness and well-being.
May Indra, the thunderbolt wielding god of rain,
And Bṛhaspati, lord of prayer and devotion,
Grant us happiness and well-being.
May the far-stepping Viṣṇu, grant us happiness and well-being.
Salutations to *Brahman*, the eternal Spirit.
Salutations to Vāyu, god of the wind.
You alone are the perceptible *Brahman*.
I will declare you alone as the perceptible *Brahman*.
I will declare you as divine law.
I will declare you as truth.
May that protect me.
May that protect the speaker.
Protect me!
Protect the speaker!
*Oṃ*, Peace, Peace, Peace!

11 (20N)

Having taught the Vedas, the teacher then advises the student:
"Speak the truth.
Act with justice.
Do not neglect your studies.
Having given to the teacher a valuable gift,
Do not cut off the line of descendants.

Truth is not to be neglected.
Justice is not to be neglected.
Your welfare is not to be neglected.
Your prosperity is not to be neglected.

Your study and teaching are not to be neglected.
Actions for the gods and the ancestors are not to be neglected.

Treat your mother as a god.
Treat your father as a god.
Treat your teacher as a god.
Treat your guest like a god.
Those actions which are irreproachable, those are to be followed.
Not any others.
Those virtuous actions of mine, those are to be esteemed by you.
Not any others.
One who is more distinguished among the learned, is to be comforted with a seat by you.

Give with faith.
Do not give without faith.
Give with dignity.
Give with modesty.
Give with fear.
Give with understanding.

Now, if you ever have uncertainty about your actions or uncertainty about your practices,
If there should be learned people who are able to judge,
Who are experienced, accredited, gentle, and justice loving.
Just as they might act in those circumstances,
So, too, you should act.

And with respect to those accused falsely,
If there should be learned people who are able to judge,
Who are experienced, accredited, gentle, and justice loving.
Just as they might act in those circumstances,
So, too, you should act.

This is the rule.
This is the teaching.
This is the hidden meaning of the Vedas.
This is the instruction.

Thus it is to be respected.
Thus you should respect it in this way."

12 (20C)

May Mitra, the Sun God, grant us happiness and well-being.
May Varuṇa, god of the oceans, grant us happiness and well-being.
May Aryaman, who presides over the Milky Way, grant us happiness and well-being.
May Indra, the thunderbolt wielding god of rain,
And Bṛhaspati, lord of prayer and devotion,
Grant us happiness and well-being.
May the far-stepping Viṣṇu, grant us happiness and well-being.
Salutations to *Brahman*, the eternal Spirit.
Salutations to Vāyu, god of the wind.
You alone are the perceptible *Brahman*.
I declared you alone as the perceptible *Brahman*.
I declared you as divine law.
I declared you as truth.
May that have protected me.
May that have protected the speaker.
May I have been protected!
May the speaker have been protected!
*Oṃ*, Peace, Peace, Peace!

2.1 (7C)

May it protect us both together,
May it nourish us both together.
May we work together with vigor,
May our study be illuminating.
May we be free from discord.
*Oṃ* Peace, Peace, Peace!

4.1 (21D)

Who is most excellent among sacred hymns, manifold,
Born from sacred hymns, who arose from beyond the immortal.
That is Indra.
May he bestow me with intelligence,

May I keep a memory of the immortal, O God.
May my body be very active,
May my tongue be rich in honey,
May I hear abundantly with my ears.
You are the sheath of *Brahman*,
Covered with intelligence.
Protect what I have heard.

## *Vivekamārtaṇḍa*

8 (10G)

There are as many *āsanas*,
As species of living beings.
All of these different varieties,
The Great Lord Śiva knows.

55 (10F)

Very rich, sweet food,
Leaving the fourth quarter empty.
It is said that one who eats a moderate diet,
Eats well-flavored food for the sake of satisfaction.

66 (11Q)

One is not tormented by sorrow,
One is not smeared by action.
One is not oppressed by Death,
Who knows *khecarī mudrā*.

108 (21G)

The yogī, seated in *baddhāpadmāsana*,
Having bowed to the guru Śiva.
Alone, gazing at the tip of his nose,
Should practice *prāṇāyāma*.

112 (8M)

By *āsana*, disease is destroyed,
By *prāṇāyāma*, vice.

By *pratyāhāra*, the yogī is freed of,
Disturbances of the mind.

### *Yogabīja*

148–49 (12P)

From uniting the breath in the *suṣumnā nāḍī*, the western path,
Clear knowledge arises.
The sun is indicated by the syllable "*ha*,"
The moon by the syllable "*ṭha*."

From the union of the sun and the moon,
"*Haṭhayoga*" is so named.
By *haṭhayoga*, apathy is devoured,
The origin of all disease.

### *Yogāñjalisāram*

32 (10K)

Bind the breath, rejoice in life,
Place the mind in the supreme in the heart.
The yogī Tirumalai Krishnamacharya,
Teaches this saying, which is known as his message.

### *Yogarahasya*

#### Chapter 1

21 (11K)

If, abandoning this sequence,
One practices according to desire.
For this person, the attainment of fruits will not arise,
By the practice of *aṣṭāṅgayoga*.

32–33 (14Q)

Then, having ascertained what is suitable,
The means are explained by the teacher.

The *āsanas* to be practiced, have been taught by the seers,
According to people's differences.

At the time of practice,
Exhalation, inhalation, and retention, always,
Should be done slowly, according to one's capacity,
By means of the *ujjāyī* method.

39 (14F)

People who are ill, even though they might be wealthy,
Or kings, or even very wise.
Will not at any time obtain,
Peace of mind on this earth.

## *Yogasūtra*

### Chapter 1

1 (12A)

Now, there is instruction on yoga.

3 (6D)

Then there is stability of the Seer in its own true nature.

5 (5F)

The fluctuations of the mind are fivefold and are afflicted or unafflicted.

13 (5G)

Among those, practice is the effort toward stability.

36 (13I)

Or there is clarity of mind, when free from sorrow and luminous.

### Chapter 2

29 (11D)

The eight limbs are restraints, observances, postures, breath control, withdrawal of the senses, concentration, meditation, and meditative absorption.

42 (12J)

From contentment, there is the attainment of happiness that is unsurpassed.

46 (11E)

The *āsana* should be steady and comfortable.

### Chapter 3

23–24 (15K)

By *saṃyama* on friendliness and such things, strengths are attained.
By *saṃyama* on strengths, one attains the strength of an elephant, and so forth.

30 (17E)

By *saṃyama* on the hollow of the throat, there is the cessation of hunger and thirst.

## *Yogatattvopaniṣat*

3–4 (16A)

The Grandfather, Brahmā, honoring Viṣṇu, the Lord of the universe,
And bowing respectfully to him,
Asked him, "Tell me the true nature of yoga,
Together with its eight limbs."

Viṣṇu, the lord of the senses, answered him:
"Listen, I will tell you truly.
All living beings are enveloped with happiness and suffering,
Through the net of illusion."

14–16 (12Q)

Therefore, I will teach you the means,
For the purpose of removing these disturbances.
Without yoga, how can there be knowledge,
Which surely bestows liberation.

But yoga, without knowledge, is not enough,
As an action leading toward liberation.

Therefore, one desiring freedom,
Should steadily practice both yoga and knowledge.

From ignorance, alone, there is the cycle of worldly existence,
From knowledge, alone, one is freed.
In the beginning, one's natural state is knowledge,
Knowledge is the one practice to be known.

71 (9K)

Whatever taste he savors with the tongue,
May he consider that to be the Soul.
Whatever the yogī might touch with the skin,
May he consider that to be the Soul.

134cd–136ab (15A)

Three worlds, three Vedas,
Three junctures of the day, three sounds.

Three fires and three *guṇas*,
Everything is resting in the three letters.
One who understands even a half syllable,
Among these three letters.

By that person, this whole universe is strung.
This is the truth. This is the highest state.

## *Yogavāsiṣṭha*

2.14.22 (21F)

The light born from that which has been discerned,
Is able to cool everything in the body,
And to decorate completely,
Just as moonlight ornaments the earth.

2.16.10 (10C)

For one who has been bathed,
By the cool and bright river Gaṅgā, meeting place of sages.

What is the need for giving donations? What is the use of pilgrimages?
What is the need for austerities? What is the use of sacrifices?

## *Yogayājñavalkya*

### Chapter 1

20 (18L)

Looking at me, with a gracious nature,
Brahmā spoke about knowledge and action:
There are two paths of knowledge to be investigated,
As taught by the Vedas.

43 (13D)

Know that knowledge is composed of yoga,
And yoga consists of eight limbs.
It is said that yoga is the union,
Of the individual Soul and the universal Spirit.

46–49 (4F)

यमश्च नियमश्चैवासनं च तथैव च ।
प्राणायामस्तथा गार्गि प्रत्याहारश्च धारणा ॥

ध्यानं समाधिरेतानि योगाङ्गानि वरानने ।
यमश्च नियमश्चैव दशधा संप्रकीर्तितः ॥

आसनान्युत्तमान्यष्टौ त्रयं तेषूत्तमोत्तमम् ।
प्राणायामस्त्रिधा प्रोक्तः प्रत्याहारश्च पंचधा ॥

धारणा पंचधा प्रोक्ता ध्यानं षोढा प्रकीर्तितम् ।
त्रयं तेषूत्तमं प्रोक्तं समाधिस्त्वेकरूपकः ॥

*Yama* and *niyama*,
And likewise *āsana*.
*Prāṇāyāma*, too, O Gārgī,
*Pratyāhāra* and *dhāraṇā*.

*Dhyāna* and *samādhi*,
These are the limbs of yoga, O lovely-faced woman.
*Yama* and *niyama* are both,
Designated as tenfold.

There are eight excellent *āsanas*,
And among those three are most excellent.
*Prāṇāyāma* is threefold, it is taught,
And *pratyāhāra* is fivefold.

*Dhāraṇā* is said to be fivefold,
*Dhyāna* is sixfold, it is explained.
Among those, three are declared most important,
But *samādhi* has only one form.

2.15cd–16 (12I)

And a mantra uttered in a low voice,
Is said to be a thousand times more powerful than loud mantra repetition.

However, similarly, mental recitation,
Is said to be a thousand times more powerful than a mantra uttered in a low voice.
And, likewise, meditation,
Is said to be a thousand times better than mental recitation.

4.49 (15G)

Among these *prāṇas*, these two are the most important,
*Prāṇa* and *apāna*, O Gārgī, best among women.
And of the two, *prāṇa* is most important,
For all living beings, always.

12.33 (15Q)

Subtler than the subtle, vaster than the vast,
The Soul is entrusted in the heart of this living being.
Look at that which is beyond desire, with clear understanding,
And at the time of death, you will be free from sorrow.

# ABBREVIATIONS

| | |
|---|---|
| abl. | ablative |
| acc. | accusative |
| caus. | causative |
| dat. | dative |
| denom. | denominative |
| desid. | desiderative |
| du. | dual |
| f. | feminine |
| gen. | genitive |
| ind. | indeclinable |
| inst. | instrumental |
| loc. | locative |
| m. | masculine |
| mfn. | masculine, feminine, or neuter |
| n. | neuter |
| nom. | nominative |
| p. | person |
| pass. | passive |
| pl. | plural |
| sg. | singular |
| voc. | vocative |

# Glossary

Note that numbers after each entry refer to the chapter(s) in which the word is first referenced. Sometimes a word is introduced in more than one chapter with variant meanings, in which case the glossary will reference multiple chapters.

अंशः m. a share, portion, shoulder 10, 13
अकर्मन् m. inaction 9
अकृतात्मन् mfn. ignorant, foolish, having an uncontrolled mind 19
अक्रतु mfn. free from desire, beyond understanding 15
अक्लिष्ट mfn. unafflicted, untroubled 5
अक्षन् mfn. the eye 18
अक्षर mfn. imperishable, unchangeable II Rev
अक्षरम् n. letter, syllable 15
अक्षि n. eye 15
अखण्ड mfn. unfragmented 7
अखिल mfn. without a gap, complete, whole 10
अगस्त्यः m. name of a famous sage 6
अग्निः m. fire 4
अग्रम् n. tip, the beginning 4
अग्र्य mfn. foremost 9
अङ्ग ind. a particle implying attention, assent, or desire, and sometimes impatience, "Now, come on . . ." 20
अङ्गम् n. limb, the body 11, 14
अङ्गीकृत mfn. "made a limb," assented to, recommended 21
अचल mfn. motionless, steady, not moving 7, 11
अचिरात् ind. not long, soon 13
अचेतस mfn. unconscious, unthinking, insensible 19
अजयः m. defeat 11
अजस्रम् ind. always, constantly, perpetually, forever 12
अजिनम् n. the hairy skin of a black antelope, skin (of an animal) 10, 21
अज्ञानम् n. ignorance 10
अञ्जनम् n. kohl, kajal, black pigment applied to eyelashes 7
अणिमन् n. the smallest particle, finest essence 17

अणु mfn. minute, small, subtle 15
अतस् ind. than this 15
अतः ऊर्ध्वम् ind. from then forward II Rev
अतः परम् ind. from this point forward, henceforth 7
अतन्द्रित mfn. free from lassitude, unwearied, vigilant, alert, not lazy 9
अति ind. beyond, too much, excessive (used as a prefix) 13
अतिग्राहः m. overgrasper, object of an organ of apprehension 17
अतिजन mfn. "beyond men," uninhabited 21
अति√वृत् 1Ā, to pass beyond 17
अतिवृद्ध mfn. very old 9
अतीव ind. exceedingly II Rev
अत्यन्तम् ind. absolutely, completely 21
अत्य्√अश् 1Ā, to eat too much 13
अत्याहारः m. eating too much 3
अत्र ind. here 7
अथ ind. then, also, now (a particle used at the beginning, mostly as a sign of auspiciousness) 6, 8
अथितिः m. guest 5
√अद् 2P, to eat 8
अदस् mfn. that 17
अदारञ्च् mfn. southern, below 21
अद्भुत mfn. extraordinary, supernatural, wonderful, marvelous 20
अद्रिः m. mountain 5, 9
अद्वेष्टृ mfn. one who has no hatred II Rev
अद्वैतम् n. nonduality 8
अधन mfn. poor, without wealth 5
अधर्मः m. injustice, unrighteousness 3
अधस् ind. below, under 13
अधि ind. above, over, besides 21
अधिक mfn. surpassing, superior, more, additional, excellent 14
अधिकतर mfn. greater II Rev
अधिकारः m. authority, right 9
अधि√गम् 1P, to attain 19
अधि√इ 1Ā, to learn, understand 15
अधीत mfn. studied, read, understood 7
अधुना ind. now, at this time 7
अध्यर्ध mfn. having an additional half, one and a half 15
अध्वरः m. sacrifice 10

अनघ mfn. faultless, sinless 9
अनन्तर mfn. uninterrupted, continuously, immediately following II Rev
अनन्तवत् mfn. eternal, infinite III Rev
अनन्द mfn. joyless, cheerless 16
अनन्य mfn. no other II Rev
अनपेक्ष mfn. indifferent, impartial II Rev
अनर्घ्य mfn. priceless, invaluable I Rev
अनलः m. fire 9
अनवद्य mfn. irreproachable, faultless 20
अनश्नन् mfn. not eating 17
अनसूय / अनसूयु mfn. not spiteful, not envious 13, 15
अनागत mfn. not come, not arrived, future 11
अनामय mfn. free from disease 10
अनायास mfn. ease, absence of exertion 14
अनारम्भः m. noncommencement, nonundertaking 9
अनिकेत mfn. houseless, having no fixed abode II Rev
अनित्य mfn. not everlasting, transient 17
अनिमिषः m. a fish 9
अनिर्देश्य mfn. undefinable II Rev
अनिर्विण्ण mfn. not downcast, depressed, despondent 14
अनुग्रहः m. favor, kindness 21
अनुच्छित्तिः f. indestructibility 20
अनुत्तम mfn. unsurpassed 3
अनुध्यानम् n. meditation 15
अनु√पश् 1P, to look, to perceive 2
अनुप्रभूत mfn. penetrated 17
अनुमानम् n. inference 11
अनु√वच् 2P, to cause to repeat/recite, teach 20
अनु√वद् 1P, to repeat 20
अनु√वृत् 1Ā, to follow 15
अनु√शास् 2P, to teach, advise 20
अनुशासनम् n. instruction 12
अनु√शुच् 1P, to mourn, lament 6
अनुसं√व्रज् 1P, to look after, attend to III Rev
अनु√स्था 1P, to carry out, perform, practice 16
अनु√स्मृ 1P, to remember 7
अनूचान mfn. well versed in the Vedas, knowledgeable 21

अनृतम् n. falsehood, lie 8
अनेक mfn. not one, many 21
अनेकधा ind. in various ways 21
अन्तः m. end, limit, boundary, certainty 13
अन्तर् ind. within, inside 19
अन्तर mfn. interior, in the middle, between 10
अन्तिकम् n. vicinity, proximity, near 9
अन्तेवासिन् m. a pupil who dwells near or in the house of his teacher 20
अन्ध mfn. blind 7, 17
अन्नम् n. food 15
अन्य mfn. other 7
अन्यथा ind. otherwise 5
अन्वित mfn. endowed with, possessed of 14
अन्व्√इष् 1P, to desire, seek 5
अप् f. water 18
अपमान mn. dishonor, disgrace 11
अपर mfn. other, latter, lower 7
अपरिहार्य mfn. unavoidable, inevitable 6
अप√वह् 1P, to carry off, lead away 16
अपानः m. exhalation, downward breath 8, 11
अपायिन् mfn. going 17
अपि ind. even, also, and, moreover 4, 5
अपि√इ 2P, to go to, enter into, join, merge 20, 21
अपुत्र mfn. sonless 5
अपेत mfn. escaped, departed, gone 17
अप्ययः m. entering into, vanishing, absorption, dissolution 9
अप्रमत्त mfn. not careless or inattentive, careful, attentive 9
अप्रिय mfn. disagreeable, unkind 8
अप्सरस् f. nymph 10
अब्धिः m. ocean, receptacle of water 8
अभय mfn. fearless 21
अभावः m. nonexistence
अभिक्रमः m. undertaking, effort 4
अभि√चक्ष् 2Ā, to look at, view, perceive 17
अभिजात mfn. born 8
अभि√ज्ञा 9P, to recognize 18
अभिज्ञानम् n. token of remembrance/recognition 16

अभि√धा 3P, to set forth, explain, declare; pass. to be named or called 11, 12
अभिनद्ध mfn. tied round 21
अभिनहनम् n. a bandage over the eyes, blindfold 21
अभिप्र√स्था 1P, to start or advance toward; caus. to drive (as the cattle to pasture) III Rev
अभिप्र√अस् 4P, to throw 20
अभिसायम् ind. about evening, at sunset III Rev
अभीप्सिन् mfn. wishing for, desirous of obtaining 17
अभ्यन्तर mfn. interior, inside 7
अभ्य√हन् 2P, to strike 17
अभ्याख्यात mfn. accused falsely 20
अभ्यागत mfn. arrived, approaching, imminent 6
अभ्यासः m. practice, repeated practice, study 3, 15
अभ्युत्थानम् n. rising up, emerging 3
अमर्षः m. impatience, indignation II Rev
अमूलम् n. rootless, without a root 18
अमृतत्वम् n. immortality 16
अमृतम् n. immortality, nectar, ambrosia 10, II Rev
अम्बकम् n. an eye 21
अम्बरम् n. clothes, garment 13
अम्बु n. water 18
अम्भस् n. water 13
अम्भोधिः m. ocean 9
अयुक्तः m. one who is not concentrated/yoked/attentive, unsuitable, inappropriate, improper 5, 12
अरण्यम् n. a forest I Rev
अरम्भः m. undertaking, beginning, commencement 8
अरविन्दम् n. lotus 3
अरिः m. enemy 5
अरिष्टनेमिः m. the protector 15
अरे ind. interjection of affection or calling, "my dear" 16, 20
अरोगता f. health, the state of being disease-free 9
अर्जवम् n. honesty 7
अर्जुनः m. hero of the *Bhagavadgītā* 3
अर्णवः m. sea, ocean 15
अर्थः m. purpose, aim, worldly prosperity, object, affair, concern, value 3, 6, 7
अर्ध mfn. half 15

अर्पणम् n. offering, the act of offering, entrusting 9
अर्पित mfn. fixed 7
√अर्ह् 1P, to be able, should, ought 6
अर्हत् m. Jain 9
अलम् ind. able 21
अलंकारः m. ornament 21
अलाभः m. loss 11
अलूक्ष mfn. not hard, soft, gentle 20
√अव् 1P, to protect 7
अव√धा 3P, to place down, plunge into, deposit 20
अवबोधः m. awakening 17
अव√मृश् 6P, to touch, reach for 20
अवर mfn. inferior, below 5
अवलोकिनी f. looking 12
अवश mfn. not having one's free will, doing something against one's desire, unwillingly 17
अवश्य mfn. disobedient 13
अवश्यम् ind. inevitably, certainly, by all means 14
अव√सद् 1P, to sink down, become disheartened 7
अव√स्था 1P, to remain standing 6
अवस्थानम् n. residing, dwelling, stability 6
अवस्थित mfn. standing near 17
अव√आप् 5P, to attain, obtain 11
अविद्या f. ignorance 4
अविनाशिन् mfn. imperishable 20
अव्यक्त mfn. unmanifest 14
अव्यय mfn. imperishable, undecaying, eternal 13
√अश् 5Ā, to eat, enjoy, obtain 9
अशक्त mfn. unable, incapable II Rev
अशनम् n. eating 14
अशान्तः m. one who is unpeaceful 5
अशीर्य mfn. indestructible 21
अशुभ mfn. unpleasant, disagreeable II Rev; n. inauspiciousness, misfortune 15
अश्रु n. tears 18
अश्वः m. horse 13
अश्वत्थः m. the holy fig tree 13
अष्टन् mfn. eight 15

√अस् 2P, to be 2
असक्त mfn. unattached 16
असत् n. nonexistence, the unreal, untruth 10
असमर्थ mfn. unable, incapable II Rev
असंमूढ mfn. not confused 12
असंशयम् ind. without doubt, undoubtedly 3, 7
असिः m. sword 17
असित mfn. unbound 21
असिद्धिः f. failure 11
असुरः m. demon 20
असुरी f. demonic 8
अहन् n. day 18
अहम् mfn. I 2
अहंकारः m. "I-maker," egotism 13
अहिः m. snake 21
अहिंसा f. nonviolence 4

आकारः m. form, shape, appearance, figure 4, 7
आकाशः m. ether, sky 3
आख्य mfn. named, called (at the end of compounds) 10
आगत mfn. come, arrived 5
आ√गम् 1P, to come 2
आगम mfn. coming, approaching 17
आगमः m. verbal testimony 11
आ√चम् 1P, to sip, to sip water from the palm of the hand for purification 6
आ√चर् 1P, to act, undertake, practice, perform 15
आचार्यः m. teacher 6
आज्यम् n. clarified butter, ghee 21
आतपः m. sunshine, light 16
आतुर mfn. suffering, diseased, or pained by 8
आत्मज mfn. born from oneself, son, daughter 16
आत्मता f. Soul, Soul-ness, Self-hood 17
आत्मन् m. the Soul, individual Soul, Self 9
आदर्शः m. a looking glass, mirror 16
आदिकर्तृ m. the original Creator 15
आदित्यः m. the sun 6
आ√दृ 1Ā, to regard with attention, attend to, be careful about 16

आदेशः m. rule, symbolic rule, instruction 20
आदौ in the beginning, at first 12
आद्य mfn. first 13
आ√धा 1Ā, to place II Rev
आधारः m. support, vessel, receptacle 13, 14
आनकः m. drum 6
आनन्दः m. happiness, joy, delight 4
आ√नी 1P, to lead toward or near, bring 21
आन्त mfn. end, settlement 16
√आप् 5P, to get, obtain 9
आपद् f. calamity, misfortune, danger 19
आपनेय mfn. to be obtained, reached 20
आ√पॄ 9U, to fill up 17
आबाहु mf. up to the arms 17
आम mfn. unbaked 13
आ√मन्त्र् 10Ā, to speak, say III Rev
आयतनम् n. resting place, home, support 18
आयतनवत् mfn. having a seat or home or support III Rev
आयुक्त mfn. accredited 20
आयुस् n. life 10
आरम्भः m. beginning, commencement, undertaking 9
आ√राध् 5P, to honor, worship, propitiate 16
आरामः m. delight, pleasure 19
आ√रुह् 1P, to ascend, mount, climb, attain 17
आरोग्यम् n. absence of disease, health 19
आर्त mfn. afflicted, pained, disturbed 19
आलम्बनम् n. foundation, support 17
आलस्यम् n. laziness, idleness 10
आ√लोक् 1Ā, to look at 18
आवली f. a range 9
आवह mfn. brings, produces 15
आ√विश् 6P, to enter, approach; caus. to cause to enter or approach II Rev
आवृत mfn. covered, surrounded, enveloped 5
आवेशित mfn. entered into II Rev
आशा f. hope, expectation, wish 16
आशु ind. quickly, immediately, directly 4
आश्चर्यवत् ind. wondrously, as a wonder 19

आश्रमपदम् n. a hermitage 16
आ√श्रि 1P, to inhabit, dwell in, reside, exist in 11
आश्रित mfn. resorting to II Rev
आ√श्वस् 2P, to breathe again, calm, console 16
√आस् 2Ā, to sit 8
आसक्त mfn. attached to II Rev
आसनम् n. posture, seat 3
आसाद्य mfn. attainable, to be attained 13
आ√स्था 1P, to undertake, perform, practice 19
आहारः m. food 10

√इ 2P, to go 8
इक्ष्वाकुः m. first king of the solar dynasty, son of Manu Vaivasvata 13
√इङ्ग् 1U, to move or agitate, flicker 13
इच्छा f. desire, wish, endeavor II Rev
इज्या f. sacrifice, ritual 18
इतरद् n. other 12
इति ind. quotative particle, "thus" 5, 9
इदम् mfn. this 17
इदानीम् now, at this moment 12
इन्दुः m. moon 5
इन्द्रः m. Vedic lord of the gods, god of rain, who wields a thunderbolt 7
इन्द्रियम् n. sense, sense organ, faculty of sense 3, 10
इव ind. like, as, in the same manner as, just as 3
√इष् 6P, to desire, wish for 14
इह ind. here, to this place, in this world 4, 5, 7

√ईक्ष् 1Ā, to see 4
ईदृश् mfn. endowed with such qualities, such 7
√ईर् 10U, utter, pronounce, proclaim 17
√ईश् 2Ā, to command, allow 20
ईशः m. lord, ruler 13

उक्त mfn. spoken, taught 9
उक्तवाक्यम् n. sayings I Rev
उग्र mfn. powerful, mighty, formidable 17
उच्च mfn. high, elevated 11

उच्चैस् ind. loud 12
उच्छ्रित mfn. raised up, high, tall 10
उज्जायी f. victorious breath 14
उड्√डी 4Ā, to fly up, soar 11
उड्डीयनः / उड्डीयानः m. abdominal energy lock 11
उत ind. and, even, indeed, could it be that 21
उत्तम mfn. best, greatest, highest, end, ultimate stage 4, 5
उत्तरम् n. the upper surface or cover 10
उत्तान mfn. stretched out, lying on the back 5
उत्√पत् 1P, to jump 15
उत्पतित mfn. sprung up, arisen 15
उत्√सद् 1P, to sink down, fall into ruin or decay 18
उत्√सृज् 6P, to let loose, pour forth 10
उत्साहः m. effort, perseverance 3
उदकम् n. water 7, 16
उदञ्च् mfn. northern, above 21
उदधिः m. the ocean 16
उदपान mn. a well 7
उदयः m. rise up, increase 9
उदरम् n. belly, stomach, abdomen 9
उदार mfn. great, noble 15
उदासीन mfn. sitting apart, indifferent, neutral, open-minded II Rev
उदित mfn. born, produced 21
उद्गारः m. belching 15
उद्दिश्य ind. with regard to, for the sake of 5
उद्√धृ 1P, to raise up, uplift 9
उद्√विज् 1Ā, to tremble, fear, shrink from II Rev
उद्वेगः m. agitation, anxiety II Rev
उद्√स्था 1P, to stand up, arise 19
उन्√मिष् 6P, to open the eyes 13
उन्मीलनम् n. opening the eyes, raising the eyelids 15
उन्मीलित mfn. opened 7
उपकरणवत् mfn. furnished with means 16
उप√जन् 4Ā, to be born or produced, originate, arise 4
उपदिष्ट mfn. taught 14
उपदेशः m. teaching 20
उप√निपत् 1P, to fly down III Rev

उपनिषद् f. sitting down at the feet of another to listen to their words, secret knowledge, hidden meaning 20
उप√नी 1P, to initiate III Rev
उप√पद् 1Ā, to be suitable, possible, fit 20
उपमा f. comparison, simile 13
उप√रम् 1U, to give up, renounce 13
उप√रुध् 7P, to lock in, shut up III Rev
उप√लिप् 6P, to defile, besmear 19
उप√विश् 6P, to sit down 6
उपशान्तम् n. pacifying, quelling, tranquillity, peace 13
उप√श्रि 1P, to lean against, go toward 19
उपसमा√धा 3P, to kindle (a fire) III Rev
उपसं√पद् 1Ā, to come to, arrive at 21
उप√हन् 2P, to destroy 18
उपा√गम् 1P, to come near, approach 6
उपादानम् n. material cause 7
उपांशुः m. a prayer/mantra uttered in a low voice 12
उपायः m. means, expedient 10
उप√आस् 1Ā, to honor, worship, meditate on II Rev
उपासितव्य mfn. to be revered, honored, respected 20
उपास्य mfn. to be revered, honored, esteemed 20
उपे = उप√इ 2P, to approach a teacher, become a student III Rev
उपेत mfn. accompanied by, endowed with, possessing II Rev
उभ mfn. both 8
उरुक्रमः m. far-stepping 7
उर्वारुकम् n. cucumber, gourd 21
उशन् m. father of Naciketas, "desirous" 16
उष्ण mn. heat 11

ऊर्ध्व mfn. rising upward, elevated, above 13

ऋतम् n. divine law, custom, truth 7
ऋत्विज् m. priest 8
ऋषभः m. a bull, the best or most excellent of any kind or race 16
ऋषिः m. sage 5

एक mfn. one 7, 15
एकम् n. unity 7

एकता f. oneness, unity 11
एकाकिन् mfn. alone, solitary 21
एकाग्र mfn. one-pointed, concentrated on a single object 7, 10
एकान्तम् ind. absolutely, solely, at all 13
एनम् mfn. him, it, her, this 19
एव ind. only, indeed (particle of emphasis) 3
एवम् ind. thus 6
एवंविध mfn. of such a kind, in such a form or manner 6

ऐश्वर mfn. powerful, majestic 8

ओजस् n. vitality, energy, strength 10
ओम् ind. yes, verily, so be it 15

कण्ठः m. throat 17
कतर mfn. which of two 17
कति ind. how many 15
√कथ् 10P, to tell 2
कथम् ind. how 5
कथा f. story 4
कथित mfn. told, related, taught 7
कदाचन ind. at any time 9
कमल mn. lotus 13
कम्पः m. trembling, shaking 5
कम्बल mn. a woolen blanket 21
कम्बु mn. conch shell 13
कंसः m. king of Mathurā, brother of Devakī 4
करः m. hand, the doer 4
करुणा f. compassion 4
कर्तृ m. doer, maker 6
कर्मन् n. action 9
कर्श्यम् n. thinness 9
कर्षकः m. one who plows, farmer 18
कलत्रम् n. wife I Rev
कला f. one-sixteenth III Rev
कलिलम् n. a large heap, thicket, confusion 16
कलेवर mn. the body 14
कल्मषम् n. stain, dirt, impurity, sin 9

कविः m. poet, seer 5, 15
कश्चिद् ind. someone, anyone 13
√काङ्क्ष् 1P, to desire, lust II Rev
काङ्क्षिन् mfn. desiring, longing for 18
काञ्चनम् n. gold 12
कान्तः mfn. desired, loved, dear I Rev; m. beloved, lover, husband 13
कान्तार mn. large or dreary forest 19
कान्तिः f. loveliness, beauty 14
कापालिकः m. follower of a particular Śaiva sect that carries skulls 9
कामः m. desire 3
कायः m. the body 10
कारः m. a letter or sound 12
कारक mfn. making, doing, creating, who or what produces or creates 5, 14
कारणम् n. cause, means 5, 14
कार्य mfn. to be done I Rev
कार्ष्णायस mfn. made of black iron 21
कालः m. Time, Death, Fate, season, proper time or season 5, 7, 16
कालतः ind. in the course of time 8
कावेरी f. a river in the south 4
किञ्चित् ind. somewhat, a little 13
किम् ind. what, how 3, 5
किल ind. as they say, reportedly 17
कीटः m. worm, insect 11, 18
कुक्कुटः m. rooster 10
कुटिल mfn. curled, coiled 4
कुटीर mn. hut 11
कुण्डली f. Kuṇḍalinī 4
कुतः ind. from where? how can there be? 5
कुमारः m. a child, boy, youth 16
कुम्भः m. jar, pot 13
कुम्भकः m. a pot, stopping the breath 14
कुलाचलः m. mountain 15
कुशः m. a kind of grass considered holy and used in religious ceremonies 10
कुशलम् n. welfare, well-being 20
कूटस्थ mfn. immovable, unchangeable II Rev
कूपः m. well, hollow, throat 11, 17
कूर्मः m. a tortoise 11
√कृ 8U, to do, make 9

कृच्छ्र mn. difficulty, trouble, hardship 19
कृत mfn. done 9
कृत्स्न mfn. all, whole, entire 20
कृपण mfn. pitiable, miserable, wretched 5
कृश mfn. lean, emaciated, feeble III Rev
कृष्णायसम् n. black iron 21
√कृत् 10U, to praise 19
केचित् ind. some 7, 10
केचित् . . . केचित् ind. some . . . others 7
केदारः m. a field or meadow, especially one underwater 18
केवल mfn. only, merely, solely, pure, absolute 10, 14
केवलकुम्भकः m. pure/absolute breath retention 14
केशवः m. Viṣṇu, Kṛṣṇa 3
केषाञ्चित् ind. of some 9
कोशः m. sheath 21
कौन्तेयः m. son of Kuntī, Arjuna 5
कौशलम् n. skillfulness, ease 8
क्रमः m. order, sequence, method 11, 12
क्रिया f. action, practice 5
√क्री 9U, to buy 10
क्रोधः m. anger 3
√क्लिद् 4P, to be wet 10
क्लिष्ट mfn. afflicted, distressed 5
क्लेशः m. affliction II Rev
क्लैब्यम् n. cowardice 20
क्षण mn. an instant, moment 14
क्षम mfn. adequate, enough, appropriate 12
क्षमा f. patience, the earth 6, 7, I Rev
क्षमिन् patient, possessing patience II Rev
क्षयः m. loss, wane, diminution 12
√क्षिप् 6P, to throw 2
क्षिप्रम् ind. quickly 7
क्षीरम् n. milk 21
क्षुद्र mfn. low, base, minute, small 20
क्षुध् f. hunger 17
√क्षुभ् 1Ā, to shake, tremble 16
क्षेत्रम् n. field 3

क्षेमेण ind. easily, with ease 13
क्षोभः m. agitation, disturbance 5

खम् n. ether, space 13
खलु ind. indeed, certainly, as you know 12
√खाद् 1P, to eat 2
खेचर mfn. moving in the air, creature of the air 18
√ख्या 2P, to tell, narrate 8

गङ्गा f. the Ganges River 4
गगनम् n. sky, the atmosphere 13
गजः m. elephant 5
√गण् 10P, to count 2
गणः m. a group 2
गत mfn. gone to, situated in, contained in, connected to, spread 4, I Rev
गतिः f. movement, path 14
गद्यम् n. prose I Rev
गन्तव्य mfn. to be attained 9
गन्धः m. smell, fragrance 11
गन्धर्वः m. a celestial musician 16
गन्धारः m. ancient kingdom 21
√गम् 1P, to go 2
गम्य mfn. approachable, attainable 13
गरीयस् mfn. heavier, greater, preferable 17
गव्य mfn. coming from a cow 3
गाण्डीव mn. name of Arjuna's bow, give to him by Agni 6
गात्रम् n. body, limbs 5
गार्गी f. belonging to the Garga lineage, Yājñavalkya's wife 4
गिरिः m. mountain 5
गुणः m. characteristic, quality, a good quality, virtue 13
गुणिन् mfn. virtuous, one who possesses virtue 14
√गुप् 4P, to hide, conceal, guard, protect, preserve 21
गुरुः m. teacher, heavy 4, 5
गुल्म mn. cluster of trees, thicket, bush 18
गुह्यतमम् n. most hidden, secret 9
गुह्यम् n. secret, mystery 3
गृध्रः m. vulture 16
गृहः m. a house, home I Rev

गेहम् n. a house I Rev
गो mf. bull, cow 18
गोचरः m. range, field for action 14
गोत्रम् n. lineage, family name III Rev
गोदावरी f. a river in the south 4
गोमयम् n. cow dung 12
गोमुखः m. trumpet, "cow-faced" 6
गौरी f. the goddess Parvatī 4
ग्रन्थिः m. knot 7
√ग्रस् 1U, to swallow, devour 12, 17
√ग्रह् 9U, to grasp 10
ग्रहः m. grasper, organ of apprehension 17
ग्रामः m. a multitude, class, collection, village II Rev, 21
ग्रीवः m. the neck 11
ग्लानिर् f. decrease, waning 3

घटः m. large earthen water jar, pot, vessel, the body 7, 19
√घ्रा 3P, to smell 13
घ्राणम् n. nose 11

च ind. and 2
चक्रम् n. wheel, discus 17
चक्षुस् n. eye, seeing 2, 10
चञ्चल mfn. moving to and fro, unsteady, shaky 13
चतुर् mfn. four 13, 15
चतुर्थ mfn. the fourth 10
चरण mn. foot 17
चराचरम् n. all created things, moving and unmoving, the world 7
चल mfn. moving, unsteady, fluctuating 3, 14
चलित mfn. tremulous 9
चाणूरः m. a wrestler in Kaṃsa's service, slain by Kṛṣṇa 4
चाप mn. a bow 6
चारु mfn. pleasing, lovely, beautiful I Rev
चार्वाकः m. follower of Cārvāka, a philosopher who propounded materialism 9
चिकीर्षु mfn. intending to do, desiring to make 16
चित् f. understanding, true knowledge, consciousness 17
चित्तम् n. mind, consciousness, thought, thinking 3, 17
चित्र mfn. excellent, manifold I Rev

√चिन्त् 10P, to think, contemplate 2
चिन्तनम् n. meditation, reflection 12
चिन्ता f. thought, care, anxiety 6
चिरम् ind. for a long time, after a long time 21
चिह्नम् n. mark, sign, characteristic 14
√चुर् 10P, to steal 2
चेत् ind. if I Rev
चेतना f. consciousness, understanding, intelligence 4
चेतस् n. mind 10
चैलम् n. a piece of cloth 10
चोदित mfn. urged, impelled, put forward, enjoined, taught 16, 18

छन्दस् n. sacred hymn, Vedic hymn 13
छाया f. shadow 16
√छिद् 7U, to cut, pierce, divide 10, 14

√जक्ष् 2P, to eat, consume 16
जगत् n. the world, universe 4, 8
जठरम् n. stomach, belly, abdomen 9
√जन् 4Ā, to be born 4
जनः m. person, people 3
जननम् n. birth 21
जनाधिपः m. "ruler of people," king 7
जन्तुः m. person 10
जन्मम् n. birth 6
√जप् 1P, to utter in a low voice, mutter 6
जपः m. repetition of a mantra, muttering prayers 12
जयः m. victory 11
जलम् n. water 4, 5
√जागृ 2P, to be awake 8
जाङ्गलिकः/जाङ्गुलिकः m. snake doctor 17
जाङ्गलिकायते denom. to act like a snake doctor 17
जाड्यम् n. apathy, sluggishness, inactivity, dullness, stupidity 12
जात mfn. born, present, existent 5, I Rev; m. one who has been born 6; created 7
जातिः f. species, type, kind 10
जातु ind. ever 7
जालम् n. a net 9
√जि 1P, to conquer 2

जित mfn. controlled, conquered, subdued 13
जिह्वा f. tongue 9
जीर्ण mfn. old, worn-out 10
√जीव् 1P, to live 5
जीवः m. life, individual Soul, living essence, sap 10, 17
जीवनम् n. life 7
जीवात्मन् m. individual Soul 13
जृम्भः m. yawning 15
√जॄ 1, 4U, to grow old, decay 13
√ज्ञा 9U, to know 10
ज्ञानम् n. knowledge 10
ज्ञेय mfn. to be known, to be investigated or understood 12, 18
ज्योतिष्मत् mfn. luminous, possessing light 13
ज्योतिस् n. light, star 5, 10
ज्योत्स्ना f. moonlight 21
√ज्वल् 1P, to burn brightly, blaze 17

तडागः m. tank, pool 11
ततः ind. from that, therefore, then, after that 5, 6
ततः m. father 16
ततः परम् ind. besides that, thereupon, afterward 15
तत्त्वतः ind. truly, really, accurately 16
तत्त्वम् n. real truth, true nature 13
तत्र ind. there, with respect to that, among those 4, 5
तथा ind. so, in that way 4, 5
तथैव ind. similarly, in a like manner 19
तदा ind. then 3, 6
√तन् 8U, to extend, stretch 9
तनुः / तनूः f. body, self, form, manifestation 5, 10
तन्त्री f. wire or string of a lute, strings of the heart, stringed instruments 19
√तप् 1P, to give out heat, shine 10
तपस् n. discipline, burning devotion, austerity 2, 10
√तपस्य 10P, to undergo religious austerities 9
तपस्विन् mfn. one who practices austerities, m. ascetic 14
तमस् n. inertia (one of the three *guṇas* or qualities of mind) 10
तरुः m. tree 5
तर्कः m. reasoning, speculation, inquiry 20
तर्पणीय mfn. to be satisfied 20

तर्हि ind. then, in that case 16
तस्मात् ind. from that, therefore 6
तादृक् ind. in such a manner 21
तार्क्ष्यः m. Garuḍa 18
√तिज् 1U, to be or become sharp; √तितिक्ष् desid. to desire to become sharp, to bear with firmness or courage, endure 17
तिमिरम् n. darkness 7
तिर्यञ्च् mfn. horizontal, diagonal 21
तिलः m. sesame seed 11
तीरम् n. shore, bank 16
तु ind. but 3
√तुद् 6P, to push 2
तुमुल mfn. tumultuous, noisy 6
तुरीय mfn. fourth part 15
तुल्य mfn. equal to I Rev
√तुष् 4P, to be pleased/content 2
तृणम् n. grass 16
तृतीय mfn. third part 15
तृष्णा f. thirst 10
√तॄ 1P, to cross over 8
तेजस् n. splendor, brilliance, fire 10, 13
तेजस्विन् mfn. one who possesses light, brilliant, energetic, powerful, illuminating 14
तैलम् n. sesame oil 11
तोयम् n. water 3
तोरणम् n. arch, arched doorway 16
√त्यज् 1P, to abandon 2
त्यागः m. giving up, abandoning II Rev
त्रयः ind. threefold 4
त्रि mfn. three 15
त्रिधा ind. threefold 4
त्रिर् ind. three times, thrice 6
√त्रै 1Ā, to protect 4
त्वच् f. skin 8
त्वम् mfn. you 2
त्वादृश् mfn. like you 20

दक्ष mfn. right, situated on the right side, able, adroit, dexterous 4, II Rev
दक्षिण mfn. right, southern 21

दक्षिणा f. cows presented as donation to the priest 16
√दम् 4P, to be tamed, subdued, self-controlled 20
दमः m. self-control 20
दंशः m. gadfly, gnat 18
√दय् 1Ā, to be compassionate 20
दया f. compassion 6
दर्दुरः m. frog 15
दर्दुरी f. frog-like 15
दर्शनम् n. looking at, seeing, aspect, appearance, vision 4, 12
दर्शित mfn. shown, revealed
दशधा ind. tenfold, in ten parts 4
दशन् mfn. ten 15
√दह् 1P, to burn 10, 14
दहरः m. the heart 10
√दा 3U, to give 8
दातृ m. giver, donor, generous person 6
दानम् n. the act of giving, generosity, donation I Rev, 10
दायक mfn. giving, granting, bestowing 14
दिदृक्षु mfn. desirous of finding 16
√दिव् 4P, to play 2
दिव्य mfn. divine 8
√दिश् 6P, to show 2
दिश् f. direction 8
दीपः m. a light, lamp, lantern 13
दीपित mfn. set on fire, illuminated, kindled 12
दुःखम् n. suffering 2, 3
दुर्बल mfn. weak 9
दुष्ट mfn. bad
√दुह् 4P, to give milk 16
दुहितृ f. daughter 6
दूर mfn. distant, remote, far, a long way 9, 16
दूरम् ind. far from 17
दूरेण ind. by far 5
दृढ mfn. firm, strong II Rev
दृढता f. firmness, solidity, strength, steadiness 5
दृढम् ind. steadily 12
√दृश् 1P, to see 2
दृष्टिः f. seeing, gaze 5

देवः m. god 3
देवकी f. mother of Kṛṣṇa 4
देवदेवः m. God of gods 7
देवी f. goddess 4
देशः m. place, country 5
देह mn. the body 4, 10
देहवत् m. living creature, man, embodied being, one who identifies with the body II Rev
दैवतम् n. deity, god 6
दैवी f. divine 8
दोषः m. fault, deficiency, defect, disease, the three humors when in a disordered state 5, 12
दोषा f. darkness, night 20
दोहः m. milk 16
दौर्बल्यम् n. weakness, impotence 20
द्युतिः f. splendor, brightness, luster 13
√द्रम् 1P, to wander about 17
द्रविणम् n. wealth 6
द्रष्टृ m. seer, Soul 6
द्वि mfn. two 15
द्विजः m. twice-born, a man of the first three classes, especially a Brahmin (born for the second time after the *upanayana*) 13
द्वितीय mfn. second 13
द्विधा ind. twofold 13
द्विविध mfn. twofold, of two kinds 11
√द्विष् 2U, to hate 8
द्वीप mn. continent, island 15
द्वैतम् n. duality 8

धनम् n. wealth, riches 5
धनंजयः m. name for Arjuna, "conqueror of wealth" 5
धनवत् mfn. wealthy, possessing wealth 13
धनिन् mfn. wealthy, one who possesses wealth 14
धनुस् mn. a bow 10
धन्य mfn. fortunate, happy I Rev
धर mfn. holding, bearing, wearing 13
धर्मः m. right action, duty, practice, discipline, law, nature 3, 4, 8, 20
धर्म्य mfn. just, righteous, fair II Rev

√धा 3U, to put, place, create, make, compose 8
धातुः m. constituent element (seven according to Āyurveda) 3
धातृ m. establisher, supporter 6
धान mfn. holding II Rev
धानी f. receptacle, seat, home 9
धारण mfn. keep in remembrance, memory 21
धारणा f. concentration 4
धी f. understanding, intelligence, wisdom, thought, meditation, prayer 18
धीमत् mfn. intelligent, possessing intelligence 13
धीर mfn. strong-minded, persevering, resolute, steady, composed, calm, intelligent, wise 10, 17
धृतः mfn. resolved 6
धृतिः f. constancy, resolution 13
धेनुः f. cow 5
धैर्यम् n. constancy, calmness, patience 3
ध्मात mfn. blown, fanned 13
ध्यानम् n. meditation 4
√ध्यै 1P, to meditate on, contemplate, think of 12, II Rev
ध्रुव mfn. certain, fixed, immovable, unchangeable, eternal 6, II Rev
ध्रुवम् ind. certainly, surely 8, 12

न no/not 2
नख mn. fingernail. toenail 21
नचिरात् ind. shortly, soon II Rev
नदी f. river 4
√नन्द् 1P, to rejoice, delight, be pleased 10
√नम् 1P, to bow 2
नमः m. a bow, salutations 5
नमस्कारः m. salutation 21
नयनम् n. eye 13
नरः m. man, person 10
नर्मदा f. river 4
नव mfn. new 10
√नश् 4P, to be lost/destroyed 2
नष्ट mfn. lost, destroyed 12
नागः m. one of the five winds of the body 15
नाडी f. subtle channel 4

नाथः m. lord 13
नादः m. internal resonance, sound 11
नानात्यय mfn. various, manifold 18
नाभ mfn. navel 13
नाम ind. by name, called, named 4
नामधेयम् n. a name, title, appellation 21
नामन् n. name 9
नारी f. woman 4
नाशः m. loss, disappearance 4
नाशन mfn. destroying 12
नासिका f. the nose 11
निकृन्तनम् n. an instrument for cutting 21
नि√ग्रह् 9P, to hold back 10
निग्रहः m. restraining, holding fast 15
नित्यम् ind. constantly, continually, always, regularly, steadily 3, 4, 7
निद्रा f. sleep 4
निधनम् n. settling down, residence, end, death 15
निन्दा f. blame, reproach II Rev
निबन्धः m. chain, fetter, bondage 8
निबर्हण mfn. crushing, destroying, removing 13
नि√भल् 10U, to see, perceive 20
नि√मिष् 6P, to close the eyes 13
निम्न mfn. low, deep 11
नियत mfn. restrained, controlled 13
नियतम् ind. always, surely 11
नियमः m. observance 3
निरहंकार mfn. free from egotism, unselfish II Rev
निरामयः m. freedom from disease, health 5
निरिन्द्रिय mfn. barren 16
नि√रुध् 7P, to control, hold back, stop, restrain 14
निरोधः m. restraint, control, stilling, destruction 3
निर्देशः m. description, statement 19
निर्भय mfn. free from fear 5
निर्मम mfn. unselfish, free from worldly attachment II Rev
निर्मलत्वम् n. stainlessness, clearness, purity 10
निर्लिप्तः m. untaintedness, unsmeared, indifference, unobscured awareness 19
निर्वाणम् n. liberation 14

निर्वीर्य mfn. powerless, impotent 14
निर्वेदः m. disgust, loathing, complete indifference to worldly objects 16
निवातम् n. a place sheltered from the wind, calm, stillness 13
निवासः m. dwelling place, abode 15
नि√विद् 2P, to tell, communicate; caus. to offer, present, give, deliver 16
निविद् f. ritual invocation 15
नि√विश् 6Ā, to enter, be fixed on; caus. to put, place, keep 10
नि√वृत् 1Ā, to disappear, be ineffective, vanish, not exist 8
नि√शम् 4 P, to hear 21
निशा f. night 8
निश्चयः m. resolution, fixed intention 3
निश्चल mfn. motionless, steady 7
निःश्रेयसम् mn. ultimate refuge, final beatitude, having no better, best, most excellent 17
निष्क्रान्तिः f. going out, departure 7
नि√ष्ठा 1U, to fix in, give forth, emit, yield 18
निहित mfn. placed, situated, entrusted 15
नीच mfn. low 10
नीतिः f. conduct, propriety, prudence 13
नु ind. so now, indeed (indicates a question) 16
नूनम् ind. now, at present 21
√नृत् 4P, to dance 2
नृपः m. king 8
नेतृ m. leader 6
नैकधा ind. manifoldly, in various ways 12
नैमिषम् n. a sacred forest 18
नैष्कर्म्यम् n. inactivity, exemption from acts and their consequences 9
न्यायः m. justice, virtue 3

पञ्चन् mfn. five 15
पञ्चतय mfn. fivefold 5
पञ्चधा mfn. fivefold 4
√पठ् 1P, to read, learn, study 2
पणवः m. small drum or cymbal 6
पण्डितः m. wise person, scholar, philosopher, learned, wise 6, 21
√पत् 1P, to fall, to fly 2, 19
पतङ्गः m. moth 18

पतिः m. lord, husband, master, ruler 5, 18
पतित mfn. fallen 3
पत्त्रम् n. leaf 3
पत्नी f. wife 6
पथिन् m. path 18
पदम् n. foot, word, grammar, state 3, 7
पद्म mn. lotus 7
पयस् n. milk 12
पर mfn. highest, supreme, further, higher 5, 7
परतरम् n. higher than, superior 12
परम् ind. highest, supreme, after that, thereupon, simply, nothing but, merely, in a high degree, absolutely, completely 8, 11, 14
परम mfn. highest, best, greatest 4
परमात्मन् m. universal Soul, Supreme Spirit 13
परंतप mfn. enemy-scorcher 12
परम्परा f. succession, tradition 12
पराञ्च् mfn. turned away 21
परिकरः m. attendants, retinue 21
परिचारिणी f. a maid, moving about, attending on, serving III Rev
परिणामः m. change, transformation 19
परि√त्यज् 1P, to leave, abandon, give up 20
परित्यागिन् mfn. renouncing, unattached II Rev
परित्राणम् n. protection 3
परि√भ्रम् 1, 4P to rove, ramble, wander about 18
परिव्राज् m. wandering mendicant 8
परि√शुष् 4P, to dry up, wither 2
परि√ष्वज् 1Ā, to embrace, clasp, nestle 17
परि√इ 2P, to go around, move in a circle 17
परोपकारः m. helping others 3
पर्जन्यः m. rain cloud, god of rain 5
पर्णम् n. leaf 13
पर्यङ्कः m. bed, couch, sofa 8
पर्यव√स्था 1Ā, to become firm or steady 4
पर्युत्सुखि√भू 1P, to become restless 21
पर्युप√आस् 1Ā, to approach respectfully, attend upon, worship, meditate on II Rev
पर्वतः m. mountain 18
पलितम् n. gray hair 12

पवनः m. vital air, breath, wind, "purifier" 9, 11
पवित्रम् m. a means of purification, the purifier 6
पश्चात् ind. westward, afterward 14, 21
पश्चिमतानः m. stretch of the western part of the body, i.e., the back 9
पश्चिम mfn. western 5
√पा 2P, to protect 8
पाण्डवः m. son/descendant of Pāṇḍu 3, 5
पातकम् n. sin, crime, vice 8
पादः m. a quarter, fourth part 3
पापम् n. evil, misfortune, sin 11, 12
पार्थः m. son of Pṛthā, matronymic name for Arjuna 6
पालित mfn. guarded, protected 16
पावकः m. fire 10
पाशः m. chain, fetter, noose 2
पाषाणः m. stone 12
पिंगला f. name of the right-hand *nāḍī* (subtle channel) 4
पिण्डः m. roundish mass or heap, lump 21
पितामहः m. grandfather 6, 16
पितृ m. father 6
पितृलोकः m. world of the ancestors 16
पिपासा f. thirst 17
पिप्पलः m. sacred fig tree 17
पिहित mfn. covered 21
√पीड् 10U, to pain, torment 11
पीत mfn. drunk, sipped 16
पुत्रः m. son 6
पुनः / पुनर् ind. again 9, 20
पुरः ind. in front 8
पुरम् n. city, town 9
पुरस्तात् ind. before, eastward 16, 21
पुरा f. city 16
√पुष् 4P, to be nourished 2
पुष्ट mfn. nourishing 3
पुष्पम् n. flower 3
पुस्तकम् n. book 3
√पू 9U, to purify, sanctify 10
√पूज् 10P, to honor, worship 2, 7

पूजनम् n. honoring 15
पूजित mfn. honored, worshipped, adored 7
पूर्णम् n. full, whole, entire, complete 3
पूर्व mfn. before, eastern 5, 7
पूषन् m. a Vedic deity connected with the Sun, the surveyor of all things 18
पृथिवी f. earth 5
पृथ्वी f. the earth 13
पृष्ट mfn. asked 5
पृष्ठतः ind. behind 8
√पॄ 3P, to fill; caus. to fill with wind, inhale 14
पौत्रः m. grandson 6
पौरुषम् n. manhood 19
प्रकाशक mfn. clear, bright, shining, illuminating 10
प्रकाशवत् mfn. bright, brilliant, shining III Rev
प्रकाशीत mfn. displayed, revealed 14
प्रकृतिः f. Nature, woman 5, 8
प्रकीर्तित mfn. proclaimed, declared, said 4
प्रक्षीण mfn. destroyed, diminished 21
प्रग्रहः m. rein, bridle 14
प्र√चुद् 1P, to set in motion, impel, inspire 21
√प्रछ् 6P, to ask 21
प्रजल्पः m. talking too much 3
प्रजा f. people, subjects, offspring 4
प्रजातन्तुः m. a line of descendants 20
प्रजापत्यः m. a descendant of Prajāpati 20
प्रज्ञा f. wisdom, knowledge, intelligence, discrimination 5
प्र√णम् 1P, to bow 6
प्र√णश् 4P, to be lost, destroyed 2
प्रणि√पत् 1P, to bow respectfully to, to throw oneself down before 16
प्र√तप् 1P, to give forth heat, shine, set on fire 17
प्रतापः m. prowess, splendor, brilliance, majesty I Rev
प्रति√गम् 1P, to go toward, go back, return 3
प्रति√ष्ठा 1P, to stand firm 11
प्रति√ज्ञा 9P, to acknowledge, promise 21
प्रतिष्ठम् n. support 18
प्रतिष्ठित mfn. is situated, resides in, stands firm 10
प्रति√इ 2P, to recognize; pass. to be recognized 13

प्रतीत mfn. glad, pleased 16
प्रतीतिः f. clear apprehension, complete understanding 12
प्रत्यक्ष mfn. present before the eyes, perceptible 7
प्रत्यक्षम् n. direct perception, clear vision 11
प्रत्यञ्च् mfn. western, behind 21
प्रत्ययः m. trust, faith, proof, confidence 14
प्रत्यवायः m. contrary course, harm 4
प्रत्याहारः m. withdrawal of the senses 4
प्रथम mfn. first 15
प्र√दिश् 3P, to point out, indicate, teach 10
प्र√ध्मा 1P, to blow into, to be tossed about, wander about 16, 21
प्रबद्ध mfn. bound, tied, fettered 19
प्र√ब्रू 2P, to say, tell, relate 21
प्रभवः m. origin, birth, cause of existence, production, source 9, 18
प्रभा f. light, splendor, radiance 19
प्रभातम् n. daybreak, dawn, morning 4, 15
प्र√भाष् 1Ā, to speak 5
प्र√मद् 4P, to neglect 20
प्रमाणम् n. right knowledge, measure, standard 11, 15
प्रमादः m. intoxication, madness 10
प्रमिताहारः m. a measured diet 15
प्रमुक्त mfn. released, freed 16
प्रमुखम् n. before the face of, in front of, before 17
प्र√मुच् 6P, to set free, liberate 21
प्रयत्नः m. great care, effort 4
प्रयत्नेन ind. with special effort, diligently, carefully 13
प्र√यम् 1P, to offer 3
प्रयाणम् n. departure, death 15
प्रयासः m. overexertion 3
प्रयोज्य mfn. to be used, employed, or practiced 14
प्र√लप् 1P, to talk idly 13
प्र√वच् 2P, to teach, explain 12
प्रवचनम् n. teaching 20
प्रविभागतः ind. proportionately, according to differences 14
प्रवि√ली 1P, to melt away, disappear 18
प्र√वृत् 1Ā, to occur, happen 4
प्रवृत्त mfn. came from, occurred 19

प्रवृत्तिः f. news, tidings 16
प्र√शंस् 1P, to proclaim, praise 7
प्र√शुष् 4P, to dry up, be extinguished, eliminated 9
प्रश्वसितव्य mfn. to be comforted 20
प्रश्वासः m. inhalation 14
प्रष्टृ m. one who asks or inquires, questioner 20
प्रसन्न mfn. pure, bright, clear, pleased, delighted, gracious, propitious, kindly disposed 8, 18
प्रसादः m. calmness, graciousness, kindness, favor, tranquillity 4, I Rev, 18
प्र√सिध् 4P, is accomplished, succeeds 3
प्रसूतिः f. bringing forth 21
प्रसृष्ट mfn. let loose, dismissed, set free 16
प्र√स्था 1U, to set out; caus. to send out 16
प्र√हा 3P, to give up, forsake, abandon, avoid 11
प्राचीर mn. an enclosure 11
प्राजापत्यः m. descendant of Prajāpati 20
प्राञ्च् mfn. eastern, ahead, in front 21
प्राञ्जलि mfn. joining and holding out the hollowed open hands as a mark of respect and humility 6
प्राणः m. breath, inhalation, upward breath 11
प्राणभृत् mfn. filled with *prāṇa* (i.e., a living being) 15
प्राणायामः m. breath control 4
प्रातर् ind. in the early morning, at daybreak, at dawn, tomorrow 20
प्र√आप् 5P, to obtain, attain 11
प्राप्त mfn. obtained, received 12
प्रासादः m. palace 8
प्रिय mfn. pleasant, agreeable, dear, beloved 8
प्रीत mfn. pleased, delighted 20
प्रीतिः f. pleasure, satisfaction, joy 10, 21
√प्रेक्ष् 1Ā, to look at, behold 6
प्रेष्ट mfn. dearest, most beloved 20
प्रोक्त mfn. declared, said, taught, told 4, 8
प्रोत mfn. sewed, strung, contained in, pervaded by 12, 15
प्रौढ mfn. mighty, strong 14
√प्लु 1Ā, to leap, jump, spring 16

√फल् 1P, to bear fruit 3
फलम् n. fruit 3, 9

बत ind. particle expressing astonishment 20
√बन्ध् 9P, to bind 10
बन्धः m. binding, bondage 7
बन्धनम् n. binding, bond, stalk, stem 19, 21
बन्धुः m. relative, friend 2, 6, 9
बलम् n. power, strength 2, 15
बलवत् mfn. strong, possessing strength 13
बलिन् mfn. strong, one who possesses strength 14
बहु mfn. much, many 8
√बाध् 1Ā, to harass, oppress 11
बान्धवः m. relative 6
बारः (वारः) m. time 14
बालः m. boy 3
बाला f. girl 4
बाहुः m. arm 5
बाह्य mfn. exterior, outside, outer part 7, 8
बिन्दुः m. seed, semen, dot, drop 11, 12
बुद्धिः f. understanding, discernment, wisdom, intelligence, intellect 5
बुद्धिमत् mfn. endowed with understanding, wise, possessing wisdom 13
√बुध् 1U, 4Ā, to know 2
बृहस्पतिः m. lord of prayer and devotion 7
बौद्धः m. Buddhist 9
ब्राह्मणः m. Brahmin, one who has divine knowledge, a person belonging to the priestly class 5, 7
ब्रह्मन् n. the one, self-existent Spirit, universal Spirit 9
ब्रह्मचर्यम् n. religious studentship, the first stage of life for a Brahmin boy, spent in celibacy, studying the Vedas 20
√ब्रू 2U, to speak 8

भक्त mfn. attached to, devoted to; m. a worshipper, adorer, devotee II Rev
भक्तिः f. devotion, love 5
भक्तिमत् mfn. filled with devotion II Rev
भगवत् mfn. possessing fortune, glorious, divine II Rev
√भज् 1Ā, to pursue, practice 13
भद्रम् n. good fortune, auspiciousness, welfare 5, 18
भयम् n. fear, danger 4
भर्गस् n. radiance, splendor 21
भर्तृ m. bearer, sustainer, preserver 6

भवः m. existence 13
√भा 2P, to shine, exist, manifest 8, 11
भावः m. being, existence, object, thing, state, state of being 13, 15, 18, 19
भावना f. meditation, imagination, thought 5
√भाष् 1Ā, to speak 4
भाषा f. description, language, speech 5
भासः m. brightness, light, luster 17
√भिद् 7P, to split, break, pierce, destroy 10, 12
√भी 3P, to fear, be afraid of 8
भीः f. fear, apprehension 20
भीत mfn. frightened 16
√भुज् 7U, to eat, enjoy, experience 10
भुजः m. arm 13
भुजगः m. snake, serpent 4, 13
भुजगी f. a female snake, serpent 4
भुवः m. the air, atmosphere, place between heaven and earth 21
√भू 1P, to be, to become 2
भूः f. the earth 15
भूचर mfn. moving on the earth, creature of the earth 18
भूतम् n. living being 3, 8
भूतलम् n. the earth, ground 14, 15
भूतिः f. wealth, fortune, prosperity 20
भूपतिः m. king I Rev
भूमिः f. earth 5
भूयस् ind. again, besides, then, more, most, very much, exceedingly 14
भूर् ind. the earth 15
भूरि ind. much, abundantly 21
√भृ 3U, to support, hold 8
भेदः m. distinction, variety, difference, breaking open, piercing 10, 12
भेरी f. kettle drum 6
भोगः m. enjoyment, pleasure, fruition, rewards, results I Rev, 10
भोजनम् n. food 3
√भ्रम् 1P, to wander about 6
भ्रातृ m. brother 6
भ्रान्तिः f. wandering or roaming about, mistaken perception 8, 12

मङ्गलम् n. happiness, auspiciousness 7
मज्जनम् n. immersion, bathing 17

मठ mn. a hut, cottage 6
मणिः m. jewel, gem, pearl 12, 21
मण्डलम् n. circle, globe, orb 7
मत mfn. thought, believed 8
मतम् n. thought, opinion, belief, doctrine, ideology 8, 15
मतिः f. thought, mind, intelligence 5, 20
मद्गुः m. a diver bird III Rev
मधु n. honey 18
मधुकृत् m. making honey, a bee 18
मधुमत् mfn. sweet, rich in honey 21
मधुर mfn. sweet, pleasant, charming 10
मध्य mfn. middle 4
मध्यम mfn. middle 5
√मन् 4Ā, 8Ā, to think, consider 4, 9
मनस् mn. mind 10
मनीषिन् mfn. teacher, one who is wise 14
मनुष्यः m. a man, human being 11
√मन्त्र् 10Ā, to advise 4
मन्त्रः m. sacred prayer 4
√मन्थ् 9P, to churn, agitate 10
मन्युः mfn. rage, fury, anger 16
मय / मयी mfn. made up of, consisting of (at the end of a compound) 12
मरणम् n. death 7
मरुत् m. wind 8
मर्दन mfn. destroying 4
मलम् n. dirt, filth, dust, impurity 3
मशकः m. mosquito 18
महत् mfn. great, large, long 12
महामनस् mfn. arrogant, swollen-headed 21
मही f. earth 4
महीशः m. ruler, king 3
महेश्वरः m. Śiva, God of Destruction, "The Great Lord" 5
मा ind. don't, not 9
√मा 3Ā, to measure 8
मातुलः m. maternal uncle 6
मातृ f. mother 6
मात्र mfn. having the measure of 12

मात्रा f. material, measure 17
माधवः m. descendant of Madhu, Kṛṣṇa 16
मान mn. respect, honor 11
मानस mfn. pertaining to the mind, mental, spiritual, expressed only in the mind, performed in thought, silent 8, 12
मानसम् n. the mind, heart, soul 6
मानिन् mfn. thinking oneself to be 21
मान्य mfn. to be respected or honored I Rev
मामक mfn. mine 3
माया f. illusion 4
मायाविन् mfn. possessing illusion or magical powers, master of illusion 16
मारुतः m. wind 10
मार्गः m. path, right way, custom 3
माला f. garland 4
मासः m. a month 12
मित mfn. measured, moderate 14
मिताहारः m. moderate diet 3
मित्रः m. friend, the Sun God 7, 11
मुक्त mfn. liberated, set free 7, 8
मुखम् n. mouth, face 3
मुख्य mfn. first, principal, best 3
√मुच् 6U, to let go, free oneself of, to let loose, liberate, bestow 8
√मुद् 1Ā, to rejoice 4
मुद्रा f. various bodily actions such as the *bandhas*, described as tenfold in the *Haṭhapradīpikā* 19
मुनिः m. sage, seer, one who is moved by inward impulse, an inspired person 5, 17
मुमुक्षु mfn. desiring freedom 12
मूढः m. a fool 17
मूढमतिः m. foolish person 14
मूर्धन् m. head, forehead, highest or first part of anything 9
मूलम् n. root 4
मृतम् n. one who has died, dead 6
मृत्तिका f. earth 21
मृत्युः m. death 6
√मृद् 9P, to crush, smash 16
मृद् f. earth, clay 21
मेघः m. cloud 13

मेधा f. intelligence, mental vigor 21
मेधाविन् m. learned, wise man 21
मैत्र mfn. friendly II Rev
मोक्षः m. liberation 3
मोहः m. delusion 17
मोहनम् n. confusing, deluding 10
मोहान्तः m. deep bewilderment of mind 20
मोहित mfn. deluded 18
मौनिन् mfn. observing silence, silent, taciturn II Rev

√यज् 1U, to worship, sacrifice 4
यजत्र mfn. worthy of worship or sacrifice 18
√यत् 1Ā, to persevere 19
यत mfn. controlled, restrained 10
यतः ind. from which, wherefore, for which reason 8
यतिः m. ascetic I Rev
यत्नः m. effort 5
यथा ind. in the same way as, just as, in which way 3, 5
यदा ind. when 3
यदा यदा ind. whenever 3
यदि ind. if 11, 12
यद्यत् ind. whatever 10
√यम् 1P, to bestow 11
यमः m. restraint 3
यमुना f. the Jumna/Jamuna River 4
यशस् n. fame I Rev, 10
√या 2P, to go, to disappear 8, 12
याजिन् mfn. worshipping, sacrificing 21
यामः m. a period of three hours, an eighth of the day 12
युक्त mfn. joined, united, yoked to, engaged in, absorbed in, fit, suitable, appropriate, proper, endowed, possessed of, experienced 5, 12, 15, 20
युक्ततम mfn. most intent upon, most devoted II Rev
युक्तिः f. junction, application, plan 19
युगम् n. yoke, pair, age of the world 3
√युज् 7U, to join, yoke, unite, engage 10
युद्धम् n. battle, fight, war 6
√युध् 4P, to fight, engage in battle 7

युवन् m. youth, young 9
योक्तव्य mfn. to be joined, yoked, united, concentrated, absorbed, to be practiced 14
योक्तृ m. one who yokes, joins, unites 19
योक्त्रम् n. a cord, rope, the tie of the yoke of a plow 19
योगः m. the act of yoking, union, concentration of the mind, system of philosophy established by Patañjali 3
योगिन् m. practitioner of yoga 14
योगिनी f. female yogī 14
योग्य mfn. useful, fit, proper, suitable 3, 18
योग्यता f. fitness, propriety 19
योजनम् n. measure of distance equal to eight to nine miles, league, joining, uniting 16
योजनीय mfn. to be joined, united 19
योधवीरः m. hero, warrior 16
यौक्तिक mfn. suitable, fit, proper 19
यौगः m. a follower of the yoga system of philosophy 19
यौवनम् n. youth III Rev

√रक्ष् 1P, to protect, save 14
रजस् n. activity (one of the three *guṇas* or qualities of mind) 10
रज्जुः/ रज्जू f. rope 5
रणम् n. battle, conflict 6
रत mfn. delighting in, intent upon II Rev
रथः m. chariot 14
रन्ध्रम् n. hole 12
रम्य mfn. enjoyable, pleasing, delightful, beautiful 21
रविः m. sun 5
रसः m. taste, essence, nectar 10, 14
रसना f. tongue 11
रागः m. passion 10
राघवः m. descendant of Raghu 19
राजन् m. king 9
रात्रिः f. night 5
रामः m. hero of the *Rāmāyaṇa* 3
राशिः m. a heap, mass 21
√रिच् 7U, 1, 10P to empty; caus. to make empty (of breaths), exhale 14
रिपुः m. enemy 2, 9
√रिष् 1,4P, to be hurt or injured 21

रीतिः f. custom, practice, method 14
रुज् mfn. pain, illness, disease 8
√रुध् 7U, to obstruct, restrain 10
रूपम् n. form, shape I Rev, 11
रेणुः f. dust 5
रोगः m. disease 4, 8
रोमहर्षण mfn. causing the hair to stand on end or bristle (through joy or terror) 20
रौप्य mfn. silver 12

लक्षणम् n. mark, sign, characteristic, attribute 8, 13
लक्ष्मी f. goddess of wealth 4
लग्न mfn. attached to I Rev
लघु mfn. small, light 2, 15, 19
लघुता f. lightness 5, 19
लता f. creeper 4, 18
√लभ् 1Ā, to obtain 4
लयः m. melting, dissolution, absorption in, percussion instruments 19
लवण mfn. salt, salty 16
लाघवम् n. lightness 19
लाभः m. gain, attainment 11, 12
√लिप् 6U, to smear, stain 11
लिप्त mfn. smeared 12
लिप्सा f. the desire to gain, wish to obtain, longing for 18
√लिह् 2U, to lick 17
√लुप् 4P, to disturb, bewilder, perplex, confound 17
लोकः m. world, inhabitants of the world 3
लोह mfn. gold, made of copper 13, 21
लौल्यम् n. restlessness 3

वंशः m. lineage 13
वक्तृ m. eloquent speaker, orator 6
वक्त्रम् n. mouth, face, head 21
√वच् 2P, to speak 8
वचनम् n. advice, instruction, direction 16
वत्सः m. calf, child 3
√वद् 1P, to speak 2
वदनम् n. the face, mouth 13

√वध् 1P, to slay, kill 14
वधः m. killing 6
वनम् n. forest 15
वनिका f. little wood, grove 16
√वन्द् 1Ā, to salute, honor, bow, to greet 4
वपुस् n. form, figure 16
वयस् n. energy, strength, youth 10
वरः m. wish, request, boon 20
वरणीय mfn. to be chosen 20
वरानना f. lovely-faced woman 4
वराहः m. boar 18
वरुणः m. god of the oceans 7
वरेण्य mfn. desirable, excellent 21
वर्ज्य mfn. to be avoided 8
वर्णः m. appearance, form, letter 13, 15
वर्य mfn. excellent, eminent, best of 18
वर्षः m. rain 10
वर्षगणः m. a long series of years III Rev
वलित mfn. wrinkles 12
वल्लभ mfn. beloved above all, dear to 14
वल्ली f. vine 18
वशिन् mfn. possessing self-control 14
वश्यः mfn. subdued, tamed 5
√वस् 1U, to live 4
वसन्तः m. spring 8
वसुदेवः m. father of Kṛṣṇa 4
वस्तु n. thing 18
√वह् 1P, to flow 3
वह्निः m. fire, digestive fire 14
वाच् f. speech 8
वाञ्छित mfn. wished, desired I Rev
वाजश्रवसः m. son of Vājaśravas 16
वातः m. wind, breath 14
वादः m. speech, discourse, talk 8
वानरः m. monkey 16
वापी f. pond, large reservoir of water 11
वाम mfn. left, situated on the left side 4

वायुः m. wind, air, breath, god of the wind 4, 5, 7
वारि n. water 18
वार्त्मन् n. path 9
वाव ind. indeed, just, even 17
वासवः m. name of Indra, Vedic chief of gods 3
वासस् n. garment, clothes 10
वासुदेवः m. son of Vasudeva, name for Kṛṣṇa
विकारः m. disturbance, disease, change of form or nature, transformation 8, 13
वि√कृ 8P, to change, transform 14
विगुण mfn. deficient, imperfect 15
विग्रहः m. individual form, figure, the body 15
विघ्नः m. obstacle 3
विचर्षण mfn. very active or busy 21
विचारः m. reflection, inquiry, consideration 7
विचिकित्सा f. doubt, uncertainty 20
विच्छेदः m. cutting off 14
विजानत् m. wise man, sage, one who knows 20
वि√जि 1P, to succeed, conquer 7
वि√ज्ञा 9P, to discern, observe, know, understand 18
विज्ञानम् n. the act of discerning, understanding, experience 13
विज्ञेय mfn. to be known 17
वित्तम् n. wealth, acquisition, money, power I Rev, 16
वित्तम mfn. most knowing, having the best knowledge II Rev
√विद् 4Ā, to exist; 2P, to know, feel, consider; 6P, to find; caus. to feel, experience 4, 8, 17, 20
विदेशः m. another country, abroad I Rev
विद्या f. knowledge 4
विद्यावत् mfn. learned, possessing knowledge 13
विद्युत् f. lightning 4
विद्वांस् mfn. wise, learned; m. a seer 16
वि√द्विष् 1Ā, to be hostile, hate, argue 7
वि√धा 3P, to make, render 10
विधिः m. practice, method, rule, injunction 8
विनयः m. education, moral training, decency 18
वि√नश् 4P, to perish, to be utterly lost 3
विनष्टिः f. loss, ruin, destruction 20
विनाशः m. utter loss, destruction, death 3, 8

चिनाशनम् n. removal, destruction 4
विनिर्णयः m. certainty, a settled rule 13
विपरीत mfn. turned around, reversed, contrary 17
विपुल mfn. large, extensive, wide 13
वप्रतिपन्न mfn. confused, bewildered, perplexed 7
विभागः m. share, division, role 9
विमल mfn. spotless 21
वि√मुच् 6U, to release, set free, liberate; pass. to be freed, liberated 12
विमूढ mfn. deluded, confused, foolish 20
विमूढात्मन् mfn. bewildered, perplexed in mind 13
विमृत्यु mfn. free from death, immortal 20
विमोक्षः m. liberation 8
वियोगः m. disjunction, separation, absence of 8, 14
विरज mfn. free from dust, clean, pure 13
विलम्बित mfn. slowly 14
विलीन mfn. immersed, dissolved 20
विलुलित mfn. moving hither and thither 9
विवर्जित mfn. free from 8
वि√वस् 1P, to live, spend time, enter into an apprenticeship 21
विविध mfn. of various sorts, manifold 6
विवेकित mfn. discernment 21
√विश् 6P, to enter 6
वि√शिष् 7P, to be better than, distinguish, excel II Rev
विशुद्धिः f. purification, true knowledge 10
विशेषः m. distinction, difference 13
विश्रान्तिः f. rest, repose 5
विश्वञ्च् mfn. facing in all directions, pervading 21
विश्वम् n. the whole world, universe 13
विश्वरूप mfn. manifold, with various forms 21
विश्ववेदस् mfn. all-knowing, omniscient 18
विश्वासः m. confidence, trust, belief in 15
विषधरः m. containing poison, venomous, a snake 21
विषम् n. poison 19
विषम mfn. dangerous 21
विषयः m. an object of sense 11
विष्णुः m. God of Preservation, the all-pervader, god of light and sun, all-pervading 5, 7, 13
वि√सृज् 6P, to throw down, cast aside, eliminate, release 6, 13, 21

विसृष्ट mfn. left, let go 21
विस्तीर्ण mfn. spread out, extending, expanded, broad 12, 16
वि√हा 3P, to abandon, cast off 10
वि√ईक्ष् 1Ā, to look at, see, behold 21
वीचीचयः m. a multitude of waves 9
वीत mfn. gone away, departed 16
वीर्यम् n. strength, energy, vigor, power 7
√वृ 9U, to choose 10
वृकः m. wolf 18
वृक्षः m. tree 3
√वृत् 1Ā, to be, exist, live, dwell 4, 7
वृत्तम् n. mode of life 16
वृत्तिः f. fluctuating state, mode of life, profession, occupation 5, 12
वृद्ध mfn. old, great 9, 18
√वृध् 1Ā, to grow, increase 4
√वृष् 1P, to rain down, shower down 5
वृष्णिः m. family from which Kṛṣṇa descended 5
वेदः m. sacred knowledge, the *Vedas*, divided into three or four works, known as the *Ṛg-veda*, *Yajur-veda*, *Sāma-veda*, and *Atharva-veda* 3
वेदस् n. property, wealth 16
वेद्य mfn. to be learned or known 6
वेधस् m. creator 10
वेषः m. dress, clothing, assumed appearance 5
वेष्टित mfn. enveloped, covered with, veiled in 16
वै ind. indeed, truly (particle of emphasis) 7
वैदेही f. name for Sītā, daughter of Janaka, the king of Videha 16
वैद्यकम् n. the science of medicine 3
वैराग्यम् n. detachment 3
वैश्वदेव mfn. relating or sacred to all the gods 15
व्यति√तृ 1P, to completely cross over 16
√व्यथ् 1Ā, to tremble, waver 20
व्यथा f. agitation, anguish, fear II Rev
व्यपेत mfn. gone away, disappeared, freed from 20
व्यव√च्छिद् 7P, to cut off, separate 20
व्यवस्थित mfn. situated 4
व्यू√अश् 1Ā, to attain 18
व्याघ्रः m. tiger 5

व्याधित mfn. sick, afflicted with disease 9
व्याप्त mfn. pervaded 7
व्यासः m. "compiler, arranger" of the Vedas, author of the *Mahābhārata* and *Purāṇas* 5
व्योमन् m. sky 10
√व्रज् 1U, to go, wander, move, take 5, 20

√शक् 5P, to be able or capable 9
शकुनिः m. a bird 19
शक्तिः f. power 5
शङ्खः m. conch shell (used as horn or trumpet in battle) 6
शतम् n. a hundred 5
शत्रुः m. enemy 11
शनैः शनैः ind. softly, gently, gradually 5
शब्दः m. sound, noise 6
शम् ind. happiness and well-being 7
शमः m. tranquillity, equanimity, calmness 7, 17
शयनम् n. act of lying down, rest, repose, bed, sleeping place 5, 13
शरः m. an arrow 6
शरणम् n. refuge 5
शरद् f. autumn 8
शरीरम् n. body 3
शलाका f. pencil 7
शवासनम् n. corpse pose 5
शशिन् m. "containing a hare, rabbit," the moon 13, 14
शश्वत् ind. perpetually, continually, always 20
शस्त mfn. praised, recommended 21
शस्त्रम् n. weapon 10
शाखा f. a branch 13
शान्त mfn. tranquil 13
शान्तिः f. peace 5
√शास् 2P, to teach 8
शास्त्रम् n. an instrument of teaching, sacred text 7
√शिक्ष् 1Ā, to learn, study, practice 20
शिथिल mfn. relaxed 16
शिरस् n. the head 11
शिव mfn. auspicious, favorable, benevolent 10
शिशुः m. baby, child 5

शिष्यः m. a pupil, scholar, disciple, student 18
√शी 2Ā, to lie down, rest, sleep 8
शीत mfn. cold, cool 10
√शीतलय denom. to cool 21
शीलम् n. habit 13
शुक्तिः f. pearl oyster 12
शुक्ल mfn. white 13
शुङ्गम् n. sheath or calyx of a bud, effect 18
√शुच् 1P, to grieve 6
शुच् f. grief 8
शुचि mfn. clear, pure, radiant, shining, glowing, bright 6
शुद्धिः f. purification, purity, true knowledge 10
शुभ mfn. good fortune, auspiciousness, beautiful, pleasant 3, 13, II Rev
√शुष् 4P, to be dry 10
शून्यम् n. a void, empty place, vacuity, nonentity 19
शूरः m. hero 6
√शॄ 9P, to break; pass. to be broken, worn-out, decay 21
शैलः m. mountain 12
शोकः m. sorrow, grief 6
शोधनम् n. purifying, purification 19
श्रद्धा f. faith 4
श्रद्धावत् mfn. full of faith 13
श्रमः m. fatigue, exertion 5
श्रमणः m. ascetic, devotee 9
श्रवस् n. glory, fame, renown 18
श्री f. radiance, beauty, grace 13; mfn. sacred, holy, revered, splendor, dignity II Rev, 20
श्रीगुरुः m. sacred/revered teacher 5
√श्रु 5P, to hear, listen 9
श्रुत mfn. known, famous, celebrated 13
श्रुतिः f. a Vedic or sacred text 7
श्रेयस् mfn. better II Rev
श्रोत्रम् n. ear, act of hearing 10
श्लोकः m. verse, poetry 19
श्वन् m. a dog 18
श्वपाकः m. "dog cooker," untouchable 18
√श्वस् 2P, to breathe 8
श्वस् ind. tomorrow, on the following day III Rev
श्वासः m. breath, exhalation 13, 14
श्वेत mfn. white 16

षड् m. six 6
षष् mfn. six 15
षोढा ind. in six ways, sixfold 4

संयञ्च् mfn. turned together or in one direction, proper, in one line, straight 21
संयमः m. *dhāraṇā* + *dhyāna* + *samādhi*, profound contemplation, control, restraint 3, 12
सं√या 2P, to come to or into, attain 10
संयुक्त mfn. endowed with, full of 12
संयुत mfn. endowed with, contains, consists of 13
संयोगः m. conjunction, union, combination 13
सं√रक्ष् 1P, to protect, preserve, keep 15
संवादः m. speaking together, conversation, dialogue 20
संविग्न mfn. agitated, disturbed, overcome by 6
संवित्त्वम् n. consciousness 21
संविद् f. understanding 20
संशयः m. uncertainty, doubt 3, 7
संसारः m. cyclic existence, transmigration, worldly illusion 8
संसिद्धिः f. complete accomplishment or fulfillment, attainment, success 11
सं√स्था 1Ā, to dwell or live in, stand close, together; caus. to establish, settle, raise up 10
सं√हृ 1U, to draw together, unite 11
सकल mfn. with parts, whole, entire 8
सक्त mfn. attached 16
सखः m. friend 17
सखिः m. friend 18
संकर m. mixing together, confusion 18
संकल्पः m. intention, thought 11
संकेतः m. secret practice of *layayoga*, the yoga of cosmic absorption 16
संक्षेपतः ind. briefly, concisely, shortly 14
संख्यम् n. battle, conflict 16
सङ्गः m. attachment, association, desire 3, 9
संगतिः f. meeting 10
संग्रहः m. holding together 16
√सञ्ज् 1U, to be attached to 9
संज्ञित mfn. known as, called, named 14
सत् n. existence, the real, truth 10
सततम् ind. constantly, always, ever II Rev
सत्त्वम् n. equilibrium, luminosity, purity, goodness (one of the three *guṇas*) 10

सत्त्वस्थ mfn. resolutely, energetically 13
सत्यम् n. truth 3
√सद् 1P, to sit 2
सदा ind. always 7
सदाचारः m. virtuous conduct, good manners I Rev
सदृश् mfn. like, resembling 13
सदोष mfn. having faults, deficiencies 5
सद्यस् ind. on the same day, in the very moment, at once, immediately 14
सधन mfn. wealthy, with wealth 5
सनातन mfn. eternal, everlasting, primeval 3, 14
सन्तत mfn. extended, stretched 10
संतुष्ट mfn. quite satisfied or contented II Rev
सन्तोषः m. contentment 3
सन्दर्शित mfn. shown, displayed, manifested 17
सं√दह् 1U, to burn up, bake 13
सन्देशः m. message 10
सन्ध्या f. juncture of the three divisions of the day (morning, noon, and night) 15
संनिभ mfn. like, similar, resembling 4, 16
संनि√यम् 1P, to hold together, restrain, control II Rev
संनिहित mfn. near, at hand 14
सं√न्यस् 2P, to place together II Rev
संन्यसनम् n. renunciation 9
सपत्नः m. rival, adversary, enemy 16
सप्तन् mfn. seven 15
सबीजः m. type of *samādhi* or meditative absorption in which *samskāras* (past impressions) still exist, "with seed" 8
सम mfn. same, equal, even, straight, on a level 11
समग्र mfn. all, entire, whole 17
समता f. equanimity 15
समत्वम् n. equanimity 11
समधि√गम् 1P, go toward, approach 9
समन्तात् ind. on all sides, wholly, completely 14
समन्वित mfn. connected with, endowed with 19
समभ्यु√अस् 4P, to practice 6, 14
समम् equal to 2
समयः m. proper time 14
समरः m. battle, struggle 3

समवहारम् ind. by gathering 18
समवेत mfn. come together, assembled 3
समा√कृष् 1P, to draw together, draw in 14
समा√गम् 1P, to come together with 6
समा√चर् 1P, to act, practice 8
समा√धा 3P, to place, direct, keep II Rev
समाधिः m. meditative absorption 5
समान mfn. same 17
समा√नी 1U, to collect, assemble 16
समा√सद् 1, 6P, to approach, arrive 16
समासाद्य ind. by means of, on account of 15
समासीन mfn. sitting 21
समिधः m. fuel, wood III Rev
समुदा√हृ 1U, to call, pronounce, declare, teach 11
समुद्धर्तृ mfn. one who lifts up or raises or extricates from II Rev
समुद्भवः m. origin, arising 12
समुद्रः m. the sea, ocean 16
समुप√गम् 1P, to approach 6
सं√पद् 1Ā, meet or unite with, enter into, come together, attain, arrive, become complete 18, 21
संपद् f. fate, destiny 8
संपन्न mfn. endowed with, possessed of 18
सम्पातिः m. name of a vulture, elder brother of Jaṭāyu 16
संपूर्ण mfn. completely filled or full 14
संप्रकीर्तित mfn. mentioned, designated, called 4
सम्प्राप्त mfn. attained, reached, arrived 14
सं√प्रेक्ष् 1Ā, to look at, concentrate the eyes, gaze 11
सम्प्लुत mfn. flooded over, overflowing 7
संभवः m. origin, source 10
सं√भू 1P, to arise, be born 3
संमत mfn. agreed or consented to, approved of 9
संमर्शिन् mfn. able to judge 20
सम्मुख mfn. facing, being in front of 18
सम्मोहः m. delusion 3
सम्यक् ind. completely 12
सम्राज् m. king, emperor 8
सयुज् mfn. a companion 17

सरस्वती f. goddess of knowledge; legendary river, part of which dried up and part that joins the Ganges and the Jumna at Allahabad 4
सरित् f. river, stream 8
सर्पः m. snake, serpent 12
सर्व mfn. all, every, everything 7
सर्वगत mfn. all-pervading, omnipresent 19
सर्वतः ind. from all sides, in every direction, everywhere 7
सर्वत्र ind. everywhere, in all places, at all times 2
सर्वत्रग mfn. all-pervading, omnipresent II Rev
सर्वदा ind. always, at all times 3
सर्वशस् ind. wholly, completely, entirely, always, universally 11, 13
सलिलम् n. water 13
सवितृ m. the Sun God, the divine influence and vivifying power of the sun 21
सस्यम् n. crop 5
सह ind. together, with 7
सहज mfn. inborn, innate, natural 5, 17
सहसा ind. suddenly, quickly, all at once 6
सहस्र nm. a thousand 6
सहित mfn. possessed of, accompanied by 9
साक्षात् ind. clearly, right before one's eyes 5
सागरः m. ocean 3
सांख्यम् n. one of the six systems of Hindu philosophy, followers of Sāṃkhya 11
सात्त्विक mfn. endowed with clarity and calmness 18
साधनम् n. accomplishment, attainment, mastery 4
साधकः m. practitioner 5
साधुः m. holy man, sage, seer 5, 10
सामवेदः m. the *veda* of songs 3
सारथिः m. charioteer 13
साहसम् n. boldness, daring, courage 3
सित mfn. bright, white, pure 10, 21
सिद्ध mfn. attained, perfected, established 8, 14, 19; m. an inspired sage or seer, a semi-divine being of great perfection and purity, perfected one 3, 15
सिद्धिः f. fulfillment, accomplishment, attainment, success 5
सिंहः m. lion 5
√सु 5U, to press out, extract 9
सुकल्प mfn. very qualified or skilled 10
सुखम् n. happiness 2, 3

सुखितः mfn. happy, contented 21
सुखिन् mfn. happy, one who possesses happiness 14
सुखेन ind. easily, comfortably, joyfully 12
सुचरितम् n. virtuous actions 20
सुज्ञान mfn. easy to be known or understood 20
सुतः m. son 4
सुदुर्दर्श mfn. very difficult to be seen or discerned 18
सुपद्यम् n. beautiful poetry I Rev
सुपर्ण mfn. having beautiful wings, a bird 17
सुप्त mfn. sleeping 7
सुभोगिन् mfn. beautifully ringed 21
सुभोजिन् mfn. one who eats well 14
सुमधुर mfn. very sweet 3
सुरः m. a god 13, 14
सुरूप mfn. well formed, beautiful I Rev
सुषुम्णा f. the central *nāḍī* or channel of the nervous system 4, 11
सुहृद् m. friend, "good-hearted" 8
सूक्ष्म mfn. subtle 4
सूत्रम् n. thread, string 19
सूर्यः m. sun 3, 14
√सृज् 6P, to bring forth, to create, to manifest 3
सेतुः m. bridge, embankment 16, 18
सेवितः mfn. attended upon, served 5, I Rev
सेवितव्य mfn. to be followed or practiced 20
सेव्य mfn. to be resorted to, practiced 18
सोम्य / सौम्य mfn. gentle, soft, moonlike, "son," "my dear son" 16, 17
सौक्ष्म्यम् n. subtlety 19
सौहृदम् n. friendship, affection, love 21
स्तनयित्नुः m. thunder 20
स्तब्ध mfn. puffed up, proud, arrogant 21
√स्तु 2U, to praise 8
स्तुतिः f. praise II Rev
स्त्री f. woman 16, 18
√स्था 1U, to stand, stay 6
स्थाणुः m. fixed, stationary, immovable 14
स्थाणुत्वम् n. motionlessness, stableness 14
स्थानम् n. stability, place, state 5

स्थित mfn. situated, standing, abiding, or remaining in 4, 6, 7
स्थितिः f. stability 5
स्थिर mfn. steady 11
स्थूल mfn. large, big, thick 9, 21
√स्ना 2P, to bathe 8
स्नात mfn. bathed 10
स्निग्ध mfn. oily 3, 10
स्पर्शः m. touch 11
√स्पृश् 6P, to touch 2
√स्फुर् 6P, to shine, be evident or manifest, be brilliant, burst out plainly or visibly 13
स्म ind. indeed 20
√स्मृ 1P, to remember 21
स्मृत mfn. taught, considered 11
√स्यन्द् 1Ā, to flow 21
स्यन्दन mfn. chariot, "moving swiftly" 16
√स्रंस् 1Ā, to fall down, drop 6
√स्रु 1P, to flow 17
स्व mfn. one's own 11
स्वनुष्ठित mfn. performed well 15
√स्वप् 2P, to sleep 8
स्वप्नः m. dream 9
स्वयम् ind. spontaneously, of one's own accord 14
स्वर् ind. heaven 21
स्वरः m. sound, tone, accent 15
स्वरूपम् n. one's own true nature, true form, natural state 6, 12
स्वल्पः m. a little 4
स्वसृ f. sister 6
स्वस्ति fn. well-being, fortune 18
स्वात्मन् m. one's own self 17
स्वादु mfn. sweet, pleasant to the taste 17
स्वेदः m. sweat, perspiration 5

ह ind. indeed, assuredly, verily, of course 15
हत mfn. slain, killed 8
√हन् 2P, to kill 8
हनुः f. jaw 5
हनुमत् m. Hanumān, possessing a jaw 13

हन्त ind. interjection of exhortation to do something, "Look," "Listen" 16
हन्तृ mfn. a killer, slayer 8
हयः m. horse 16
हर्षः m. joy, exultation, lustfulness 6, II Rev
हविस् n. oblation, burnt offering 9, 10
हस्तः m. the hand 17
हस्तिन् mfn. elephant, one who possesses a hand 14
√हा 3U, to leave, abandon 8
हालाहलम् n. a deadly poison, produced in the churning of the ocean 17
हि ind. emphatic particle, indeed, for, because 3, 4
हिक्का f. hiccup 15
हित mfn. beneficial, wholesome 14
हिमवत् mfn. snowy, possessing snow, m. Himālaya 13
हीन mfn. without, deprived of 12
√हु 3P, to sacrifice, to offer an oblation 8
हुत mfn. poured out into the fire 9
√हृ 1U, to carry 17
हृद् n. heart 9
हृदयम् n. heart 3
√हृष् 4P, to rejoice, exult, gloat II Rev
हृषिकेशः m. Lord of the senses, Viṣṇu 16
हेतुः m. motive, cause 9
हेय mfn. to be avoided 11
ह्री f. modesty 20

# Bibliography

## PRIMARY SOURCES

The Sanskrit text used in this book has been drawn from critical editions whenever possible. In all other instances, it has been drawn from popularly printed texts.


*Abhijñānaśākuntalam*. Edited and translated by M. R. Kale. Delhi: Motilal Banarsidass, 2010.

*Amaruṣatakam*. Edited and translated by Chintaman Ramchandra Devadhar. Delhi: Motilal Banarsidass, 1984.

*Aparokṣānubhūtiḥ—Vidyāraṇyakṛtayā Aparokṣadīpikākhyaṭikayā Saṃvalitā*. Edited by Kamla Devi. Allahabad: Akshayavaṭa Prakāśana, 1988.

*The Bhagavadgītā*. Edited by Shripad Krishna Belvalkar. Pune: Bhandarkar Oriental Research Institute, 1945.

*Bhāgavatapurāṇa. Śrīmadbhāgavatapurāṇam with the Tīkā Bhāvārthabodhinā of Śrīdharasvāmin*. Edited by Jagadisalala Sastri. Delhi: Motilal Banarsidass, 1983.

*Dattātreyayogaśāstra*. Edited by James Mallinson. Unpublished edition, April 1, 2013. PDF file.

*The Early Upaniṣads: Annotated Text and Translation*. Edited and translated by Patrick Olivelle. New York: Oxford University Press, 1998.

*Gheranda Saṃhitā*. Edited and translated by James Mallinson. Woodstock, New York: YogaVidya, 2004.

*Haṭhapradīpikā of Svātmarāma*. Edited by Swami Digambaraji and Pt. Ragunatha Shastri Kokaje. Lonavla: Kaivalyadhama S.M.Y.M. Samiti, 1998.

*The Mahābhārata for the First Time Critically Edited*. Edited by V. S. Sukthankar, S. K. Belvalkar, and P. L. Vaidya. 19 vols. Pune: Bhandarkar Oriental Research Institute, 1933–66.

*Mantrapuṣpam*. Edited by Swami Devarupananda. Mumbai: Ramakrishna Math, 2007.

*Nāthamuni's Yoga Rahasya*. Translated by T.K.V. Desikachar. Chennai: Krishnamacharya Yoga Mandiram, 1998.

*Pātañjalayogasūtrāṇi. Vācaspatimiśraviracitatīkāsametaśrīvyāsabhaṣyasmetāni*. Ānandāśrama Sanskrit Series 47. Puṇyapattane: Ānandāśrama Press, 1978.

*Śiva Saṃhitā*. Edited and translated by James Mallinson. Woodstock, New York: YogaVidya, 2007.

*Tantrāloka of Abhinavagupta with the Commentary of Rājānaka Jayaratha*. Edited by Mukund Rām Śāstrī. Allahabad: Indian Press, 1918–38.

*The Vālmīki Rāmāyaṇa: Critical Edition*. Vol. 1, *The Bālakāṇḍa*, edited by G. H. Bhatt. Vadodara: Oriental Institute, 1960–75.

*Vivekamārtaṇḍa*. Edited by Rāmalāl Śrīvāstava. Gorakhpur: Gorakanāth Mandir, 1983.

*Yogabīja of Gorakhanātha*. Edited by Rāmalāl Śrīvāstava. Gorakhpur: Gorakanāth Mandir, 1982.

*Yogāñjalisāram*. Composed by T. Krishnamacharya and edited by T.K.V. Desikachar. Chennai: Krishnamacharya Yoga Mandiram, 2001.

*Yoga Upaniṣads with the Commentary of Śrī Upaniṣadbrahmayogin*. Edited by Pandit A. Mahadeva Sastri. Chennai: Adyar Library and Research Center, 1968.

*The Yoga-Vāsiṣṭha of Vālmīki*. Edited and translated by Vihari Lal Mitra. Delhi: Parimal Publications, 1998.

*Yogayājñavalkya*. Edited by Śrī Prahlad C. Divanji. B.B.R.A. Society's Monograph, 3. Bombay: Bombay Branch Royal Asiatic Society, 1954.

## SECONDARY SOURCES

Apte, Vaman Shivaram. *The Practical Sanskrit English Dictionary*. Delhi: Motilal Banarsidass Publishers, 2007.

Doniger, Wendy. *The Hindus: An Alternative History*. New York: Penguin, 2009.

Macdonell, Arthur A. *A Sanskrit Grammar for Students*. Oxford: Oxford University Press, 1986.

Monier-Williams, Sir Monier. *A Sanskrit-English Dictionary*. New York: Oxford University Press, 2000.

## FURTHER READING

Birch, Jason. "The Meaning of *Haṭha* in Early Haṭhayoga." *Journal of the American Oriental Society* 131, no. 4 (2011): 527–54.

———. "Rājayoga: The Reincarnations of the King of All Yogas." *International Journal of Hindu Studies* 17, no. 3 (2013): 401–44.

Bryant, Edwin F. *The Yoga Sūtras of Patañjali*. New York: North Point Press, 2009.

Calasso, Roberto. *Ardor*. Translated by Richard Dixon. New York: Farrar, Straus and Giroux, 2014.

Chapple, Christopher Key. *Yoga and the Luminous: Patañjali's Spiritual Path to Freedom*. Albany: State University of New York Press, 2008.

De Michelis, Elizabeth. *A History of Modern Yoga*. London: Continuum, 2004.

Desikachar, T.K.V., and Hellfried Krusche. *Freud and Yoga: Two Philosophies of Mind Compared*. Translated by Anne-Marie Hodges. New York: North Point Press, 2014.

Feuerstein, Georg. *The Yoga Tradition: Its History, Literature, Philosophy and Practice*. Prescott, Ariz.: Hohm Press, 2001.

Jois, R. Sharath. *Aṣṭāṅga Yoga Anuṣṭhāna*. Mysore: KPJAYI, 2014.

Jois, Śrī K. Pattabhi. *Yoga Mala*. New York: North Point Press, 2002.

Larson, Gerald James, and Ram Shankar Bhattacharya, eds. *Encyclopedia of Indian Philosophies*. Vol. 12, *Yoga: India's Philosophy of Meditation*. Delhi: Motilal Banarsidass, 2008.

Mallinson, James, and Mark Singleton. *The Roots of Yoga*. New York: Penguin Classics, forthcoming.

Pollock, Sheldon. *The Language of the Gods in the World of Men*. Berkeley: University of California Press, 2006.

Sargeant, Winthrop, trans. *The Bhagavad Gītā*. Edited by Christopher Key Chapple. New York: State University of New York Press, 2009.

Tubb, Gary A., and Emery R. Boose. *Scholastic Sanskrit: A Manual for Students*. New York: Columbia University Press, 2007.

Whicher, Ian. *The Integrity of the Yoga Darśana: A Reconsideration of Classical Yoga*. New York: State University of New York Press, 1998.

White, David Gordon, ed. *Yoga in Practice*. Princeton: Princeton University Press, 2012.

# Acknowledgments

My deepest gratitude extends to all those who have taught me not only to understand but, more important, to love Sanskrit. Particularly my teachers Śrī K. Pattabhi Jois, R. Sharath Jois, Jayashree Anandampillai, Sheldon Pollock, and Gary Tubb.

Thank you to Nathan Englander for encouraging me to transform my endless teaching notes into this book and to Jeff Seroy for believing in me and patiently supporting the process.

Thank you to everyone at FSG who worked so hard to make my vision a reality, especially Steven Pfau, Debra Helfand, Jonathan Lippincott, Elizabeth Gordon, Jennifer Carrow, and Peter Richardson. Thank you to Richard Lasseigne for so generously allowing us to use his beautiful font Times Nagari.

Thank you to all those who have helped to edit along the way. A particular thanks to Jason Birch for his thorough attention to detail and for his invaluable suggestions. Also thank you to Alana Lajoie-O'Malley, Victor Davella, Isaac Murchie, Anne Pollack, Narelle Scotford, and Laura Diamond. Any mistakes that remain are completely my own.

Thank you to all of my students, particularly my Sanskrit students, for bearing with my mistakes and being part of this experiment. A special thank-you to Laura Ritter, Ciaran Jonathan Lavery, and Sarvesh Makthal for their kind eyes and helpful suggestions. Thank you also to Liana Ross, Millinee Bannister, Suzanne Malitz, and David Medvigy.

Thank you to my parents, Diane Lutwak and Don Slatoff, for always encouraging and supporting me on my unusual path. Thank you to Jenny Russo, for her unending support and friendship.

Thank you to my husband, Ben Ponté, for his continuous encouragement and inspiration, without whom I never would have finished. And for bringing alive the very Soul and Spirit of translation with his illustrations in ways I never dreamed possible.

10

# A Note About the Author

Zoë Slatoff-Ponté has spent extensive time studying yoga and Sanskrit over the past twenty years both in Mysore, South India, and in her hometown of New York City. She has an M.A. in Asian languages and culture from Columbia University and was authorized to teach Ashtanga yoga by Śrī K. Pattabhi Jois in 2002. *Yogāvatāraṇam* is her attempt to build a bridge between these two worlds. Zoë teaches yoga and Sanskrit with her husband, Ben Ponté, at their yoga shala on the Upper West Side in Manhattan. You can visit their Web site at www.ashtangayogaupperwestside.com.

Ben Ponté was born in Australia and now lives and works in New York City. He has an M.A. in fine arts from the College of Fine Arts, Sydney. He has been traveling to India and practicing yoga since the late 1990s and was authorized to teach by R. Sharath Jois. His work draws on this experience to explore the perceptual process as a moment of translation, and he is currently focusing on the use and effect of mobile media devices on the body/mind relationship in public space. You can visit his Web site at www.benponte.com.